**Single Best
Answers for
Medical Students**

Single Best Answers for Medical Students

Basic Science

Stuart Kyle MEng (Hons), PhD MBChB (Hons), MRCGP
GP Partner with special interests in medical education
Honorary Senior Lecturer
Swansea University Medical School
Swansea, UK

WILEY Blackwell

Registered Offices
John Wiley & Sons, Inc., 111 River Street, Hoboken, NJ 07030, USA
John Wiley & Sons Ltd, The Atrium, Southern Gate, Chichester, West Sussex, PO19 8SQ, UK

For details of our global editorial offices, customer services, and more information about Wiley products visit us at www.wiley.com.

Wiley also publishes its books in a variety of electronic formats and by print-on-demand. Some content that appears in standard print versions of this book may not be available in other formats.

Library of Congress Cataloging-in-Publication Data
Names: Kyle, Stuart - author.
Title: Single best answers for medical students : basic science / Dr. Stuart Kyle MEng (Hons) PhD MBChB (Hons) MRCGP, GP Partner
   with special interests in medical education, Honorary Senior Lecturer, Swansea University Medical School, Swansea, UK.
Description: Hoboken, NJ : John Wiley & Sons, 2024. | Includes bibliographical references and index.
Identifiers: LCCN 2023041022 (print) | LCCN 2023041023 (ebook) | ISBN 9781119691112 (paperback) | ISBN 9781119691099 (pdf) |
   ISBN 9781119691075 (epub)
Subjects: LCSH: Medical sciences--Miscellanea. | Human biology--Miscellanea.
Classification: LCC R129 .K95 2024 (print) | LCC R129 (ebook) | DDC 612--dc23/eng/20231025
LC record available at https://lccn.loc.gov/2023041022
LC ebook record available at https://lccn.loc.gov/2023041023

Cover image: © Viaframe/Getty Images
Cover design by Wiley

Set in 9/11.5pt Meridien LT Std by Integra Software Services Pvt. Ltd, Pondicherry, India

SKY10063588_122923

To my three children – Sophia, Olivia, and Alice – you have grown into strong, independent women, and you make me proud every day
To my husband – Anthony – thank you for your unwavering support; you make me a better person every single day
To my family – especially my mum who sadly passed away in 2020 and who I miss more than ever – thank you for supporting me over the years; I hope I have made you proud

Contents

Preface

This book was conceived in 2019 and it has been slowly burning ever since. It is the first of a two-part series which tests basic science across a variety of disciplines that are commonly examined throughout the medical curriculum. Each chapter consists of 50 questions with some sub-questions. There is a mixture of easier and more challenging questions interspersed within each chapter. The detailed answers provide you with a good foundation of the topic. I have created figures to summarise key concepts and hopefully this gives you the impetus to research the topic in more detail.

I have been at the coalface of exams for several years and therefore understand first-hand the stresses that exams can cause the learner. What I have learnt over the years from writing this book, in addition to writing questions for national exams, and examining and teaching students, is that there are several variations of common themes in medical school exams. The key is to do as many questions as possible. I have written the solutions to each question with explanations to the correct answer, but also, and what I think is far more important, an explanation on why other options are incorrect answers. I have included topics which are often scantily taught or poorly understood by students such as histology and histopathology, pharmacology, medical ethics, and statistics. There is no doubt that some of the questions are more challenging than others, and perhaps quite esoteric, and this has not been done to simply distinguish the distinction level candidates, but to encourage you to dig deeper into your understanding of the topic. More importantly, the foundations laid down in this book, together with clinical scenarios in the second book, will hopefully help you develop the knowledge and skills required to treat patients.

I am indebted to the many who have taught me over the years, those who I have worked with and absorbed knowledge from, those students who have given me vital feedback in my teaching and, without a shadow of a doubt, every patient I have cared for. The best aspect of my job is being able to communicate complex medicine into bite-size chunks that patients can understand which hopefully improves their care. I hope this book fulfils its aim in being a useful revision tool and it provides a stepping stone in helping you reach your potential. If you have any feedback or suggestions, please let me know (SBAforMedStudents@gmail.com).

Finally, I wish you the very best of luck in your exams and future career as clinicians of tomorrow.

Acknowledgements

I am extremely grateful to Mrs Sue Routledge, a retired school Art teacher and my Head of Year in Secondary School between 1994 and 1999. Using pastels, she artfully drew two figures in the book – blood vessels supplying the kidneys and adrenals (Q6.5.26), and a renal corpuscle (Q6.5.48). She remains a dear friend. I would also like to thank Dr Rory Mcnair, Consultant Radiologist, Swansea Bay University Health Board who scrupulously checked annotated radiographic figures. I am indebted to Prof Paul Griffiths, Consultant Histopathologist, Swansea Bay University Health Board who provided histology images and feedback for Chapter 5.

For every life saved
For a smile on a face
For a hope in a heart
There is a doctor who works tirelessly

Hippocrates

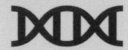

CHAPTER 1

Biochemistry, Cell and Molecular Biology

Molecular biology is essentially the practice of biochemistry without a licence.
Erwin Chargaff

Single Best Answers for Medical Students: Basic Science, First Edition. Stuart Kyle.
© 2024 John Wiley & Sons Ltd. Published 2024 by John Wiley & Sons Ltd.

1.1 In the Krebs cycle, which of the following is formed during the conversion of succinate to fumarate?
 A Reduced NAD
 B Reduced FAD
 C Carbon dioxide
 D ATP
 E GTP

1.2 The influx of which of the following ions is responsible for neurotransmitter release from pre-synaptic neurones?
 A Sodium
 B Calcium
 C Potassium
 D Chloride
 E Magnesium

1.3 Which of the following is **not** correct regarding apoptosis?
 A The process is ATP-dependent
 B Cell shrinkage occurs
 C Cell contents are packaged into apoptotic bodies
 D Can be physiological and pathological
 E Karyolysis is a typical feature

1.4 Antimitochondrial antibodies are the main serological marker for which disease?
 A Autoimmune hepatitis
 B Primary biliary cirrhosis
 C Sjögren's syndrome
 D Systemic lupus erythematosus
 E Goodpasture's syndrome

1.5 Which of the following sequence of events is correct with regard to haematopoiesis?
 A Haemocytoblast → Myeloid progenitor → Plasma cell
 B Haemocytoblast → Lymphoid progenitor → Macrophage
 C Myeloid progenitor → Erythrocyte → Basophil
 D Lymphoid progenitor → Megakaryocyte → Thrombocytes
 E Monoblast → Monocyte → Macrophage

1.6 Which of the following shifts the oxyhaemoglobin dissociation curve to the left?
 A Increase in temperature
 B Increase in pH
 C Increase in carbon dioxide concentration
 D Increase in 2,3-DPG
 E Increase in altitude

1.7 In control of metabolic processes, which of the following is **not** a second messenger system?
 A Binding of glucagon to hepatocytes
 B Diffusion of nitric oxide which stimulates cGMP synthesis
 C cAMP activating protein kinases
 D Binding of calcium ions to calmodulin
 E G protein activating phospholipase C

1.8 Phenylketonuria is a genetic disorder in which the enzyme phenylalanine hydroxylase cannot convert phenylalanine into which amino acid?
 A Tryptophan
 B Methionine
 C Histidine
 D Tyrosine
 E Proline

1.9   Which of the following is **not** an enzyme involved in glycolysis?
A   Aldolase
B   Hexokinase
C   Enolase
D   Isomerase
E   Oxidase

1.10   Which of the following is a Gram-positive bacterium?
A   *Haemophilus influenzae*
B   *Neisseria meningitidis*
C   *Salmonella typhi*
D   *Clostridium difficile*
E   *Helicobacter pylori*

1.11   In molecular biology, which of the following techniques can be used to detect methylated sites in a DNA sequence?
A   Northern blot
B   Western blot
C   Eastern blot
D   Southern blot
E   Southwestern blot

1.12   Which of the following hormones is secreted by most carcinoid tumours?
A   Dopamine
B   Adrenaline
C   Noradrenaline
D   Aldosterone
E   Serotonin

1.13   Which of the following amino acids is present in all types of collagen?
A   Arginine
B   Aspartate
C   Alanine
D   Glutamate
E   Glycine

1.14   Which of the following is **not** a component of the extracellular matrix?
A   Chondroitin sulphate
B   Versican
C   Fibronectin
D   Laminin
E   Glycophorin

1.15   In the polymerase chain reaction, which of the following statements is correct?
A   Magnesium is an essential cofactor for DNA polymerase
B   Elongation is performed at a temperature of 60 °C
C   Extension occurs in the 3′ to 5′ direction on each strand
D   The annealing temperature is typically 10 °C below the primer T_m
E   DNA polymerase synthesises a new DNA strand using deoxynucleoside diphosphates

1.16   Which of the following is a diagnostic test for pheochromocytoma?
A   Human chorionic gonadotrophin
B   Alpha fetoprotein
C   Vanillylmandelic acid
D   5-hydroxyindoleacetic acid
E   Cortisol

1.17   Which of the following disorders is caused by a deficiency of the enzyme hypoxanthine-guanine phosphoribosyltransferase?
   A   Ehlers-Danlos
   B   Tay-Sachs
   C   Lesch-Nyhan
   D   Budd-Chiari
   E   Peutz-Jeghers

1.18   Which of the following is **not** a human herpes virus?
   A   Varicella zoster
   B   Cytomegalovirus
   C   Epstein-Barr
   D   Coxsackievirus
   E   Kaposi's sarcoma-associated virus

1.19   Which of the following statements regarding coagulation is correct?
   A   Coeliac disease can cause vitamin K deficiency
   B   Disseminated intravascular coagulation is associated with thrombocytosis
   C   Warfarin affects the synthesis of factors 2, 7, 8 and 10
   D   The prothrombin time is prolonged in von Willebrand's disease
   E   The APTT is normal in haemophilia A

1.20   Which of the following statements regarding glucagon is correct?
   A   Released by beta cells
   B   Inhibits gluconeogenesis
   C   Secretion is stimulated by hyperglycaemia
   D   Secretion is inhibited by increased free fatty acids
   E   Composed of a 29-amino acid dimer

1.21   Which of the following statements regarding muscle contraction is correct?
   A   An action potential causes calcium ions to diffuse into sarcoplasmic reticula
   B   Calcium ions bind to tropomyosin
   C   During the power stroke, ADP and P_i dissociate from myosin
   D   Actin and myosin bind together to form disulphide bridges
   E   At the neuromuscular junction, noradrenaline binds to the sarcolemma

1.22   Which of the following carcinogens is associated with bladder carcinoma?
   A   Asbestos
   B   Aflatoxin
   C   2-naphthylamine
   D   Chromium
   E   Benzopyrene

1.23   Which of the following viruses and their associated diseases are correctly matched?
   A   Herpes simplex type 1 – shingles
   B   Mumps – pancreatitis
   C   Coxsackie A – yellow fever
   D   Epstein-Barr – cervical cancer
   E   Varicella zoster – lymphoma

1.24   Which of the following regarding the sarcomere is correct?
   A   Thick filaments are composed mainly of the protein myosin
   B   H-zones and I-bands represent overlap between myosin and actin
   C   A-bands contain thin filaments only
   D   Within H-zones are Z-lines which represent the middle of the sarcomere
   E   Upon muscle contraction, Z-lines do not change their length

1.25   Which of the following statements regarding the ultrastructure of a single sarcomere (shown below) found in skeletal muscle is correct?

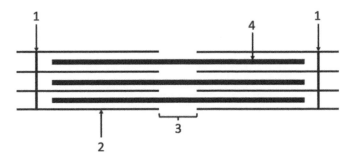

A   Sarcomere length is the distance between each M line which corresponds to lines labelled 1
B   Structure labelled 2 contains actin-binding sites
C   Region labelled 3, the A band, shortens with muscle contraction
D   Calmodulin and creatine kinase are found in region labelled 3
E   Calcium ions bind to structure labelled 4

1.26   Which of the following regarding stages of mitosis is **not** correct?
A   During prophase, microtubules of the cytoskeleton disaggregate
B   During metaphase, duplicated chromosomes attach at the kinetochore
C   During anaphase, chromosomes are positioned at opposite poles
D   During telophase, chromosomes condense and cleavage furrows form
E   During cytokinesis, two daughter cells are produced

1.27   Which of the following cells does omeprazole act on the surface of?
A   Delta
B   Gamma
C   Chief
D   Parietal
E   Foveolar

1.28   Phosphatidylinositol is a phospholipid found on the cytosolic side of some eukaryotic cell membranes. Which of the following regarding phosphatidylinositol is **not** correct?
A   It is amphiphilic
B   It contains a glycerol backbone, two fatty acids and a modified phosphate polar head
C   At physiological pH, it is zwitterionic
D   Common fatty acids within its structure include arachidonic and stearic acid
E   Inositol rings are commonly phosphorylated by kinases

1.29   Which of the following regarding Michaelis-Menten kinetics (shown below) is correct?

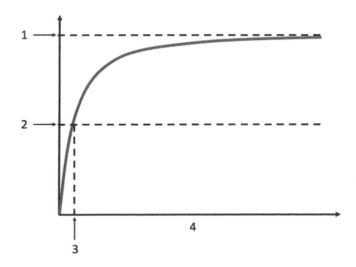

	1	2	3	4
A	V_{max}	$\frac{1}{2}V_{max}$	K_m	[E]
B	K_m	V_{max}	$\frac{1}{2}V_{max}$	V
C	$\frac{1}{2}V_{max}$	[S]	K_m	V
D	V_{max}	$\frac{1}{2}V_{max}$	K_m	[S]
E	K_m	$\frac{1}{2}V_{max}$	V_{max}	[S]

1.30   Which of the following diseases and causative organisms are matched correctly?

	Tuberculosis	Malaria	Measles	Tinea cruris	Schistosomiasis
A	Adenovirus	Fungus	Bacterium	Parasite	Fungus
B	Bacterium	Protist	Paramyxovirus	Fungus	Parasite
C	Rhinovirus	Bacterium	Bacterium	Parasite	Fungus
D	Bacterium	Protist	Adenovirus	Fungus	Parasite
E	Bacterium	Parasite	Paramyxovirus	Fungus	Parvovirus

1.31   Which of the following regarding adult haemoglobin is **not** correct?
A It is composed of two alpha and two beta chains
B It contains a porphyrin ring with a central Fe^{3+} which binds oxygen
C It has a quaternary structure
D Hydrophobic and hydrophilic groups face inwards and outwards, respectively
E It has four oxygen binding sites

1.32   Which of the following enzymes helps anneal DNA fragments through the formation of phosphodiester bonds?
A Ligase
B Polymerase
C Helicase
D Endonuclease
E Kinase

1.33   Which of the following is correct regarding this biochemical pathway?

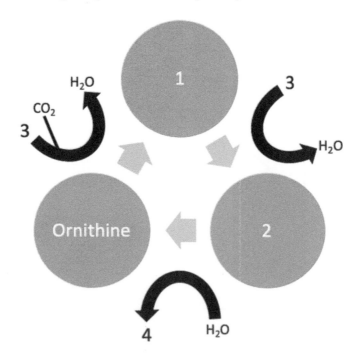

	1	2	3	4
A	Citrulline	Asparagine	Urea	Ammonia
B	Asparagine	Citrulline	Ammonia	Urea
C	Citrulline	Arginine	Ammonia	Urea
D	Methionine	Arginine	Urea	Ammonia
E	Arginine	Citrulline	Ammonia	Urea

1.34 Which of the following regarding organelles is correct?
A The endoplasmic reticulum transports lysosomes
B Mitochondria are approximately 300 nm in diameter
C Nuclei contain 80S ribosomes
D Peroxisomes contain the enzyme reductase
E Golgi bodies contain cristae

1.35 Which of the following techniques is used to determine 3D protein structure?
A Mass spectrometry
B X-ray crystallography
C Ion-exchange chromatography
D Gel electrophoresis
E Protein sequencing

1.36 Which of the following statements regarding this protein structure is **not** correct?

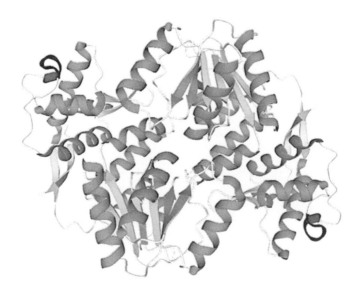

A It is homodimeric
B α-helices and β-pleated sheets are evident
C No random coils are evident
D Level of protein organisation is quaternary structure
E Prosthetic groups are not present

1.37 Which of the following amino acids would **not** form ionic bonds with lysine at physiological pH?
A Aspartate
B Glutamate
C Arginine
D Histidine
E Proline

1.38 Which of the following regarding the *trp* operon is correct?
  A It encodes three structural genes
  B Tryptophan acts as an activator
  C Transcriptional attenuation occurs when tryptophan concentration is high
  D It was first characterised in *Saccharomyces cerevisiae*
  E The trp repressor is a pentamer, structurally similar to CRP

1.39 Which of the following proteins usually coat endocytic vesicles?
  A Clathrin
  B Actin
  C Laminin
  D Desmin
  E Tubulin

1.40 Which of the following metabolic processes occurs in the mitochondria?
  A Glycolysis
  B Cholesterol synthesis
  C Pentose phosphate pathway
  D Fatty acid β-oxidation
  E Fatty acid synthesis

1.41 Which of the following enzymes catalyses substrate-level phosphorylation?
  A Pyruvate kinase
  B Galactokinase
  C Hexokinase
  D Phosphofructokinase
  E Glycerol kinase

1.42 Which of the following cell junctions allow intercellular communication via connexins?
  A Gap junctions
  B Tight junctions
  C Adherens junctions
  D Desmosomes
  E Hemidesmosomes

1.43 Which of the following is the correct conversion of amino acid to neurotransmitter?
  A Tyrosine → Glutamate
  B Tryptophan → Acetylcholine
  C Tyrosine → Gamma-aminobutyric acid (GABA)
  D Tryptophan → Dopamine
  E Tyrosine → Dopamine

1.44 Which of the following is directly formed from 3-hydroxy-3-methylglutaryl-CoA (HMG-CoA) using HMG-CoA reductase?
  A Squalene
  B Ubiquinone
  C Fumarate
  D Mevalonate
  E Palmitate

1.45 Which of the following diseases is **not** caused by a spirochete?
  A Syphilis
  B Lyme disease
  C Leptospirosis
  D Relapsing fever
  E Leishmaniasis

1.46 Which of the following regarding calcium homeostasis is **not** correct?
A Thyroid gland releases calcitonin in response to hypercalcaemia
B Parathyroid glands release PTH in response to hypocalcaemia
C Increased PTH release causes direct osteoclast activation
D Increased PTH release causes hydroxylation of 25-dihydroxycholecalciferol in the small intestine
E Phosphate reabsorption is inhibited in the kidney and serum calcium increases

1.47 Which of the following regarding vitamin B_{12} metabolism is correct?
A Vitamin B_{12} is required for the conversion of methionine into homocysteine
B Vitamin B_{12} has high affinity for haptocorrin at high pH
C Methionine synthase is a folic acid- and B_{12}-dependent enzyme
D Paneth cells secrete intrinsic factor which binds vitamin B_{12}
E Intrinsic factor-vitamin B_{12} complex is absorbed by active transport

1.48 Which of the following regarding oxidative phosphorylation is correct?
A 30 ATP molecules are produced from a single glucose molecule
B There are three protein complexes found in the inner mitochondrial membrane
C Water is the final electron acceptor in the electron transport chain
D Carbon monoxide inhibits ATP synthase
E 5–6 ATP molecules are produced from 2 NADH in oxidative decarboxylation

1.49 Which of the following sequences of secretory pathways for proteins is correct?
A Smooth ER → cis-Golgi network → Golgi cisternae → Secretory vesicle → Cell surface membrane
B Rough ER → cis-Golgi network → Golgi cisternae → Secretory vesicle → Cell surface membrane
C Rough ER → trans-Golgi network → Golgi cisternae → Secretory vesicle → Cell surface membrane
D cis-Golgi network → Rough ER → Golgi cisternae → Secretory vesicle → Cell surface membrane
E Golgi cisternae → trans-Golgi network → Smooth ER → Secretory vesicle → Cell surface membrane

1.50 Which of the following is the correct DNA base triplet that corresponds to the tRNA anticodon AUG?
A UAC
B ATG
C TAC
D AUG
E TTC

Answers

1.1 B – Reduced FAD

The Krebs Cycle (or citric acid cycle/tricarboxylic acid cycle) is a series of chemical reactions in aerobic organisms that releases energy in the form of ATP. In eukaryotes, it occurs in the matrix of the mitochondria, and in prokaryotes, it occurs in the cytosol. The cycle generates reduced NAD which is used in oxidative phosphorylation (electron transport chain). In a single turn, the cycle yields three reduced NAD molecules, one reduced FAD molecule and one ATP/GTP/ITP molecule (ATP in plants, and GTP/ITP in animals). The cycle goes around twice for each molecule of glucose that enters respiration due to there being two pyruvate molecules and hence two acetyl Coenzyme A molecules for every glucose molecule.

Succinate is oxidised to the four-carbon molecule, fumerate. Two hydrogen atoms and accompanying electron are transferred to FAD producing reduced FAD. The reduced FAD can then transfer its electrons directly to the electron transport chain; hence B is the correct response. Reduced NAD and carbon dioxide are both formed during the conversions of isocitrate to α-ketoglutarate, and α-ketoglutarate to succinyl CoA. Reduced NAD is finally formed during the conversion of malate to oxaloacetate. ATP or GTP is only formed during the conversion of succinyl CoA to succinate.

1.2 B – Calcium

Intracellular ions include potassium and magnesium, whilst extracellular ions include calcium, sodium and chloride. Calcium ions are important in nerve transmission, blood clotting and muscle contraction. In neurones, an action potential arrives at the presynaptic neurone, depolarising the membrane and opening the voltage-gated calcium channels. Upon influx of calcium ions, intracellular calcium sensing proteins called synaptotagmins bind with calcium, which leads to synaptic transmission via the exocytotic release of neurotransmitters into the synaptic cleft by fusion of synaptic vesicles to the pre-synaptic membrane; hence B is the correct response.

In excitatory ion channel synapses, sodium ion channels are found on post-synaptic membranes. When neurotransmitters such as acetylcholine and glutamate bind to these ion channels, they open and sodium ions enter causing depolarisation, making an action potential more likely. In inhibitory ion channel synapses, neuroreceptors are found on chloride channels. Binding of the neurotransmitter such as GABA, opens the chloride ion channels and chloride ions flow in causing hyperpolarisation which makes an action potential less likely. Therefore, impulses arriving in one neurone at these synapses can inhibit an impulse in the next neurone. The Na^+/K^+ ATPase pump builds up an electrochemical gradient across neuronal membranes by helping to pump 3 sodium ions out of the cell and 2 potassium ions into the cell hence resulting in excess extracellular sodium ions and intracellular potassium ions. This pump helps maintain the resting membrane potential of the neurones at ca. −70 mV.

Magnesium ions are important cofactors in a variety of chemical processes in the body. They activate DNA/RNA polymerases, help in DNA synthesis and help regulate other ion and mineral concentrations inside and outside of cells. Magnesium ions help regulate calcium ions in cells by helping to pump them out of the cells, particularly in neurones. It should be remembered that in the clinical context, primary disturbances of magnesium are uncommon and deranged magnesium levels usually result from disturbances of fluid or other electrolytes.

1.3 E – Karyolysis is a typical feature

Apoptosis is programmed cell death. The process requires ATP. It has characteristic morphological features which involve single or clusters of cells, such as cell shrinkage, formation of membrane bound vesicles and a cytoplasm with organelles retained in apoptotic bodies, pyknosis (irreversible condensation of chromatin in the nucleus), karyorrhexis (destructive fragmentation of the nucleus) and blebbing of the plasma membrane. It does not involve karyolysis; hence E is the correct response. Karyolysis is the complete dissolution of chromatin of a dying cell as a result of enzymatic degradation of endonucleases. It is a common feature in necrosis. Apoptosis can be physiological or pathological. Necrosis is always pathological.

1.4 B – Primary biliary cirrhosis

Antimitochondrial antibodies are the main serological marker for primary biliary cirrhosis; hence B is the correct response. The presence of antinuclear antibody (ANA), anti-smooth muscle antibody (SMA), anti-liver kidney microsomal antibodies (LKM) and anti-soluble liver antigen (SLA) is more suggestive of autoimmune hepatitis. Anti-Ro and anti-La antibodies are suggestive of Sjögrens syndrome, in addition to ANA. Anti-dsDNA is highly suggestive of SLE. Anti-glomerular basement membrane (GBM) is suggestive of Goodpasture's syndrome.

1.5 E – Monoblast → Monocyte → Macrophage

Haematopoiesis is the continuous process by which blood cell lineages are produced from haemopoietic stem cells. The figure below highlights the important cell lineages and the mature cells formed from haematopoietic stem cells; hence E is the correct response.

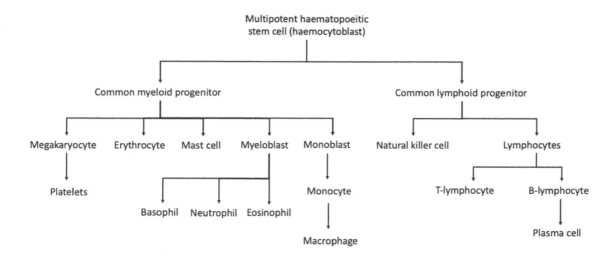

1.6 *B – Increase in pH*

The sigmoid shape of the oxyhaemoglobin dissociation curve results from interaction between oxygen and haemoglobin. The curve can be displaced such that the affinity for oxygen is altered. Factors that change the curve, shown in the figure below, include changes in temperature, pH (or hydrogen ion concentration), concentration of carbon dioxide and 2,3-diphosphoglycerate (2,3-DPG). Increasing pH shifts the curve to the left; hence B is the correct response. 2,3-DPG is a by-product made by erythrocytes during glycolysis. It reduces the affinity of deoxyhaemoglobin for oxygen and facilitates unloading in the tissues. Levels increase under hypoxaemia such as at high altitude and in congenital heart disease, in addition to conditions such as hyperthyroidism and pyruvate kinase deficiency. Interestingly, organisms living at higher altitudes, where partial pressure of oxygen is lower, have adapted and evolved to increase stores of myoglobin, which has a much higher affinity for oxygen than haemoglobin at a lower partial pressure.

The Bohr effect, through changes in carbon dioxide and hydrogen ion concentration in the blood, enables enhanced association/loading of oxygen in the lungs and dissociation/unloading of oxygen in the tissues. Carbon monoxide poisoning and hypophosphataemia can also shift the curve to the left, as can Hb variants such as foetal haemoglobin, methaemoglobin and carboxyhaemoglobin. Pregnancy, chronic anaemia and sickle cell anaemia shifts the curve to the right.

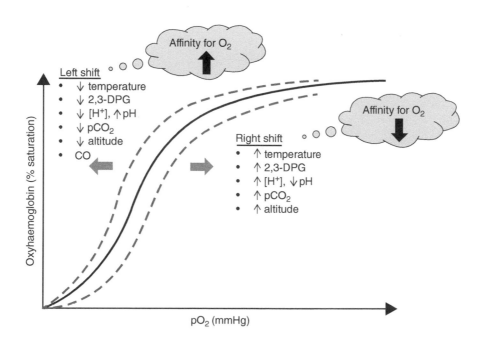

1.7 A – Binding of glucagon to hepatocytes

First messengers are any extracellular factors that elicit an intracellular response. They can range from environmental factors and small molecules, to larger proteins. Common examples include neurotransmitters, peptide hormones, cytokines, growth factors and drugs. First messengers tend not to physically cross the phospholipid bilayer; instead they need to be transduced into second messengers. Glucagon binding to hepatocytes is an example of a first messenger; hence A is the correct response. All other options are examples of second messengers. Second messengers trigger intracellular signalling cascades and may act as enzyme activators, inhibitors or cofactors. Examples include (1) activation of guanylyl cyclase (GC) by calcium or nitric oxide, which catalyses synthesis of cGMP from GTP. Subsequently, cGMP activates protein kinase G; (2) cAMP forms phosphodiesterases which are regulated through phosphorylation by protein kinase A and C. Adenylate cyclase is responsible for synthesising cAMP; (3) calcium ions bind to calmodulin which can activate nitric oxide synthase, and lead to vasodilation via nitric oxide; and (4) phospholipase C is activated through coupling to a G protein.

1.8 D – Tyrosine

Phenylketonuria is an autosomal recessive metabolic disorder (inborn error of metabolism) whereby there is a deficiency in the enzyme, phenylalanine hydroxylase which is required for the conversion of phenylalanine into tyrosine. Phenylalanine accumulates and is converted to phenylpyruvate which is excreted in the urine. Tyrosone is essential for the production of dopamine; hence D is the correct response.

1.9 E – Oxidase

Glycolysis occurs in the cytoplasm and is the process of breaking down glucose (or fructose and galactose) into two three-carbon compounds. It takes place in 10 steps. It is used by all cells in the body for the generation of energy. Glycolysis produces pyruvate and lactate in aerobic and anaerobic conditions, respectively. Pyruvate then enters the Krebs cycles for further energy generation. Glycolysis generates 2 molecules of ATP when 1 molecule of glucose is converted into 2 molecules of pyruvate. NAD^+ is an obligatory substrate in glycolysis, and if it is not generated, glycolysis will cease. In aerobic conditions, NADH is oxidised in the mitochondria to regenerate NAD^+. Anaerobically, NADH and NAD^+, and pyruvate and lactate are interconverted using lactate dehydrogenase. As shown in the following figure, the enzyme not used in glycolysis is oxidase; hence E is the correct response.

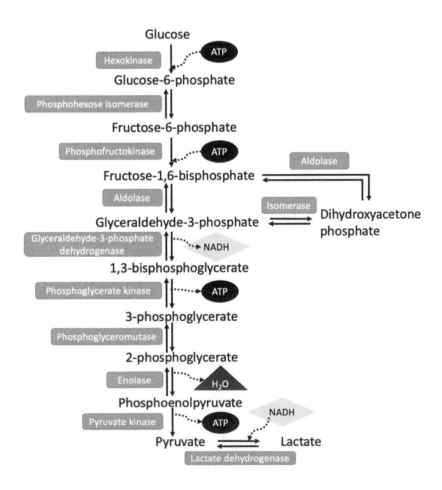

1.10 *D – Clostridium difficile*

The following table highlights common Gram-positive and -negative bacteria; hence D is the correct response, as all other options are examples of Gram-negative bacteria.

		Gram-positive	**Gram-negative**
Cocci	Aerobe	Enterococcus	Neisseria
	Facultative anaerobe	Staphylococcus Streptococcus	
	Anaerobe	Peptostreptococcus	
Bacilli	Aerobe	Bacillus	Pseudomonas
	Facultative anaerobe	Cornebacterium Lactobacillis Listeria Mycobacterium Nocardia	Bordetella Brucella Escherichia Haemophilus Klebsiella Pasteurella Proteus Salmonella Shigella Vibrio Yersinia
	Anaerobe	Actinomyces Clostridium	Bacteroides Fusobacterium Prevotella
	Microaerophile		Campylobacter Helicobacter (curved rod)
Spirochaetes	Aerobe		Leptospira
	Anaerobe		Borrelia Treponema

1.11 *D – Southern blot*

A blot is a method of transferring DNA, RNA or proteins onto a blotting membrane, often using gel electrophoresis. Transferred biological molecules are visualised using various staining methods, autoradiography or specific labelling techniques. All options in this question are techniques employed in molecular biology. Southern blot is a technique used to detect alterations in DNA, such as point mutations, translocations and DNA methylation; hence D is the correct response. Northern blots are used for analysing molecular size and abundance of mRNA, and individual gene expression. Western blot or protein immunoblotting is used to identify and locate specific proteins. Eastern blot is used to analyse post-translational modifications such as the addition of carbohydrates, lipids or phosphates to proteins. Southwestern blot, which combines aspects of Southern and Western blotting, is used to study DNA-protein interactions.

1.12 *E – Serotonin*

Carcinoid tumours are slow-growing neuroendocrine in origin, derived from enterochromaffin or Kulchitsky cells. Microscopically, a conglomerate of neuroendocrine cell types can be seen, containing many membrane-bound neurosecretory granules. These granules are composed of a variety of hormones, the most common being serotonin; hence E is the correct response. Other substances include histamine, prostaglandins, dopamine, kallikrein, substance P and corticotrophin. In addition to carcinoid-like symptoms such as flushing, wheezing and tachycardia, serology may be required to diagnose carcinoid. 5-hydroxyindoleacetic acid (5-HIAA) is a primary metabolite of serotonin which can be measured in a 24-hour urine collection. Serum chromograffin A can also be measured.

1.13 *E – Glycine*

Collagen is the main structural protein in the extracellular matrix. It is composed of amino acids that form a triple helix, consisting of two identical α1 chains and one α2 chain. The most common sequence of collagen follows the pattern Gly-X-Pro or Gly-X-Hyp, where X is any other amino acid, Pro is the amino acid proline and Hyp is hydroxyproline; hence E is the correct response. Glycine is essential in maintaining and stabilising the triple helix. It is required at every third position, as upon assembly, glycine is placed inside the helix where no other larger side groups can be inserted. This means the proline and hydroxyproline rings are placed exteriorly in the helix. Proline and hydroxyproline provide the triple helix with thermal stability.

1.14 *E – Glycophorin*

Glycophorin is a sialoglycoprotein which spans the membrane of erythrocytes. It does not form part of the extracellular matrix; hence E is the correct response. The extracellular matrix is a highly dynamic support network which surrounds all cells and tissues. It is composed of macromolecules, regulatory factors and cells. Extracellular matrix molecules form part of a tightly regulated system for the maintenance of tissue homeostasis, repair and development. The major constituents in the extracellular matrix include collagens, elastins, and non-collagenous glycoproteins and proteoglycans. Adhesive extracellular matrix glycoproteins allow cells to adhere to the matrix, such glycoproteins include fibronectin, laminins, vitronectin, tenascins, thrombospondins, entactins and many others. Proteoglycans consist of a central protein core with glycosaminoglycan side chains, and include versican, aggrecan, decorin, biglycan, fibromodulin and others. Glycosaminoglycans (GAGs) are linear polysaccharides composed of many disaccharide repeating units including chondroitin sulphate, keratan sulphate and heparan sulphate.

1.15 *A – Magnesium is an essential cofactor for DNA polymerase*

Magnesium ions function as a cofactor for DNA polymerase activity by enabling incorporation of dNTPs during polymerisation. They help catalyse phosphodiester bonds between primers and phosphates of dNTPs; hence A is the correct response. Elongation, or the extension step, is carried out at ~72 °C as this is the optimum temperature for DNA polymerase to bind to primers and catalyse replication using dNTPs. This allows for new DNA strands to be synthesised. Extension occurs in the 5′ to 3′ direction on each strand. The annealing temperature, as a general rule of thumb, is 3–5 °C below the lowest primer T_m. DNA polymerase synthesises a new DNA strand using dNTPs (deoxynucleoside triphosphates).

1.16 *C – Vanillylmandelic acid*

Pheochromocytomas are rare, catecholamine-producing neuroendocrine tumours predominantly arising from chromaffin cells of the adrenal medulla. Adrenal tumours produce both norepinephrine and epinephrine, whereas extra-adrenal tumours exclusively produce norepinephrine. Twenty-four-hour urinary metanephrine metabolites can be measured or an end-stage metabolite of catecholamines – vanillylmandelic acid (VMA); hence C is the correct response. Elevated levels of VMA are useful in diagnosing pheochromocytoma. Human chorionic gonadotrophin (HCG) is produced by a growing embryo and the placenta. Measuring HCG levels can be helpful in identifying normal and pregnancies. Detection can also be useful in evaluating various trophoblastic diseases, such as hydatidiform moles and gestational trophoblastic neoplasia (invasive moles, choriocarcinomas). Elevated levels of alpha fetoprotein are useful markers of hepatocellular carcinoma. It can also be raised in patients with non-seminomatous germ cell tumours. 5-hydroxyindoleacetic acid (5-HIAA) is the primary metabolite of 5-hydroxytryptamine (serotonin). Measurement of 24-hour urinary excretion of 5-HIAA is useful in patients with primary midgut carcinoid tumours. These tumours originate from enterochromaffin cells of the intestine. Elevated levels of cortisol are typical of Cushing's syndrome (corticosteroid excess), exercise, stress, depression, obesity and alcohol. Cortisol hypofunction can result due to Addison's disease, hypothyroidism, reduced ACTH production, long-term use of corticosteroids and congenital adrenal hyperplasia.

1.17 *C – Lesch-Nyhan*

Lesch-Nyhan syndrome is a rare, X-linked disorder of purine metabolism, caused by deficiency of the enzyme hypoxanthine-guanine phosphoribosyltransferase (HPRT). HPRT catalyses the conversion of hypoxanthine and guanine into their respective nucleotides, inosinic acid (IMP) and guanylic acid (GMP), respectively. The syndrome is also characterised by overproduction and accumulation of uric acid, which is most likely due to intracellular accumulation of phosphoribosyl pyrophosphate (PRPP) leading to hyperuricaemia; hence C is the correct response. Ehlers-Danlos is an inherited connective tissue disorder typically caused by mutations in collagen genes (*COL5A1* and *COL5A2*). Tay-Sachs disease is an autosomal recessive disorder resulting from deficiency in the lysosomal enzyme hexosaminidase A leading to accumulation of GM2 ganglioside within neuronal cells. Budd-Chiari syndrome can occur as a result of obstructive hepatic venous outflow which leads to hepatic venous congestion. The main cause being hepatic vein thrombosis with or without occlusion of the inferior vena cava. Other causes include hypercoagulable states, neoplasia, myeloproliferative disorders, pregnancy and contraceptive pills. Peutz-Jeghers syndrome is an autosomal dominant disorder characterised by the presence of multiple gastrointestinal hamartomatous polyps and skin hyperpigmentation. It is usually caused by germline mutation in the serine-threonine kinase tumour suppressor gene.

1.18 *D – Coxsackievirus*

Coxsackieviruses belong to the single-stranded positive-sense ssRNA viruses of the enterovirus family. Types A and B are pathogenic, commonly associated with pyrexial illnesses and are the causative organisms for aseptic meningitis, myocarditis, hand, foot and mouth disease and herpangina (common childhood illness characterised by ulcers in the mouth and throat); hence D is the correct response. All other options are human herpes viruses.

1.19 A – Coeliac disease can cause vitamin K deficiency

Coeliac disease is a gluten-sensitive enteropathy which can lead to malabsorption. It is a chronic, autoimmune, T-cell-mediated inflammatory disorder. Vitamin K deficiency may be due to malabsorption; hence A is the correct response. Other causes include inadequate stores and the use of oral anticoagulants. Disseminated intravascular coagulation is associated with thrombocytopenia (not thrombocytosis) due to platelets being consumed. Warfarin, a vitamin K epoxide reductase antagonist, inhibits the synthesis of vitamin K-dependent coagulation factors, including factors 2, 7, 9 and 10 (not 8!), as well as proteins C and S. Prothrombin time is normal in both haemophilia A and von Willebrand's disease. APTT is increased in both haemophilia A and von Willebrand's disease.

1.20 D – Secretion is inhibited by increased free fatty acids

Glucagon inhibits fatty acid synthesis (and glycolysis); hence D is the correct response. It is released by alpha cells of the pancreas; beta cells release insulin. Glucagon increases gluconeogenesis (rather than inhibiting it) and also glycogenolysis. It also increases ketone body production from fatty acids and stimulates lipolysis in adipose tissue. Glucagon increases blood glucose during hypoglycaemia, whereas insulin lowers blood glucose during hyperglycaemia. Glucagon is a 29-amino acid, single-chain polypeptide derived from a pre-proglucagon 180-amino acid precursor. It is not a dimer.

1.21 C – During the power stroke, ADP and P_i dissociate from myosin

The power stroke is related to the mechanical force generated by release of ADP and P_i, and to the conformational change in myosin which then exerts this force on actin. Myosin pulls the actin filament; the sarcomere shortens and the muscle contracts; hence C is the correct response. An action potential causes calcium ions to diffuse out of the sarcoplasmic reticulum (not in), which are released upon signalling from the transverse tubules (T-tubules). Calcium ions bind to troponin (not tropomyosin) which expose the actin-binding sites. Actin and myosin form cross-bridges (not disulphide bridges) and undergo cyclic binding interactions where they pull against one another. At the neuromuscular junction, acetylcholine (not noradrenaline) binds to the sarcolemma. Acetylcholine depolarises the sarcolemma and the action potential can then propagate across it and down the T-tubules.

1.22 C – 2-naphthylamine

Occupational exposure to 2-naphthylamine, an aromatic amine has been shown to increase the risk of bladder cancer, particularly those who work in the dye industry. It is also found in cigarette smoke; hence C is the correct response. High exposure to asbestos can cause mesothelioma. Aflatoxin is a mycotoxic carcinogen produced by certain strains of *Aspergillus* and has been implicated in the aetiology of hepatocarcinoma. Chromium compounds have been shown to increase the risk of lung carcinomas. Benzopyrene is a polycyclic aromatic hydrocarbon commonly found in cigarette smoke (tar). It can cause squamous cell, large and small cell and adenocarcinomas of the lungs.

1.23 B – Mumps – pancreatitis

Mumps is caused by a paramyxovirus and spread by droplets. Associated conditions or complications include CNS involvement, epididymo-orchitis, oophoritis, myocarditis, mastitis, hepatitis and pancreatitis; hence B is the correct response. Herpes simplex type 1 causes mucocutaneous lesions, predominantly of the head and neck such as herpes labialis, keratoconjunctivitis, stomatitis and encephalitis. Shingles is caused by herpes (varicella) zoster. Coxsackie A viruses are spread by the faecal-oral route and are responsible for a broad spectrum of diseases such as hand, foot and mouth, herpangina, meningitis, encephalitis, myocarditis and myositis. Yellow fever is caused by a flavivirus and mainly confined to Africa and South America. Epstein-Barr (EBV) is a gamma herpes virus and causes infectious mononucleosis, Burkitt's lymphoma, oral hairy leucoplakia in AIDS patients, nasopharyngeal carcinoma and post-transplant lymphoma. Cervical cancer is caused by sexually acquired infection with human papillomavirus (HPV), predominantly types 16 and 18. Varicella zoster is an alpha herpes virus, like HSV types 1 and 2, but causes chickenpox in children and shingles in adults. Viruses that can cause lymphoma include EBV, human T-lymphotropic virus type 1, human herpesvirus type 8 and hepatitis C.

1.24 A – Thick filaments are composed mainly of the protein myosin

A sarcomere is the smallest contractile unit of a muscle fibre, composed of two myofilaments: thick filaments are composed mainly of myosin, and thin filaments are composed mainly of actin (and titin); hence A is the correct response. The H-zone and I-band are the regions that only contain the thick and thin filaments, respectively. The A-band contains the thick filaments with some overlap of the thin filaments. The Z-lines (or discs) borders the sarcomere and contain a central M-line, which anchors the thick filaments. In a contracted muscle fibre, the distance between the Z-lines, the I-band and the H-zone decreases, but the A-band remains unchanged. In a fully contracted muscle, the H-zone is no longer visible.

1.25 *D – Calmodulin and creatine kinase are found in region labelled 3*

Region labelled 3 is the H-zone which contains a central M-line (middle of the sarcomere). It serves to arrange the thick filaments into the A-bands maintaining their alignment and controlling stress distribution along the sarcomere during muscle contraction. The M-line is a dense complex of proteins which contains important structural linkers such as myomesin, calmodulin and creatine kinase; hence D is the correct response. Sarcomere length is the distance between each Z line (not M). Structure labelled 2 is the thin filament, primarily composed of actin so actin binding sites are found on structure labelled 4, myosin. Region labelled 3 is the H-zone, not the A-band. The A-band remains unchanged in muscle contraction. Calcium ions bind to troponin (a component of the thin filament, label 2) and not myosin (label 4). The following figure illustrates the important features of a sarcomere.

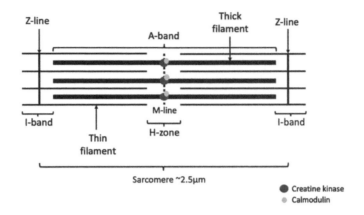

1.26 *D – During telophase, chromosomes condense and cleavage furrows form*

During telophase, chromosomes <u>de</u>condense as they arrive at opposite poles of the cell; hence D is the correct response. In addition, spindles start to break down, the nuclear envelope reforms and nucleoli reappear. In animal cells, cleavage furrows form during cytokinesis as the cytoplasm splits into two and the cell divides. All other options are correct.

1.27 *D – Parietal*

Omeprazole is a selective, irreversible proton pump inhibitor. It inhibits the H^+/K^+ ATPase pump found in parietal cells of the stomach; hence D is the correct response. Parietal or oxyntic cells are found in the lamina propria, specifically within the neck of fundic gland. They make hydrochloric acid and gastric intrinsic factor which are released into the lumen of the stomach.

Delta or D cells are somatostatin-producing cells that can be found in the stomach, pancreas and intestine. In the stomach, somatostatin acts on parietal cells and helps reduce acid secretions. In the pancreas, somatostatin has both paracrine and endocrine function. The paracrine effects are to inhibit the release of glucagon and insulin by α and β cells of the Islets of Langerhans, respectively. The endocrine effects are on reducing smooth muscle contraction in the gallbladder and alimentary canal. Another type of delta cell, D_1 produces vasoactive intestinal peptide which induces glycogenolysis and has important roles in regulating intestinal motility and the tone of smooth muscle.

Gamma, also called F or pancreatic polypeptide (PP) cells produce pancreatic polypeptide in the Islets of Langerhans of the pancreas. This hormone has roles in reducing appetite and inhibits exocrine secretions of the pancreas and the release of bile from the gallbladder. It helps stimulate the release of enzymes by chief cells and reduces the release of HCl by the parietal cells of the stomach.

Chief cells can be found in the stomach, parathyroid gland and in the carotid body. Chief or zymogenic cells make the enzymes lipase, pepsinogen and rennin and release them into the lumen of the stomach. They are found in the base of the fundic gland. They also make the hormone, leptin which inhibits the sensation of hunger.

Foveolar cells or surface mucous cells line the gastric mucosa of the stomach and secrete mucous which helps lubricate the gastric lining. Mucous neck cells are found in the neck of the fundic gland. They help reduce friction whilst food is being churned.

1.28 *C – At physiological pH, it is zwitterionic*

Phosphatidylinositol is a glycerophospholipid with an inositol head group, two fatty acid tails and a glycerol backbone. It is a precursor to inositol phosphates which are important in cell signalling. At physiological pH, the phosphate group that is substituted with the inositol polar head group renders an overall negative charge on the molecule; hence C is the correct response. It is not zwitterionic at physiological pH as there is no positive charge to balance the negatively charged phosphate. All other options are correct.

1.29 D – | V_{max} | $\frac{1}{2}V_{max}$ | K_m | $[S]$ |

Michaelis-Menten kinetics, involving a single substrate and product, is a simple model that accounts for enzyme dynamics. The Michaelis-Menten equation relates the maximum velocity at maximum substrate concentrations when all enzyme active sites are saturated with substrate, V_{max}, the substrate concentration at which the reaction velocity is $\frac{1}{2}V_{max}$, K_m (the Michaelis constant – a measure of the affinity an enzyme has for its substrate), and the substrate concentration, $[S]$, such that:

$$v = \frac{V_{max}\left[S\right]}{K_m + \left[S\right]}$$

Graphically, this can be depicted as follows; hence D is the correct response:

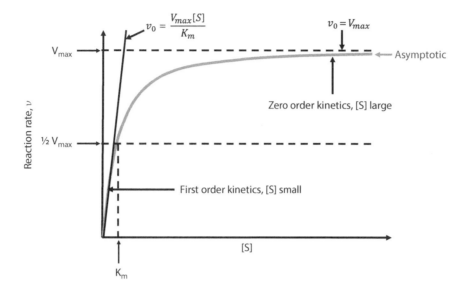

Additionally, algebraic rearrangement of the Michaelis-Menten equation yields a linear, double-reciprocal plot which is far easier to interpret than an entire rectangular hyperbola, and which facilitates estimation of K_m. Plots such as the Lineweaver-Burk are commonly employed by enzymologists as shown below:

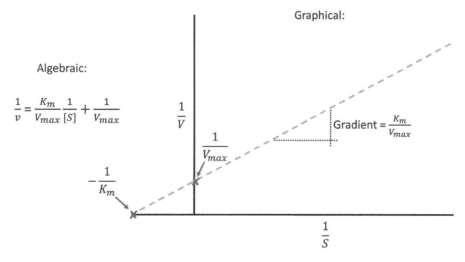

Throughout the 20th century, significant advances in enzyme kinetics were made by Haldane who introduced the concept of introducing more than one substrate into reactions, and Fersht who introduced the term *enzyme specificity*.

1.30 *B –* | *Bacterium* | *Protist* | *Paramyxovirus* | *Fungus* | *Parasite* |

Tuberculosis is caused by the bacterium *Mycobacterium tuberculosis*, malaria is caused by the parasitic protist (or protozoan) *Plasmodium*, measles is caused by the paramyxovirus, tinea cruris ('jock itch'), a fungal infection of the superficial skin of the groin is caused by a dermatophyte, and schistosomiasis (also called bilharzia) is a parasitic worm (or fluke) infection; hence B is the correct response.

1.31 *B – It contains a porphyrin ring with a central Fe³⁺ which binds oxygen*

Adult haemoglobin contains a porphyrin ring in which a central Fe^{2+} (not Fe^{3+}) co-ordinately bonds and binds oxygen; hence B is the correct response. It exists as a tetramer containing two alpha and two beta chains (subunits). Since it has more than one polypeptide chain, it has a quaternary structure. Hydrophilic groups face outwards where water is found at the surface of the protein, while hydrophobic groups face inwards and bury among hydrophobic amino acids of the protein. Haemoglobin has four separate haem groups that can each bind a molecule of oxygen and this leads to a significant increase in the affinity for oxygen at the other haem groups.

1.32 *A – Ligase*

DNA ligase (polydeoxyribonucleotide synthase) catalyses the formation of a phosphodiester bond by annealing DNA single strands; hence A is the correct response. Polymerases catalyse the polymerisation of nucleoside triphosphates into DNA or RNA in the form of dNTPs and rNTPs, respectively. A phosphodiester bond is formed between the 3′ end of the growing chain and the 5′ phosphate of the incoming nucleotide. In addition, hydrogen bonding occurs between complementary nucleotides. DNA polymerases require a primer for initiation, RNA polymerases do not. Helicase utilises energy from ATP hydrolysis to separate (unwinds) complementary strands of DNA or RNA duplexes. Endonucleases (restriction enzymes) cleave phosphodiester bonds within a polynucleotide chain, commonly doing so at specific nucleotide sequences. Kinases phosphorylate specific amino acids using the phosphate in ATP.

1.33 *C –* | *Citrulline* | *Arginine* | *Ammonia* | *Urea* |

The urea, or ornithine cycle, depicted with extra detail below, is a cyclic pathway which converts toxic ammonia into relatively inert urea. It occurs both in the cytoplasm and in mitochondria, and is the sole source of endogenous arginine, ornithine and citrulline production. Ammonia and urea are products of oxidative deamination and nitrogen metabolism, respectively; hence C is the correct response. The reaction exclusively occurs in periportal hepatocytes of the liver and urea is then transported to and excreted by the kidneys. Clinically, the major sequelae of urea cycle dysfunction are neurological, and accumulation of ammonia has been considered to play an important role in hepatic encephalopathy. The urea cycle links with the Krebs cycle, and the overall reaction can be summarised as:

$$NH_4^+ + HCO_3^- + 3ATP^{4-} + 2H_2O + aspartate \rightarrow urea + 2ADP^{3-} + 2P_i^{2-} + PP_i^{4-} + AMP^{2-} + 5H^+ + fumarate$$

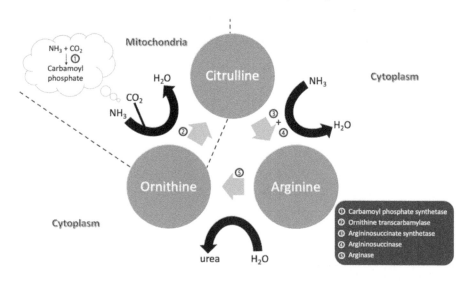

1.34 *C – Nuclei contain 80S ribosomes*

Eukaryotic cells, i.e., those that have a nucleus contain 80S ribosomes (S meaning Svedberg units, a sedimentation coefficient) composed of 40S and 60S subunits (note these are not actual masses, otherwise the maths would be completely incorrect!); hence C is the correct response. Prokaryotes contain 70S ribosomes, composed of 30S and 50S subunits. The endoplasmic reticulum synthesises membrane proteins and soluble proteins and correctly folds them. These are then transported to the Golgi where proteins are processed, packaged, modified and subsequently released in secretory vesicles. Mitochondria range in size between

1 and 10 μm (300 nm = 0.3 μm). Peroxisomes, found in all eukaryotic cells, are involved in ß-oxidation of fatty acids and hydrogen peroxide metabolism. They contain high concentrations of oxidative enzymes such as urate oxidase and catalase (whereas reductases catalyse reduction reactions). Golgi bodies (apparatus/complex) contain around 3–6 flattened sacs called cisternae (cis, medial and trans-cisternae); the inner mitochondrial membrane contains folds called cristae.

1.35 B – X-ray crystallography

Globular proteins have a well-defined 3D structure, and when crystallised, this structure can be determined by X-ray crystallography. This is done by beaming x-rays through a crystal which interact with electrons, and therefore allow atomic positions to be calculated; hence B is the correct response. In addition, 2D- and 3D nuclear magnetic resonance (NMR) spectroscopy can be used to determine protein structure in solution. Mass spectrometry is used to accurately measure molecular mass of proteins, in addition to protein sequencing and identification. Proteins can be separated and purified based on their size using gel filtration chromatography, and charge using ion-exchange chromatography and gel electrophoresis. Gel electrophoresis can also be crudely used to determine protein size. Protein sequencing is an automated yet laborious process using a technique called Edman degradation. The order of the amino acid sequence can be deduced by sequencing peptides produced by enzyme digestion, and overlapping sequences are then compared.

1.36 D – Level of protein organisation is quaternary structure

This is the protein structure for a DNA helicase, and therefore it has tertiary structure (not quaternary); hence D is the correct response. It has two polypeptide chains that are identical; therefore it is homodimeric (not heterodimeric). The structure contains both α-helices and β-pleated sheets. There are no random coils evident. There are no prosthetic groups present within the structure.

1.37 E – Proline

Ionic bonding is the electrostatic attraction between oppositely charged species. There are 20 amino acids used as protein building blocks and they differ from each other only at the R-group. R-groups render amino acids as non-polar or hydrophobic, polar or hydrophilic, acidic or basic. Basic and acidic amino acids are capable of ionic interactions. Proline is a non-polar, hydrophobic amino acid, so would not ionically bond with lysine; hence E is the correct response. Aspartate and glutamate, and arginine and histidine are acidic and basic amino acids, respectively. The 20 alpha amino acids and the R-group character which they exhibit are shown below:

Amino acid	Abbreviation		R-group character	
Glycine	G	Gly	Hydrophobic Non-polar Neutral	Aliphatic
Alanine	A	Ala		
Valine	V	Val		
Leucine	L	Leu		
Isoleucine	I	Ile		
Methionine	M	Met		
Phenylalanine	F	Phe		Aromatic
Tyrosine	Y	Tyr		
Tryptophan	W	Trp		
Serine	S	Ser	Hydrophilic Polar Neutral	
Threonine	T	Thr		
Cysteine	C	Cys		
Proline	P	Pro		
Asparagine	N	Asn		
Glutamine	Q	Gln		
Lysine	K	Lys	Hydrophilic Polar Cationic, basic	
Arginine	R	Arg		
Histidine	H	His		
Aspartate	D	Asp	Hydrophilic Polar Anionic, acidic	
Glutamate	E	Glu		

1.38 C – Transcriptional attenuation occurs when tryptophan concentration is high

The *trp* operon encodes genes involved in tryptophan biosynthesis in prokaryotes. First characterised in *E. coli*, it contains five structural genes (*trp A–E*) which encode seven protein domains, a promotor (where RNA polymerase binds) and an operator (where the repressor binds). Transcription of the *trp* operon is tightly regulated and determined by the concentration of tryptophan. At high concentration, transcription is turned off and it is turned on when tryptophan is absent (or in short supply). Attenuation is the negative feedback mechanism by which premature termination of *trp* RNA synthesis occurs. It is a mechanism for reducing operon expression when levels of tryptophan are high; hence C is the correct response. The *trp* operon is controlled by both a repressor, which interacts with the operator when tryptophan is bound (reducing transcription), and the attenuator, a terminator (leader) sequence adjacent to the *trpE* gene (which prevents completion of transcription, rather than blocking initiation). Tryptophan acts as a co-repressor (not activator) which behaves as both a sensor and a switch – it can sense when tryptophan levels are high, and then switches the operon off (an efficient process preventing unnecessary enzyme production). The trp repressor is a dimer (not pentamer), structurally similar to the CRP protein and lac repressor. Importantly, control by the *trp* repressor (70-fold) and attenuation (10-fold) serve to allow approximately 700-fold overall regulatory control of transcription of the *trp* operon as a result of tryptophan levels.

1.39 A – Clathrin

Clathrin is a three-legged scaffold protein (known as a triskelion) which forms a lattice-like coat on membranes. The connection of the clathrin lattice to the membrane is mediated by clathrin adaptor proteins. Clathrin coats transport vesicles during membrane trafficking which allows clathrin-dependent endocytosis to import extracellular molecules; hence A is the correct response. Actin is a microfilament-forming protein which plays an integral role in muscle contraction and cell movement, in addition to helping to maintain and control cell shape and architecture. Laminin is a heterotrimeric glycoprotein of the basement membrane and non-collagenous component of the extracellular matrix (ECM). Alongside collagen type IV, laminin provides mechanical support, serving as a scaffold for other ECM components. Desmin is a cytoplasmic intermediate filament protein found in cardiac, skeletal and smooth muscle. Alongside vimentin, desmin plays an essential role in maintaining muscle cytoarchitecture. Tubulin, a dimeric protein essential to the eukaryotic cytoskeleton, polymerises and assembles into microtubules needed for the cell cycle.

1.40 D – Fatty acid β-oxidation

Fatty acid β-oxidation is the process by which energy is released through breakdown of fatty acids into acetyl-CoA in the mitochondrial matrix. Acetyl-CoA is then oxidised in the Krebs cycle, releasing CoA needed to maintain β-oxidation; hence D is the correct response. Glycolysis is the process of generating energy through the breakdown of glucose into pyruvate (aerobically) and lactate (anaerobically) in the cytosol. Pyruvate then enters the Krebs cycle. Cholesterol synthesis takes place in the cytosol and endoplasmic reticulum (ER). The pentose phosphate pathway (shunt) is an alternative to glycolysis that generates NADPH (reducing power for lipid and cholesterol synthesis) and pentoses (precursor for nucleic acid synthesis). The process occurs in the cytosol. Fatty acid synthesis is initiated by carboxylation of acetyl-CoA yielding malonyl-CoA required for elongating fatty acid chains. The process also utilises NADPH. Similar to β-oxidation, the process occurs in the cytosol and ER.

1.41 A – Pyruvate kinase

Substrate level phosphorylation is the process of forming ATP from ADP and phosphorylated intermediates in coupling reactions of glycolysis and the Krebs cycle. Pyruvate kinase catalyses the transfer of phosphate from phosphoenolpyruvate to ADP yielding pyruvate and ATP (last step of glycolysis); hence A is the correct response. Step 7 of glycolysis uses phosphoglycerate kinase to convert 1,3-bisphosphoglycerate to 3-phosphoglycerate, which is another example of substrate-level phosphorylation. In contrast, oxidative phosphorylation generates ATP from oxidised NADH and FADH$_2$ using electrochemical gradients. Galactokinase catalyses the conversion of α-D-galactose into galactose-1-phosphate by means of the Leloir pathway (galactose metabolism). This results in conversion to glucose-1-phosphate which can then enter glycolysis. Hexokinase is the initial enzyme used in glycolysis for the conversion of glucose to glucose-6-phosphate by ATP. Phosphofructokinase catalyses the phosphorylation of fructose-6-phosphate to fructose-1,6-diphosphate by ATP in glycolysis. Glycerol kinase catalyses the conversion of glycerol to glycerol-3-phosphate, predominantly in the liver. This is then oxidised into dihydroxyacetone phosphate which can then enter glycolysis or gluconeogenesis.

1.42 A – Gap junctions

Gap junctions are large channels that connect the cytosol of two adjacent cells and promote intercellular communication. They are dodecameric structures composed of connexin proteins which allow passage of smaller signalling molecules such as ions, second messengers and metabolites, but not larger molecules such as proteins; hence A is the correct response. Tight junctions (zonula occludens), which include transmembrane proteins such as occludin, claudin, and cingulin, act as a continuous intercellular barrier and restrict diffusion of solutes in epithelial and endothelial cells. They regulate the passage of proteins and liquids across the cell membrane. Adherens junctions mediate cell–cell adhesions via integral membrane proteins such as cadherins and nectins. These junctions are important regulators in cell remodelling and proliferation, and tissue dynamics, architecture and morphogenesis. Desmosomes are membrane units that mediate cell–cell adhesion between adjacent cell membranes by providing structural and mechanical stability to cells subjected to physical stresses (heart, skin). They facilitate strong adhesion between adjacent epithelial cells. They are formed by two cadherin glycoproteins, desmoglein and desmocollin, which associate with other proteins such as plakoglobin, plakophilin and desmoplakin. On the other hand, hemidesmosomes connect basal epithelial cells and the underlying basement membrane or substratum via intermediate filaments. Instead of desmogleins and desmocollins in the ECM, hemidesmosomes utilise integrins to facilitate adhesion.

1.43 *E – Tyrosine → Dopamine*

The synthesis of various neurotransmitters from precursors is shown below. Phenylalanine is converted into tyrosine, which via L-DOPA, is converted into dopamine; hence E is the correct response.

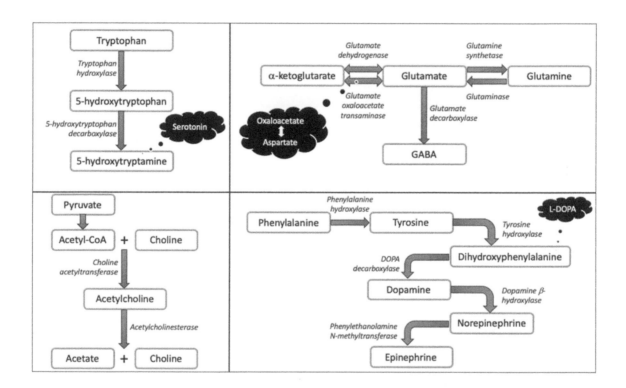

1.44 *D – Mevalonate*

HMG-CoA reductase is the enzyme that reduces HMG-CoA to mevalonate using NADPH, in cholesterol biosynthesis; hence D is the correct response. The process begins with acetyl-CoA from the mitochondria being transported to the cytosol, and with acetoacetyl-CoA, is then converted to HMG-CoA. Numerous phosphorylation and condensation reactions in the endoplasmic reticulum yield squalene which is then cyclised to lanosterol. The conversion to cholesterol then proceeds via 19 reaction steps! As shown below, there are many therapeutic targets in the process. Statins are HMG-CoA reductase inhibitors which thwart conversion of HMG-CoA to mevalonate. Bisphosphonates are pyrophosphate analogues and stimulate osteoclast apoptosis and inhibit cholesterol synthesis. They decrease prenylation of proteins by blocking farnesyl pyrophosphate synthase (FPPS) which are required for cell function and survival. There has also been growing interest in the anticancer effects of FPPS inhibition, as lack of farnesyl pyrophosphate halts protein prenylation which is required for functioning oncogenic GTPases. Interestingly as an aside, in fungi (and with minimal effects on human cholesterol biosynthesis), squalene is converted to squalene epoxide using squalene epoxidase. In dermatophyte infections, allylamines, such as terbinafine, inhibit squalene epoxidase and therefore ergosterol biosynthesis, causing a fungicidal effect (in *Candida* spp. they are fungistatic). Azoles, such as fluconazole, miconazole and clotrimazole inhibit ergosterol synthesis by inhibiting lanosterol 14-α-demethylase, which is known to play an important role in membrane permeability. In fungi, azoles prevent demethylation of lanosterol into ergosterol using fungal cytochrome P450, and the cell membrane becomes permeable.

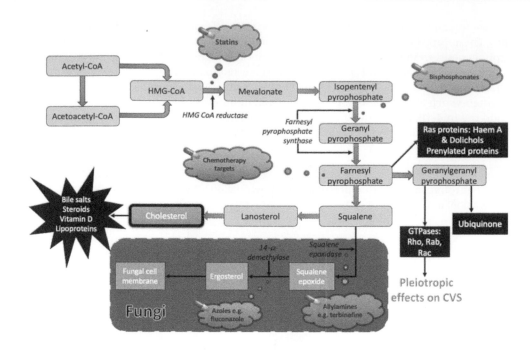

1.45 *E – Leishmaniasis*

Leishmaniasis is caused by a protozoan parasite transmitted by Phlebotomine (in the Old World) or Lutzomyia (in the New World) sand flies. It is endemic to tropics and sub-tropics and clinical manifestations include cutaneous (skin ulcers), mucocutaneous (mucosal ulcerations) and visceral (fever, weight loss, lymphadenopathy, splenomegaly, pancytopenia); hence E is the correct response. All other diseases listed are caused by spirochetes (Gram-negative, spiral bacteria): syphilis is caused by *Treponema pallidum*, Lyme disease is caused by *Borrelia burgdorferi*, leptospirosis is caused by bacteria of the genus Leptospira (primarily sp. *interrogans*) and relapsing fever is caused by various Borrelia species which can be transmitted via lice or ticks.

1.46 *D – Increased PTH release causes hydroxylation of 25-dihydroxyvitamin D in the small intestine*

PTH is released from the parathyroid gland in response to hypocalcaemia. PTH stimulates the production of active vitamin D (calcitriol, or 1,25-dihydroxycholecalciferol) in the tubular cells of the kidneys. Vitamin D_3 from sunlight or diet is converted into inactive vitamin D (calcidiol, or 25-hydroxycholecalciferol) in the liver. This is then hydroxylated in the kidneys (not 25-<u>di</u>hydroxycholecalciferol in the small intestine) by 1α-hydroxylase into active vitamin D. This increases absorption of calcium and phosphate in the intestines; hence D is the correct response. PTH also stimulates bone resorption of osteoclasts and release of calcium and phosphate from bone. Calcitonin is secreted by the parafollicular cells of the thyroid. Hypercalcaemia increases calcitonin secretion and it is known to directly inhibit bone resorption in osteoclasts. All other options are correct. Calcium homeostasis is summarised below.

Interestingly as an aside, the growth factor, FGF23, plays an important role in calcium and phosphate homeostasis. FGF23 increases urinary excretion of phosphate in the kidney. It also inhibits 1α-hydroxylase and stimulates 24-hydroxylase (which increases 1,25-dihydroxycholecalciferol inactivation). Subsequently, 1,25-dihydroxycholecalciferol levels decrease, which leads to reduced calcium (and phosphate) reabsorption in the intestines. FGF23 also inhibits PTH secretion.

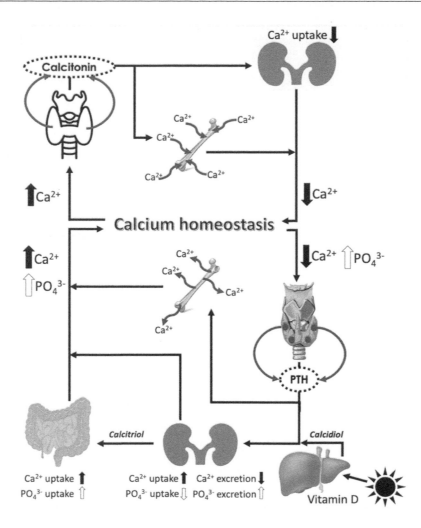

1.47 *C – Methionine synthase is a folic-acid and B$_{12}$-dependent enzyme*

The water-soluble vitamin B$_{12}$ (cobalamin) is an important cofactor in many biochemical pathways. The physiologic mechanism of absorption is complex. Salient processes involved in absorption and metabolism are highlighted below. Vitamin B$_{12}$ is key to the (re)methylation of homocysteine to methionine using methionine synthase in the cytosol. Methionine synthase also uses 5-methyltetrahydrofolate as a one-carbon donor; hence C is the correct response, as methionine synthase inexorably links folate and vitamin B$_{12}$ metabolic pathways. In addition, vitamin B$_{12}$ (adenosylcobalamin) is required for the conversion of methylmalonyl-CoA to succinyl-CoA using methylmalonyl-CoA mutase in the mitochondria (important in replenishing key intermediates in the Krebs cycle). As an aside and to a much lesser extent (as if the process was not complicated enough!), homocysteine can also be converted back into methionine via a folate-independent pathway using betaine-homocysteine methyltransferase in the liver and kidneys.

As illustrated below, vitamin B$_{12}$ is bound to protein in the diet and upon digestion, released B$_{12}$ binds to haptocorrin (previously known as R-binder or transcobalamin I) secreted by salivary glands. In the stomach (low pH), haptocorrin binds free B$_{12}$ with much greater affinity than intrinsic factor (IF) (secreted by parietal cells of the stomach, not Paneth cells – secretory epithelial cells of the crypts of Lieberkühn which contribute to enteric innate immunity). In the small intestine, pancreatic proteases partially degrade the B$_{12}$-haptocorrin complex at neutral pH (not high pH), releasing B$_{12}$ which then binds to IF. The B$_{12}$-IF complex binds to cubilin (an endocytic receptor for B$_{12}$-IF complexes) on enterocytes of the ileal mucosa and is internalised via endocytosis (not active transport). IF is then degraded. The B$_{12}$-transcobalamin II complex (active form of B$_{12}$) binds to and transports the newly internalised B$_{12}$ in the circulation and to target cells where it is needed.

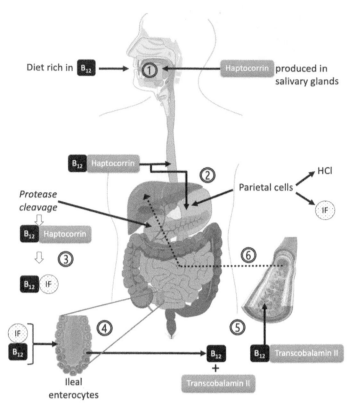

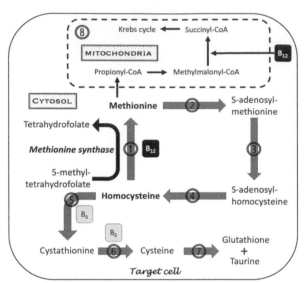

Methylation of homocysteine uses 5-methyl-tetrahydrofolate as a methyl donor and is catalysed by methionine synthase to methionine. ① B₁₂ is an essential cofactor. Tetrahydrofolate is essential in purine and pyrimidine synthesis

Methionine is catalysed by methionine adenosyltransferase into *S*-② adenosyl-methionine, a methyl donor critical for gene regulation and protein methylation

③ *S*-adenosyl-methionine is converted to *S*-adenosyl-homocysteine by methyl-transferases as a result of transmethylation

④ *S*-adenosyl-homocysteine is then converted to adenosine and homocysteine by hydrolase

Via trans-sulphuration with serine in the presence of vitamin B₆, ⑤ homocysteine can be converted to cystathionine using cystathionine β-synthase

⑥ Cystathionine is then converted to cysteine using cystathionase

Cysteine is involved in glutathione biosynthesis which has roles as an antioxidant, immune system enhancer and in detoxification ⑦ Cysteine can also be converted to taurine, which also functions as an antioxidant and is protective in cancer, heart disease and diabetes

Catabolised methionine, β-oxidation of odd-chain fatty acids and propionic acid from the gut flora produce propionyl–CoA. This is ⑧ converted to methylmalonyl-CoA, and then succinyl-CoA using methylmalonyl-CoA mutase and B₁₂ (adenosylcobalamin). This then enters the Krebs cycle

① B₁₂ is released from protein-bound foods in the diet and haptocorrin (a B₁₂ binder) is made in salivary glands

② B₁₂ binds to haptocorrin. Gastric parietal cells produce HCl and intrinsic factor (IF)

③ Pancreatic proteases digest the B₁₂-haptocorrin complex, releasing B₁₂ which forms a complex with IF

④ B₁₂-IF complex is recognised by the cubilin IF-receptor and is endocytosed into enterocytes of the distal ileum. IF is degraded, and B₁₂ is released

⑤ Free B₁₂ then binds to transcobalamin II and enters the portal circulation. It is then transported to tissues where the B₁₂-transcobalamin II complex is endocytosed, degraded in lysosomes and B₁₂ is released into the cytosol

⑥ B₁₂ is stored in the liver as adenosylcobalamin and released into the circulation when needed

1.48 *E – 5–6 ATP molecules are produced from 2 NADH in oxidative decarboxylation*

In eukaryotic respiration, the total yield of ATP per glucose molecule has often been conflicting. Earlier studies showed a yield of 36–38 ATP per glucose molecule. However, more recent studies have shown this to be closer to 30–32 ATP per glucose molecule. The reason for this difference is based on electrochemical gradients in the mitochondria, as a result of electron carriers (NADH and FADH₂ from the Krebs). Four protons are needed to synthesise 1 ATP. In oxidative phosphorylation, 10 protons are pumped for every NADH, so therefore 1 NADH yields 2.5 ATP molecules; and 6 protons are pumped for every FADH₂, so therefore 1 FADH₂ yields 1.5 ATP molecules. This is in contrast to earlier studies where the ATP:NADH and ATP:FADH₂ were 3:1 and 2:1, respectively (yielding 36–38 ATP per glucose molecule). The maximum number of NADH and FADH₂ per glucose molecule is 10 and 2, respectively. Therefore, in oxidative phosphorylation, 28 ATP molecules are produced. Together with the 4 ATP molecules from substrate level phosphorylation, this yields a maximum of 32 ATP per glucose molecule. So why does the number range from 30 and 32? The electrons of the 2 NADH produced via glycolysis in the cytosol are transported into the mitochondria (as the mitochondrial membrane is impermeable to NADH) via two shuttle systems in the inner mitochondrial membrane: malate-aspartate and glycerol-phosphate. In the malate-aspartate shuttle, 2.5 ATP are produced when hydrogen from cytosolic NADH + H⁺ is transferred to mitochondrial NAD⁺. In the glycerol-phosphate shuttle, 1.5 ATP are produced when hydrogen from cytosolic NADH + H⁺ is transferred to mitochondrial FAD. Hence the ATP yield depends on the electron carrier. The tables below show ATP yield depending on the ratio between ATP and electron carriers.

Assuming ATP : NADH = 2.5 : 1 and ATP : FADH$_2$ = 1.5 : 1					
Stage	Carbon flow	Molecules of reduced coenzymes produced	Net ATP molecules produced by substrate-level phosphorylation	Net ATP molecules produced by oxidative phosphorylation	Theoretical maximum yield of ATP molecules
Glycolysis	6C → 2 x 2C	2 NADH	2	3 ATP from 2 NADH■ or 5 ATP from 2NADH●	5 or 7
Link reaction	2 x 3C → 2 x 2C + 2CO$_2$	2 NADH	0	5 ATP from 2 NADH	5
Krebs cycle	2 x 2C → 4CO$_2$	6 NADH 2 FADH$_2$	2	15 ATP from 6 NADH 3 ATP from 2 FADH$_2$	20
TOTAL:	6C → 6CO$_2$	10 NADH 2 FADH$_2$	4	26–28	**30–32**

■: glycerol-phosphate shuttle
●: malate-aspartate shuttle

Assuming ATP : NADH = 3 : 1 and ATP : FADH$_2$ = 2 : 1					
Stage	Carbon flow	Molecules of reduced coenzymes produced	Net ATP molecules produced by substrate-level phosphorylation	Net ATP molecules produced by oxidative phosphorylation	Theoretical maximum yield of ATP molecules
Glycolysis	6C → 2 x 2C	2 NADH	2	4 ATP from 2 NADH■ or 6 ATP from 2NADH●	6 or 8
Link reaction	2 x 3C → 2 x 2C + 2CO$_2$	2 NADH	0	6 ATP from 2 NADH	6
Krebs cycle	2 x 2C → 4CO$_2$	6 NADH 2 FADH$_2$	2	18 ATP from 6 NADH 4 ATP from 2 FADH$_2$	24
TOTAL:	6C → 6CO$_2$	10 NADH 2 FADH$_2$	4	32–34	**36–38**

■: glycerol-phosphate shuttle
●: malate-aspartate shuttle

Hence, as shown in the tables, oxidative decarboxylation (the link reaction) results in between 5 and 6 ATP molecules being produced from 2 NADH; E is therefore the correct response. Depending on the ATP:electron carrier, the net ATP molecules produced by oxidative phosphorylation is either 26–28, or 32–34 (not 30). There are four protein complexes in the inner membrane of the mitochondria (not three): *Complex I* – NADH ubiquinone oxidoreductase, *Complex II* – succinate ubiquinone reductase, *Complex III* – ubiquinol cytochrome c reductase, and *Complex IV* – cytochrome c oxidase. These function to translocate the 10 proteins from the mitochondrial matrix to the intermembrane space. In addition, ATP synthase is also present in the membrane, which pumps protons from the intermembrane space to the matrix, generating ATP. Complex IV receives electrons from cytochrome c and passes them to oxygen (the final electron acceptor, not water), which is reduced to water. Carbon monoxide (in addition to cyanide, sodium azide and hydrogen sulphide) inhibits cytochrome c oxidase (complex IV) in the respiratory chain, not ATP synthase. An example of an ATP synthase inhibitor (and oxidative phosphorylation) is the antibiotic, oligomycin.

1.49 *B – Rough ER → cis-Golgi network → Golgi cisternae → Secretory vesicle → Cell surface membrane*

Ribosomes synthesise proteins and become attached to the rough ER, where translation is finalised. Proteins can be inserted into the ER membrane, remain in the ER or get transported in transport vesicles. These fuse together to form *cis*-Golgi vesicles (nearest the ER) which progress into Golgi cisternae and *trans*-Golgi (farthest from the ER). During this stage, protein modifications occur. Some proteins remain in the *trans*-Golgi cisternae, while others are transported in secretory vesicles to the cell surface membrane, releasing contents by exocytosis; hence B is the correct response. The figure below summarises the secretory pathway of proteins.

Smooth ER are not involved in protein synthesis. Instead, they synthesise lipids (and cholesterol), phospholipids, steroids and carbohydrates. The lumen of the smooth ER is also an important storage site for intracellular calcium ions. The figure below summarises the secretory pathway of proteins.

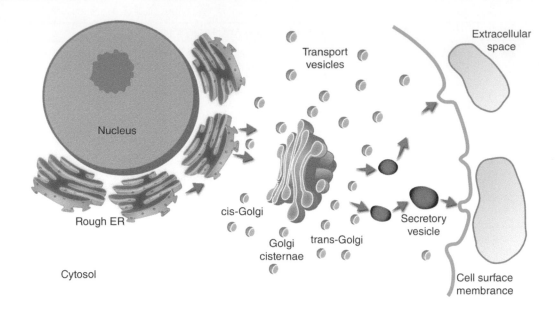

1.50 *B – ATG*

Complementary base pairing is the formation of linear hydrogen bonds between adenine (A) and thymine (T), i.e., A=T, and cytosine (C) and guanine (G), i.e., C≡G, creating a stable DNA double helix. In addition, the distance between the base pairs is virtually identical at ca. 3.4 Å which enables the DNA double helix to form with the correct spatial geometry. It is the precision of base pairing that allows nucleic acids to act as templates for the synthesis of new complementary strands. The non-transcribed, coding or sense strand, read in the 5′→3′ direction, is identical to the pre-mRNA sequence (except uracil (U) in RNA replaces T in DNA). Whereas the transcribed, non-coding or antisense strand, read in the 3′→5′ direction, acts as the template and is complementary to the 5′→3′ strand. The resulting mRNA formed in transcription is transported to the ribosome where, together with tRNA, it directs protein synthesis in translation. Each codon on mRNA interacts with a specific tRNA anticodon which carries an amino acid. Hence, in this example (working in reverse), the anticodon on tRNA is AUG; therefore this is complementary to UAC of the mRNA codon. So, the sense DNA sequence would be ATG and the non-coding (antisense template) sequence would be TAC; hence B is the correct response, such that:

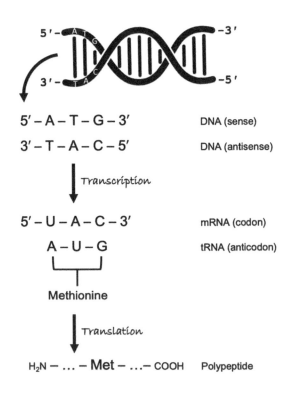

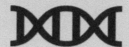

CHAPTER 2
Genetics

The art of medicine consists in amusing the patient, while nature cures the disease.

Voltaire

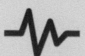

2.1 Which of the following regarding the Hardy-Weinberg equilibrium is **not** correct?
  A Consanguinity will lead to an increase in affected homozygotes
  B The frequency, p^2, is related to a homozygous genotype
  C Approximately, a disease incidence of 1/1000 equates to a carrier frequency of 1/36
  D Gene flow will lead to a change in allele frequency
  E $p + q = 1$

2.2 Which of the following factors can interfere with Hardy-Weinberg equilibrium?
  A Large population sizes
  B Random mating
  C Heterozygote advantage
  D No mutation
  E No gene flow

2.3 Which of the following regarding heterozygote advantage is **not** correct?
  A In sickle cell anaemia, heterozygotes are more resistant to effects of malaria than normal homozygotes
  B In autosomal dominant traits, homozygotes for a mutant allele have reduced biological fitness when compared with heterozygotes
  C It may explain the high frequency of Tay-Sachs disease in Ashkenazi Jews
  D It is one explanation for single locus polymorphisms
  E It may distort Hardy-Weinberg equilibrium

2.4 What is the expected incidence of affected homozygous females if an X-linked recessive disorder is in Hardy-Weinberg equilibrium and the incidence in males equals 1 in 50?
  A 1 in 250
  B 1 in 500
  C 1 in 2500
  D 1 in 5000
  E 1 in 25,000

2.5 Which of the following statements regarding Mendelian patterns of inheritance is correct?
  A In X-linked dominant inheritance, affected males transmit the disorder to their sons
  B In Y-linked inheritance, males are only affected
  C In autosomal recessive inheritance, parents cannot be related
  D In X-linked recessive inheritance, there is male-to-male transmission
  E In autosomal dominant inheritance, males are more affected than females

2.6 In pedigree drawings, the symbol represents
  A Stillbirth
  B Consanguinity
  C Spontaneous abortion
  D Termination of pregnancy
  E Infertile marriage

2.7 Which of the following symbols is used to represent an affected person of unknown sex when drawing pedigree diagrams?
  A
  B
  C
  D
  E

2.8 Which chromosome has the lowest total number of gene loci?
  A 1
  B 13
  C 21
  D X
  E Y

2.9   The formation of a pachytene quadrivalent is a feature of which of the following chromosomal abnormalities?
   A   Reciprocal translocations
   B   Robertsonian translocations
   C   Deletions
   D   Mosaicism
   E   Chimaerism

2.10 Which of the following descriptions regarding chromosomes are **not** correctly matched?
   A   Acrocentric – short p arm with the centromere located near one end of the chromosome
   B   Telocentric – no p arm is present, and the centromere is on the end
   C   Metacentric – p and q arms are approximately the same length and the centromere is in the middle
   D   Submetacentric – q arm is longer than the p arm and the centromere is located between the middle and the end
   E   Satellites – secondary constrictions at the end of a chromosome

2.11 The following definition is best described by which of the following terms?
   Sets of closely linked alleles on the same chromosome that tend to be inherited together. Evolutionary studies can then be performed.
   A   Haplotyping
   B   Single nucleotide polymorphism
   C   Epigenetics
   D   Imprinting
   E   Hybridization

2.12 Which of the following regarding the *p53* gene is correct?
   A   It is an RNA-binding protein
   B   Mutations in *p53* are rarely found in breast carcinomas
   C   In colorectal carcinomas, the mutant *p53* is longer lived than the normal allele
   D   *p53* is likely to act as a pentamer
   E   The protein encoded by it is a ribonucleoprotein

2.13 Which of the following tumour suppressor genes is associated with renal cell carcinoma?
   A   *p53*
   B   *APC*
   C   *Rb1*
   D   *VHL*
   E   *NF2*

2.14 Which of the following genetic disorders is **not** autosomal recessive?
   A   Tay-Sachs
   B   Cystic fibrosis
   C   Wilson's disease
   D   Thalassaemia
   E   Noonan syndrome

2.15 Which of the following gene mutations causes multiple endocrine neoplasia type 2 (MEN2)?
   A   *n-myc*
   B   *c-myc*
   C   *Ras*
   D   *Src*
   E   *RET*

2.16 Which of the following is **not** a sex chromosome aneuploidy syndrome?
   A   Turner syndrome
   B   Klinefelter syndrome
   C   Triple X
   D   XYY
   E   Patau syndrome

2.17 Which of the following syndromes is **not** caused by microdeletion?
A Williams
B Angelman
C Prader-Willi
D Fragile X
E DiGeorge

2.18 A baby born with cataracts caused by congenital rubella would be classified as having a
A malformation
B disruption
C deformation
D dysplasia
E syndrome

2.19 Which two chromosomes undergo a balanced reciprocal translocation in chronic myeloid leukaemia?
A 2 and 5
B 11 and 14
C 14 and 21
D 9 and 22
E 11 and 22

2.20 Which of the following statements regarding familial cancer syndromes is correct?
A Neurofibromatosis type 1 is one of the most common autosomal recessive disorders
B Neurofibromatosis type 2 can present with schwannomas in early adulthood
C Mutations in *BRCA2* account for 70% of all autosomal dominant breast cancers
D Von Hippel-Lindau is caused by mutations in DNA mismatch repair genes
E Desmoid tumours are a common feature of retinoblastomas

2.21 Which of the following autosomal dominant disorders results from a gene defect in fibrillin-1?
A Ehlers-Danlos
B Hypertrophic cardiomyopathy
C Achondroplasia
D Charcot-Marie-Tooth
E Marfan syndrome

Questions 2.22 to 2.24 relate to the following pattern of inheritance.

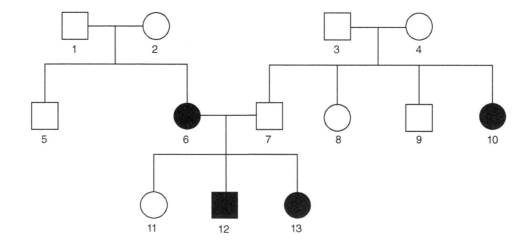

2.22 Which of the following patterns of inheritance is shown in this pedigree?
   A X-linked dominant
   B X-linked recessive
   C Autosomal dominant
   D Autosomal recessive
   E Codominance

2.23 Which of the following disorders shows this pattern of inheritance?
   A Achondroplasia
   B Hereditary haemochromatosis
   C Hereditary retinoblastoma
   D Duchenne muscular dystrophy
   E Rett syndrome

2.24 Which of the following regarding the pedigree is correct?
   A If parents 1 and 2 had another child, there is a 75% risk that they will be affected
   B Individual 5 can only be heterozygous
   C Males are affected more than females
   D If individual 10 married a heterozygous male, there is a 25% risk that their children would be affected
   E If individual 13 married an affected male, all children would be affected

2.25 Which of the following disorders of amino acid metabolism is caused by a build-up in the branched-chain amino acids valine, leucine and isoleucine?
   A Alkaptonuria
   B Maple syrup urine disease
   C Tyrosinaemia
   D Cystinuria
   E Homocystinuria

2.26 Which of the following X-linked diseases results in thrombocytopenia, atypical eczema and susceptibility to opportunistic infections, often associated with Epstein-Barr virus?
   A Hyper-IgM syndrome
   B Wiskott-Aldrich syndrome
   C Agammaglobulinaemia
   D Severe combined immunodeficiency
   E Chronic granulomatous disease

2.27 Which of the following conditions can be autosomal recessive **and** X-linked?
   A Oculocutaneous albinism
   B Hurler syndrome
   C Noonan syndrome
   D Lynch syndrome
   E Alport syndrome

2.28 Which of the following patterns of inheritance is shown in this pedigree?

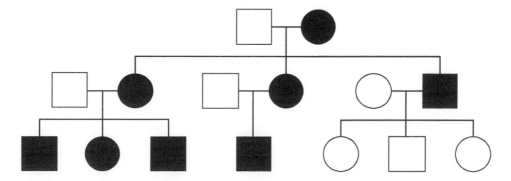

    A Mitochondrial
    B Autosomal dominance
    C Autosomal recessive
    D X-linked dominant
    E X-linked recessive

2.29 Which of the following blood types must a father have if his child is blood type A and the child's mother is blood type B?
    A A or AB or O
    B Either AB or O
    C Either AB or A
    D O only
    E AB only

2.30 Which of the following regarding trisomy 21 is correct?
    A Approximately 95% result from Robertsonian translocation
    B Mosaicism is common
    C Echocardiogram is not indicated when diagnosed
    D Risk of trisomy 21 in offspring of a mother who also has trisomy 21 is approximately 50%
    E There is an increased risk to second- and third-degree relatives, if the index case has trisomy 21

2.31 Which of the following regarding haemophilia is correct?
    A Haemophilia B is more common than haemophilia A
    B Ristocetin cofactor is useful, if diagnosis is uncertain
    C Mutations originate more in females than males
    D It shows incomplete penetrance in families
    E No known family history is found in approximately 30% of cases

2.32 The sister of an unaffected male has cystic fibrosis. The incidence of cystic fibrosis is 1 in 2500 live births. If the unaffected male has a partner who is not related and has no family history of cystic fibrosis, what is the probability that they will have an affected child with cystic fibrosis?
    A $\dfrac{1}{25}$
    B $\dfrac{1}{50}$
    C $\dfrac{1}{75}$
    D $\dfrac{1}{150}$
    E $\dfrac{1}{300}$

2.33 Which of the following regarding consent for genetic testing is **not** correct?
    A It is good clinical practice to document consent discussions in the clinical notes
    B Adults are presumed to have capacity to make decisions about testing
    C Children under 16 do not have capacity to make decisions about testing
    D Patients who lack capacity must have decisions made in their best interests
    E Consent should be broad, as many outcomes may be possible

2.34 Which of the following genetic disorders is **not** routinely screened in the new-born?
    A Down's syndrome
    B Sickle-cell anaemia
    C Hypothyroidism
    D Medium-chain acyl-coenzyme A dehydrogenase deficiency
    E Isovaleric acidaemia

2.35 Which of the following is the most likely diagnosis from these features?
Hypomelanotic macules, angiofibromas, shagreen patches and 'confetti' skin lesions
A Stickler syndrome
B Multiple endocrine neoplasia type I
C Tuberous sclerosis
D Neurofibromatosis type II
E Piebaldism

2.36 Which of the following conditions is characterised by macroglossia, gigantism and exomphalos?
A Acromegaly
B Beckwith-Wiedemann syndrome
C Hurler syndrome
D Amyloidosis
E McCune-Albright syndrome

2.37 Which of the following genetic disorders is **not** a ciliopathy?
A Kartagener's syndrome
B Retinitis pigmentosa
C Polycystic kidney disease
D Zollinger-Ellison syndrome
E Ellis-van Creveld syndrome

2.38 Which of the following diseases is **not** caused by trinucleotide-repeat mutations?
A Leber's hereditary optic neuropathy
B Fragile X syndrome
C Friedreich ataxia
D Myotonic dystrophy
E Kennedy disease (spinobulbar muscular atrophy)

2.39 During which of the following stages do chromosomes become visible and begin to condense?
A Zygotene
B Pachytene
C Diplotene
D Leptotene
E Diakinesis

2.40 Which of the following genetic disorders is shown in this karyotyping?

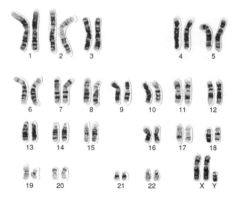

Source: Wellcome Collection

A Jacobs syndrome
B Klinefelter syndrome
C Triple X syndrome
D Patau syndrome
E Edwards syndrome

2.41   Which of the following is **not** a single-gene disorder?
A   Marfan syndrome
B   Cystic fibrosis
C   Huntington disease
D   Myotonic dystrophy
E   Cri-du-chat syndrome

2.42   Which of the following inborn errors of metabolism is **not** correctly matched to the associated deficiency?
A   Tay-Sachs disease – hexosaminidase A
B   Niemann-Pick disease – acid sphingomyelinase
C   McArdle disease – glucose-6-phosphatase
D   Cori disease – amylo-1,6-glucosidase
E   Zellweger syndrome – peroxisomal enzymes

2.43   Which of the following human leukocyte antigen (HLA) types is **not** correctly matched to the associated disease?
A   DR3 – Rheumatoid arthritis
B   B27 – Ankylosing spondylitis
C   DQ2 – Coeliac disease
D   DR15 – Goodpasture syndrome
E   DRB1 – Multiple sclerosis

2.44   Which of the following inherited causes of venous thrombosis results from a point mutation where there is a glutamine-for-arginine substitution at residue 506 or 534?
A   Protein C deficiency
B   Protein S deficiency
C   Factor V Leiden
D   Antithrombin deficiency
E   Prothrombin variant G20210A

2.45   Which of the following dinucleotide repeats can cluster in the promoter region and lead to repressed gene expression when methylated?
A   AC
B   TC
C   CG
D   TA
E   GA

2.46   Which of the following is **not** used as a method of delivering gene therapy?
A   Oncoretroviruses
B   Lentiviruses
C   Plasmid DNA
D   Antisense oligonucleotides
E   Liposomes

2.47   Which of the following regarding cancer is **not** correct?
A   Burkitt lymphoma is a high-grade nasopharyngeal carcinoma
B   Mutations in *TP53* can lead to development of small cell lung cancer
C   Men with mutations in the *BRCA2* gene have ~8% lifetime risk of developing breast cancer than men who do not
D   Men with mutations in the *BRCA1* and *HOXB13* genes are at an increased risk of developing prostate cancer
E   Melanoma affects women and men equally

2.48   Which of the following terms best describes the interaction between non-allelic genes?
A   Epigenetics
B   Epistasis
C   Eugenics
D   Ecogenetics
E   Epialleles

2.49 Which of the following terms best describes the inactivation of an X chromosome?
A Methylation
B Hemizygosity
C Lyonization
D Segregation
E Recombination

2.50 Which of the following statements is correct?
A There is a 50% chance that babies will be of equal sex in a dizygotic twin pregnancy
B The chance that an uncle of an affected individual is a carrier for an autosomal recessive disorder is 1 in 4
C In autosomal dominant disorders, a penetrance of 0.55 means that 45% of heterozygotes will manifest the condition
D Bayes' theorem is based exclusively on ancestral information
E In order to calculate posterior probability, ancestral information is not required

Answers

2.1 *C – Approximately, a disease incidence of 1/1000 equates to a carrier frequency of 1/36*

The Hardy-Weinberg principle considers an 'ideal' population where no internal factors disturb the allele distribution within a population. If there are two alleles, A and a found at an autosomal locus with allele frequencies of p and q, respectively, then $p + q = 1$ (i.e. 100%). Thus, genotypes AA, Aa and aa have allele frequencies p^2, $2pq$ and q^2 respectively, where $p^2 + 2pq + q^2 = 1$. Therefore, if a disease incidence (of an autosomal recessive disorder) is 1 in 1000 (i.e. 1/1000), then $q^2 = 1/1000$ and $q = 1/32$ so $p = 31/32$. This means the carrier frequency, $2pq = 2 \times (31/32) \times (1/32)$ which approximates to 1 in 16 or 1/16 (not 1/36); hence C is the correct response.

2.2 *C – Heterozygote advantage*

Factors which can disturb Hardy-Weinberg equilibrium include non-random mating, mutations, small population sizes, gene flow or migration and selection. Selection for heterozygotes or heterozygote advantage occurs when carriers have a biological advantage over non-carriers resulting in increased biological fitness; hence C is the correct response as in the 'ideal' population there is no selection for or against a particular genotype. There are a number of examples where this type of selection occurs including haemoglobinopathies such as sickle cell anaemia where heterozygotes are relatively immune to malaria caused by *Plasmodium falciparum*, cystic fibrosis, phenylketonuria and Tay-Sachs disease.

2.3 *B – In autosomal dominant traits, homozygotes for a mutant allele have reduced biological fitness when compared with heterozygotes*

In autosomal recessive disorders, heterozygotes show more of a biological fitness compared with unaffected homozygotes; hence B is the correct response. All other options are true for heterozygote advantage. Sickle cell anaemia highlights this where homozygotes have significant anaemia. Yet the sickle shapes of red blood cells in heterozygotes are destroyed in *Plasmodium falciparum* malaria.

2.4 *C – 1 in 2500*

In an X-linked recessive disorder, the frequency of affected males is equal to that of the mutant allele, q. Therefore, if the incidence of affected males is 1 in 50, then $q = 1/50$ and $p = 49/50$. So, the carrier frequency, $2pq = 2 \times (49/50) \times (1/50)$, which approximates to 1 in 25, and the frequency of affected females, $q^2 = 1/2500$ or 1 in 2500; hence C is the correct response.

2.5 *B – In Y-linked inheritance, males are only affected*

In Y-linked inheritance, affected males pass on traits to all sons but none are passed to daughters, and so males are only affected; hence B is the correct response. It is very rare, and interestingly hairy ears are an example. In X-linked dominant inheritance, affected males transmit the disorder to all daughters and none to sons. An example is vitamin D-resistant rickets. An enquiry into the family history of members who have rare recessive disorders may reveal that parents are related, i.e., consanguineous mating. In X-linked recessive inheritance, affected males transmit the disorder to heterozygous females (carriers), or heterozygous females transmit to affected males. There is no male-to-male transmission (although there is a very rare exception to this: uniparental heterodisomy). Examples include haemophilia A and B, Duchenne muscular dystrophy, ocular albinism and Fragile X syndrome. In autosomal dominance inheritance, alleles manifest in heterozygotes. Males and females are affected equally. Examples include Huntington's disease, Marfan syndrome, achondroplasia and hypertrophic obstructive cardiomyopathy.

2.6 *D – Termination of pregnancy*

Family trees, or pedigree drawings, are a graphical method of recording pertinent information about a family. The person in question can be referred to as the index case, proband, propositus (male) or proposita (female). As shown in the figure below, there are a variety of symbols that can be used in drawing family trees. A triangle with a line through it identifies a termination of pregnancy; hence D is the correct response.

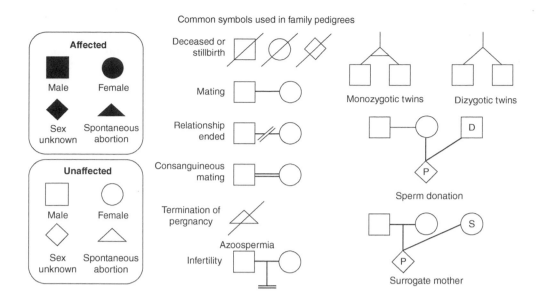

Common symbols used in family pedigrees

2.7 *E –* ◆

As shown in the figure in 2.6, a black diamond identifies an affected person of unknown sex; hence E is the correct response. Black shapes highlight that family members are affected, whereas white shapes are unaffected. Squares and circles depict males and females, respectively.

2.8 *E – Y*

Chromosome Y contains approximately 200 genes. The most noteworthy being *SRY* – testes-determining factor. Chromosome 1 contains the most genes with over 3000. Examples include *HPC1* – prostate cancer, *GLC1A* – glaucoma, *PS2* – Alzheimer's disease and *GBA* – Gaucher disease. Chromosome 13 contains approximately 800 genes. Examples include *BRCA2* – breast cancer, *RB1* – retinoblastoma and *ATP7B* – Wilson disease. Chromosome 21 contains approximately 400 genes. The most noteworthy being *SOD1* – amyotrophic lateral sclerosis. Hence E is the correct response.

2.9 *A – Reciprocal translocations*

Reciprocal translocations occur when genetic material is exchanged between two homologous chromosomes with no net loss of genetic information. Reciprocal translocation can lead to a normal phenotype, yet problems can arise at meiosis where balanced reciprocal translocations segregate, generating chromosomal imbalance. Rather than pairing in 'twos' to form bivalents, they end up pairing in 'fours' to form a pachytene quadrivalent, where each homologous chromosome aligns; hence A is the correct response. There are two patterns of segregation of reciprocal translocations:

1) 2:2 segregation – either alternate chromosomes segregate, and the gamete contains normal chromosomes or a balanced rearrangement. Or, if there is segregation of adjacent chromosomes, this results in unbalanced chromosomes leading to partial monosomy and trisomy in the zygote.
2) 3:1 segregation – three chromosomes segregate to one gamete and one chromosome in the other gamete. This unbalance leads to trisomy in the zygote with three chromosomes and monosomy in the zygote with one chromosome.

A Robertsonian translocation occurs between two acrocentric chromosomes (chromosomes which have centromeres close to one end, resulting in a small p arm). In humans, there are six acrocentric chromosomes: 13, 14, 15, 21, and 22 and in males, the Y chromosome. These translocations result in 45 chromosomes as two q long arms fuse and two p short arms are lost. In fact, there is little clinical relevance to the short p arms being lost as they only code for ribosomal RNA. These translocations are one of the most common functionally balanced rearrangements in the general population. Robertsonian translocation involving chromosomes 13 and 21 can lead to Patau and Down syndrome, respectively.

Deletions involve loss of sections of a chromosome which can result in monosomy. Clinically, the larger the deletion, the more lethal and incompatible with survival. This is certainly the case with the autosomes. However with monosomy for an X chromosome (45,X), where the other gamete loses the X or Y chromosome, this results in Turner syndrome. Other examples of disorders caused by deletions include DiGeorge, William's and Cri du chat syndromes.

When one or more cell lines differ in chromosome constitution in an individual or tissue but are derived from a single zygote, this is known as mosaicism. It usually results from non-disjunction in early embryonic mitotic division. For example, if two chromatids failed to separate in meiosis II in a human zygote, the four-celled zygote would contain two cells with 46 chromosomes (normal cell lines), one cell with 47 chromosomes (trisomy cell line) and one cell with 45 chromosomes (monosomy cell line). Clinically, mosaicism accounts for approximately 1% of cases of Down syndrome. The difference with chimaerism is that cell lines originate from different zygotes. A chimera (Think: head of a lion, body of a goat and tail of a dragon) arises from fusion of more than one zygote. Natural chimaerism is rare but can occur in utero when cells are exchanged via the placenta in non-identical twins. Parenthetically, in 1945, Dr Ray Owen described blood cell chimaerism in freemartin cattle. Gonadal chimaerism results in pseudohermaphroditism whereby a female cow is rendered infertile following exposure to male sex hormones through anastomoses between placental circulations with a male twin *in utero*. This results in XX/XY chimaeras.

2.10 D – Submetacentric – q arm is longer than the p arm and the centromere is located between the middle and the end

Morphologically, chromosomes are classified depending upon the position of the centromere, as shown in the figure below. If the centromere is centrally located, the chromosome is metacentric. If it is located at the end of one chromosome, it can result in small p arms with very small appendages called satellites (secondary constrictions) which encode ribosomal RNA. These are acrocentric chromosomes. Submetacentric chromosomes have the centromere slightly offset from the centre which leads to asymmetry in p and q arm length, i.e., it is in an intermediate position between the two; hence D is the correct response.

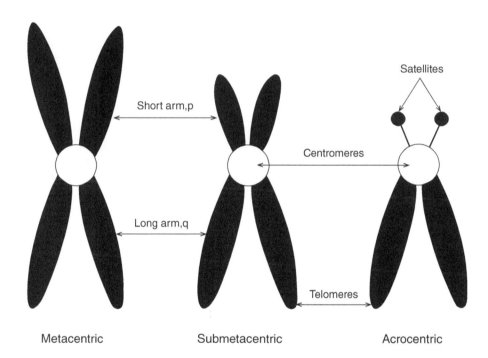

2.11 A – Haplotyping

A haplotype is the combination of alleles found on a single chromosome that were inherited together from a single parent. Evolutionary studies can be performed using haplotyping; hence A is the correct response. Single nucleotide polymorphism is a single base-pair difference in the DNA sequence. Epigenetics is the study of changes to gene function and expression that are heritable but by factors other than changes to the genetic code. Two modifications involved in epigenetics are DNA methylation and histone modification. Genomic imprinting is the ability of a gene to be expressed which depends on the sex of the parent who passed on the gene. For example, some imprinted genes are expressed when inherited only from the father, and others from the mother. A clinical example of this is when deletions occur on chromosome 15 that resulted from the father, the child will have Prader-Willi syndrome. Yet when this deletion resulted from the mother, the child will have Angelman syndrome. Hybridization is the process of combining two complementary single strands of DNA or RNA and allowing them to form single double-stranded molecules.

2.12 C – In colorectal carcinomas, the mutant p53 is longer lived than the normal allele

The *p53* gene is a tumour suppressor gene which helps control the cell cycle, DNA repair and apoptosis. Approximately 60% of patients with colorectal carcinoma show somatic mutations in *p53* and this is associated with poor clinical outcomes. Furthermore, patients with mutant *p53* are often resistant to current therapies, and this worsens the prognosis even further. In this regard, the mutant *p53* is longer lived than the normal allele; hence C is the correct response. *p53* is a tumour suppressor protein and not an RNA-binding protein. Mutations in p53 are found in breast cancers. In fact, approximately 30% are present in primary breast cancers, and mutation is associated with more aggressive disease and worse overall survival. Although not rare, mutations are lower in breast cancer compared to other solid tumours. The p53 protein (not the gene) acts as a transcription factor (not a ribonucleoprotein) and exists as a homotetramer (not a pentamer).

2.13 D – VHL

von Hippel-Lindau (VHL) is an autosomal dominant condition resulting from mutation in the *VHL* gene on chromosome 3. Tumours and/or cysts can develop in multiple locations within the body such as haemangioblastomas in the brain and eyes, pancreatic cysts/tumours, phaeochromocytoma, cystadenomas and renal cell carcinoma; hence D is the correct response. Somatic mutations in p53 can lead to bladder, lung and ovarian cancers, in addition to breast cancer, head and neck squamous cell carcinoma, melanoma and Wilms tumours. Li-Fraumeni syndrome is associated with germline mutations of *p53* and appears to be the only cancer syndrome associated with inherited mutations. Mutations in the *APC* (adenomatous polyposis coli) gene are responsible for familial adenomatous polyposis (FAP) and sporadic colorectal cancers, in addition to rarer desmoid tumours of connective tissue. Mutations in the *Rb1* gene are associated with retinoblastoma, more commonly in children. Some cases have also been reported in bladder, lung and breast cancers, melanoma, osteosarcoma and some leukaemias. The NF2 gene encodes a protein called merlin (or schwannomin). Mutations in this gene leads to neurofibromatosis type 2, whereby multiple tumours form in the nervous system as a result of the loss of merlin's function. They are particularly more common between the ears and brain, resulting in bilateral acoustic neuromas which can distort balance and hearing.

2.14 E – Noonan syndrome

Noonan syndrome is autosomal dominant (not recessive); hence E is the correct response. This condition causes abnormal development of multiple body parts including widely spaced eyes, large ears, short webbed neck, ptosis, short stature, pectus excavatum, developmental delay and cryptorchidism. All other conditions are autosomal recessive. Tay-Sachs is a lysosomal storage disorder caused by deficiency of the enzyme hexosaminidase A. Cystic fibrosis is caused by mutations of the cystic fibrosis transmembrane conductance regulator (CFTR) gene. Wilson's disease is a disorder in which excessive amounts of copper accumulates in the body, especially the liver, brain and eyes. Thalassaemia is an inherited blood disorder whereby abnormal and/or insufficient haemoglobin is formed.

2.15 E – RET

MEN2 is an autosomal dominant syndrome caused by mutation in the *RET* (rearranged during transfection) proto-oncogene; hence E is the correct response. *RET* encodes a tyrosine kinase receptor which regulates cell proliferation and apoptosis. There are three main subtypes: (1) MEN2A, which accounts for 70–80% of cases, is associated with medullary thyroid carcinoma, phaeochromocytoma and/or hyperparathyroidism; (2) MEN2B, which accounts for ca. 5% of cases, is more common in childhood and is associated with an aggressive form of medullary thyroid carcinoma and phaeochromocytoma, but no parathyroid disease; and (3) familial medullary thyroid carcinoma, which accounts for 10–20% of cases, is associated with a family history without phaeochromocytoma or parathyroid disease. The Myc (myelocytomatosis) family of genes are helix-loop-helix/leucine zipper transcription factors that regulate gene expression. Amplification of *n-myc* leads to neuroblastoma, retinoblastoma, glioblastoma and medulloblastoma. Translocation of the proto-oncogene *c-myc* from its normal position on chromosome 8 to chromosome 14 results in Burkitt's lymphoma. The *Ras* (rat sarcomas) genes encode small GTP-binding proteins which are important in cell growth, division and differentiation, and apoptosis. There are three human *Ras* genes: *H-Ras*, *N-Ras* and *K-Ras*. Mutations in *H-Ras* are associated with Costello syndrome. Individuals show developmental delay, intellectual disability, distinctive facial features and loose folds of extra skin. They may also have heart abnormalities. Mutations in *H-Ras* are also known to cause epidermal naevi, and some bladder, renal and thyroid cancers. Mutations in *N-Ras* are associated with acute myeloid leukaemia. Mutations in *K-Ras* are associated with lung, pancreatic and colorectal cancers.

2.16 E – Patau syndrome

Sex chromosome aneuploidies are characterised by the loss or gain of one or more sex chromosomes. Patau syndrome or trisomy 13 is characterised by having three copies of chromosome 13 in cells rather than the usual two. It is not a sex chromosome aneuploidy syndrome; hence E is the correct response. The more common sex chromosome aneuploidies include Turner (XO) and Klinefelter (XXY) syndromes, trisomy X (XXX), XYY and XXYY.

2.17 D – Fragile X

Microdeletions or sub-microscopic deletions involve the loss of genes at closely adjacent loci but are too small to be detected by karyotype. However, they can be detected by chromosomal microarrays. Many of the microdeletion syndromes are termed contiguous gene syndromes since the phenotype is often attributable to more or less copies of multiple genes close to one another. In some syndromes, multiple loci are involved. Fragile X results from a mutation in the *FMR1* gene on the X chromosome. This results in trinucleotide expansion of the CGG repeat region which, when several hundred repeat, leads to gene methylation causing loss of function of the FMR protein; hence D is the correct response. All other syndromes are examples of microdeletions – Williams on chromosome 7, Angelman and Prader-Willi on chromosome 15, and DiGeorge on chromosome 22.

2.18   *B – disruption*

A disruption is a morphological change due to external, destructive forces which act on the normal developmental process. This can lead to cell death or tissue destruction as a result of mechanical forces, teratogens, infections and vascular anomalies. They are usually caused by environmental factors and recurrence rate is extremely low. Examples include cataracts caused by congenital rubella, limb defects caused by amniotic bands and spina bifida caused by sodium valproate; hence B is the correct response. A malformation is a morphological change due to an intrinsic abnormality in the developing structure. There is often termination or altered tissue formation or differentiation during early development which are caused by genetic or environmental factors, or a combination of both. Examples include neural tube defects, cardiac defects, and cleft lip/palate. A deformation is due to a destructive, mechanical force which distorts normal development, such that intrinsic embryonic development is normal but mechanical compression restricts foetal movement. They usually occur late in pregnancy and convey a good prognosis. Examples include congenital dislocation of the hip, talipes, and renal agenesis. A dysplasia is abnormal organisation of cells into tissue. This usually results in a particular tissue being affected in all parts of the body. Most are caused by single-gene defects with high recurrence risks. Examples include skeletal dysplasia such as achondroplasia, osteogenesis imperfecta and thanatophoric dysplasia (short limbs); and ectodermal dysplasia, where abnormal skin, hair, teeth and nails abnormally develop, such as cranioectodermal dysplasia and Ellis-van-Creveld syndrome. A syndrome is a collection of signs and symptoms that occur together in a specific disease, where recognisable patterns of abnormalities are pathogenetically related. They can be caused by chromosomal abnormalities, single-gene defects or are multifactorial. Examples include Down syndrome, foetal alcohol syndrome and Van der Woude syndrome (cleft palate/lip and lip pits). There are many recognised causes of congenital anomalies, yet over half have no clear cause.

2.19   *D – 9 and 22*

Over 90% of patients with chronic myeloid leukaemia have an abnormal chromosome called the Philadelphia chromosome, where the *ABL* (Abelson) oncogene on chromosome 9 has been reciprocally translocated into the breakpoint cluster region (BCR) on chromosome 22; hence D is the correct response. Over 60% of patients with anaplastic large cell lymphoma have a translocation between chromosomes 2 and 5. A hallmark of mantle cell lymphoma is a translocation between chromosomes 11 and 14. Less than 5% of patients with Down syndrome have a Robertsonian translocation between chromosomes 14 and 21. Over 85% of patients with Ewing sarcoma have a reciprocal translocation between chromosomes 11 and 22.

2.20   *B – Neurofibromatosis type 2 can present with schwannomas in early adulthood*

Neurofibromatosis type 2 usually presents with bilateral vestibulocochlear nerve tumours (schwannomas or acoustic neuromas) in early adulthood; hence B is the correct response. Café-au-lait patches are also present in small numbers. It is much rarer than type 1, which is a common autosomal dominant (not recessive) disorder that also presents with café-au-lait patches (albeit in greater quantities), freckling in the axilla and groin and several cutaneous neurofibromata. Mutations in *BRCA2* account for approximately 30% (not 70%) of all autosomal dominant breast cancers. Mutations in *BRCA1* is higher at approximately 50%. However, lifetime risk in heterozygous women increases with age. Von Hippel-Lindau is caused by mutations in the *VHL* gene (not DNA mismatch repair genes). DNA repair genes include *BRCA1* and *BRCA2* which cause familial breast cancer 1 and 2, respectively, and *MLH1* and *MSH2* which cause hereditary non-polyposis colorectal cancer. Children who are treated for retinoblastoma are at a higher risk of developing osteosarcoma (not desmoid tumours) in later life. Desmoid tumours are a common feature of familial adenomatous polyposis.

2.21   *E – Marfan syndrome*

Marfan syndrome is a fibrous connective tissue disorder which is caused by mutations in the *FBN1* gene encoding fibrillin-1; hence E is the correct response. Ehlers-Danlos, another connective tissue disorder of which there are several types, is caused by abnormal collagen synthesis. Several gene mutations are known to cause various types, including *COL5A1* and *COL5A2* in types I and II, *TENXB* (which codes for tenascin, an important glycoprotein in collagen fibrillogenesis) in type III and *COL3A1* in type IV. Hypertrophic cardiomyopathy can result from several gene mutations which encode sarcomere-associated proteins, of which *MYH7* and *MYBPC3* appear to be the most common. Achondroplasia is caused by a mutation in the fibroblast growth factor receptor-3 gene (*FGFR3*). Charcot-Marie-Tooth is a disorder of the motor and/or sensory peripheral nerves. The disease shows interesting genetics as single genes can be inherited in an autosomal dominant, autosomal recessive, X-linked dominant and X-linked recessive pattern. With several genes being responsible for various forms of the disease, duplication of the *PMP22* gene appears to be the most common. Yet in many cases, the genes that are responsible have not been identified.

2.22 D – *Autosomal recessive*

Autosomal recessive inheritance is manifest only when the mutant allele is present in the homozygous state, and affected individuals have two mutant alleles. One mutant allele is inherited from each heterozygous parent who are carriers. Unlike vertical autosomal dominance inheritance, it is not possible to trace autosomal recessive traits in families since (generally) only members of a single sibship are affected. It is therefore often referred to as horizontal transmission (often at the dismay of geneticists!). This family tree shows autosomal recessive inheritance, where both males and females are affected; hence D is the correct response.

Although rare, an X-linked dominant disorder is caused by mutation in a gene on the X-chromosome which manifest in a heterozygous female and/or a male who has the mutant allele on his X-chromosome. Both males and females are affected, but only the daughters and none of the sons of an affected male are affected, hence there is no direct male-to-male transmission.

An X-linked recessive disorder is caused by mutation in a gene on the X-chromosome and usually manifest in males. Males who have a mutant allele on the X-chromosome are hemizygous; hence, the disorder resulting from the mutant allele will be expressed. Females are not affected, and all daughters of an affected male are carriers (unless they also inherited the mutant allele from their mother). There is a 1 in 2 chance of a son being affected if their mother is a carrier. This type of inheritance can often be described as a 'knights move'.

An autosomal dominant condition is one that manifests in the heterozygous state; hence an individual will be affected if they possess one normal and one mutant allele. Males and females are affected who both can pass on the disorder to sons and daughters.

Co-dominance occurs when two dominant alleles are equally expressed in the heterozygous state. ABO blood groups are a good example of this whereby the offspring with an AB blood group inherits blood group A from the father and blood group B from the mother.

2.23 B – *Hereditary haemochromatosis*

Hereditary haemochromatosis is the only option from the list which shows autosomal recessive inheritance. Achondroplasia and hereditary retinoblastoma are autosomal dominant disorders. Duchenne muscular dystrophy shows X-linked recessive inheritance. Rett syndrome shows X-linked dominant inheritance.

2.24 E – *If individual 13 married an affected male, all children would be affected*

In autosomal recessive inheritance, if individual 13 married an affected male, all children would be affected because both parents would be homozygous so all children must also be homozygous; hence E is the correct response. If parents 1 and 2 had another child, there is a 25% (not 75%) risk that they will be affected. Individual 5 could be homozygous or heterozygous. Males and females are equally affected in this inheritance pattern. If individual 10 married a heterozygous male, there is a 50% (not 25%) risk that their children would be affected since there is one homozygous affected female and one heterozygous unaffected male.

2.25 B – *Maple syrup urine disease*

Maple syrup urine disease is a rare autosomal recessive disorder that prevents metabolism of the branched-chain amino acids – valine, leucine and isoleucine caused by branched-chain α-ketoacid dehydrogenase deficiency. As the name suggests, new-born infants have a characteristic maple syrup odour of the urine; hence B is the correct response. Alkaptonuria is a rare autosomal recessive disorder which was the first to be recognised by Sir Archibald Garrod to comply with the principles of Mendelian genetics. It is a disorder of homogentisic acid (HGA) metabolism, a metabolite of tyrosine and phenylalanine, caused by deficiency of homogentisic acid oxidase. Excess HGA is excreted in the urine and upon exposure to air, the urine darkens. Dark pigment is also deposited in the sclera, cartilage and cerumen. Tyrosinaemia is an autosomal recessive disorder caused by deficiency of fumarylacetoacetate hydrolase, which is involved in tyrosine metabolism. It affects the liver, kidneys and peripheral nerves. Cystinuria (another inborn error of metabolism identified by Sir Archibald Garrod) is another rare autosomal recessive disorder caused by mutations in genes encoding transporter protein of the proximal tubule and small intestine, specifically of the dibasic amino acids – cysteine, lysine, arginine and ornithine. This results in excessive urinary secretion and the formation of urinary calculi. Hexagonal crystals on urinalysis are pathognomonic of the disease. Homocystinuria is also a rare autosomal recessive disorder usually caused by deficiency of the enzyme cystathionine β-synthase which is required for the conversion of methionine to cysteine. Diagnosis is confirmed by raised plasma homocysteine and methionine levels.

2.26 B – *Wiskott-Aldrich syndrome*

Wiskott-Aldrich syndrome is a rare X-linked recessive disorder in which affected boys have a triad of eczema, thrombocytopaenia and immunodeficiency. Other features may include petechiae, bruising, abnormal immunoglobulin isotypes, reduced T cells, recurrent infections and failure to thrive. Malignancies can also occur in young adulthood, with B cell lymphoma in Epstein-Barr virus positive patients being common; hence B is the correct response.

Hyper-IgM syndrome is an X-linked recessive condition (although there is a rare form that affects girls) which results in elevated levels of IgM (in addition to IgD), but lower levels of IgG, IgE and IgA. The CD40 ligand, normally expressed on the surface of activated T cells, is absent. This means T cells cannot bind to the CD40 on B cells, so IgM is produced continually but there is no isotype switching to IgA or IgG. Patients are susceptible to recurrent pyogenic infections, particularly *Pneumocystis* pneumonia. Agammaglobulinaemia is a primary humoral immunodeficiency which can consist of two types: (1) the X-linked variant Bruton-type which affects boys, and results from mutation in a tyrosine kinase gene specific to B cells (BTK); and (2) the autosomal recessive variant which affects boys and girls, and results from mutations in several genes that regulate B-cell development. Children develop multiple recurrent bacterial infections of the respiratory tract, and despite multiple antibiotic regimes, irreversible bronchiectasis may develop. Severe combined immunodeficiency (SCID) is the most common inherited disorder of cell-mediated specific acquired immunity characterised by defects in both B- and T-cell function. Children typically present with severe viral and/or bacterial infections, and death can be common unless bone marrow transplantation or gene therapy are performed. Most are X-linked which result from mutations in the gamma chain of the cytokine receptor interleukin-2 and result in dysfunctional B-cells (with normal number), but absent T-cells. Approximately 30–50% of children show autosomal recessive inheritance, which includes adenosine deaminase and purine nucleoside deficiency. Chronic granulomatous disease can be X-linked or autosomal recessive and is caused by a gene defect that encodes reduced nicotinamide adenine dinucleotide phosphate (NADPH) oxidase system. This results in the inability of phagocytes to generate superoxide radicals and other reactive oxygen species. Patients are susceptible to life-threatening catalase-positive bacterial and fungal infections. Routine use of prophylactic antibiotic and antifungals have significantly improved survival rates.

2.27 E – Alport syndrome

Alport syndrome is a progressive nephropathy caused by mutations encoding type IV collagen which subsequently renders glomerular basement membrane dysfunction. It is characterised by haematuria, proteinuria, worsening renal function, sensorineural deafness and multiple ophthalmic disorders (retinal detachment, cataracts and keratoconus). Alport syndrome can show X-linked dominant, autosomal dominant and autosomal recessive patterns of inheritance; hence E is the correct response. Oculocutaneous albinism is a rare autosomal recessive disorder (of which there are seven types) characterised by reduction or absence of melanin pigment in the eyes, skin and hair. This should not be confused with ocular albinism which is an X-linked recessive disorder which solely affects pigments of the eyes. Hurler syndrome, a lysosomal storage disease, is also autosomal recessive and caused by mutation in a gene that leads to the deficiency of the α-L-iduronidase enzyme with an accumulation of dermatan and heparan sulfate in the lysosomes. Diagnosis is based on detection of these glycosaminoglycans in the urine. Noonan syndrome is predominantly an autosomal dominant disorder caused by multiple gene mutations, but mutations in the *LZTR1* gene cane be inherited in an autosomal dominant or recessive pattern. It is a multisystem disorder characterised by webbed-neck, low-set ears, short stature, ptosis, down-slanting palpebral fissures, delayed puberty, conductive hearing loss, pectus excavatum and right-sided heart disease, often with pulmonary stenosis. Lynch syndrome, or hereditary non-polyposis colorectal cancer, is an autosomal dominant condition which results from mutations in multiple genes involved in DNA repair. It causes an increased risk of developing cancers of the colon and rectum, as well as stomach, small intestine and liver.

2.28 A – Mitochondrial

In humans, mitochondrial DNA is exclusively inherited from the mother via the oocyte. Sperm do not contribute any mitochondria to the developing zygote. Therefore, mitochondrial inheritance is maternal in origin. There is often phenotypic diversity seen in individuals with mitochondrial disorders and an explanation for this relates to the proportion of normal and abnormal mitochondria inherited. Most mitochondrial DNA is identical and free from mutations (homoplasmy). However, abnormal mitochondria can also be present, as seen in mitochondrial disorders, which skew the distribution (heteroplasmy). When a higher threshold of abnormal mitochondria is reached, an abnormal phenotype is present. This pedigree shows mitochondrial inheritance; hence A is the correct response as both males and females are affected and the disorder is transmitted from mother to offspring. In addition, an affected father and unaffected mother have children without the disorder. In some instances, not all children in mitochondrial inheritance will be affected, and this is a result of how expression can vary depending on the proportion of abnormal mitochondria inherited. Leber hereditary optic neuropathy shows this pattern of inheritance characterised by sudden bilateral, painless loss of vision during early adulthood. Another example is MELAS (mitochondrial encephalopathy, lactic acidosis and stroke-like episodes) which begins in childhood and results in widespread dysfunction of muscles and nerves.

2.29 C – Either AB or A

The four major ABO blood groups are A, B, AB and O. Individuals who are blood group A and B possess either antigen A and B on the surface of red blood cells, respectively. Individuals who are blood group AB have both antigens A and B, and individuals who are blood group O have neither. Individuals of blood group A and B have anti-B antibodies and anti-A antibodies in their blood, respectively. Individuals of blood group O have both. The genes for A and B in the ABO system show co-dominance inheritance. Individuals with blood group AB are referred to as *universal recipients* as they can receive red blood cells from any ABO blood type. Individuals with blood type O are referred to as *universal donors* as they can give red blood cells to any ABO blood type. The table below summarises the possible blood types of a child and the blood-type combinations of their parents.

If a child is blood type A and the mother is blood type B, the only possible blood type the father could be is either AB or A; hence C is the correct response. A father with blood type O and mother with blood type B could only have a child with blood type B or O. Therefore, A, B and D are not possible options. Option E is also not feasible as the father could be A or AB.

Parent 1		A	A	A	A	B	B	B	AB	AB	O
Parent 2		A	B	AB	O	B	AB	O	AB	O	O
Possible blood types of child	A	✓	✓	✓	✓		✓		✓	✓	
	B		✓	✓		✓	✓	✓	✓	✓	
	AB		✓	✓			✓		✓		
	O	✓	✓		✓	✓		✓			✓

2.30   D – Risk of trisomy 21 in offspring of a mother who also has trisomy 21 is approximately 50%

People with trisomy 21 rarely reproduce. Up to one-third of women are fertile and have a risk of approximately 50% of having a child with trisomy 21; hence D is the correct response. Although there have been very few reported cases of parenting fathers with trisomy 21, men are usually infertile. Over 90% of Down syndrome cases are caused by trisomy, where the extra chromosome is maternal in origin, and usually a result of non-disjunction in meiosis I. Robertsonian translocation accounts for 3–4% of all cases and approximately 70–80% of these arise *de novo*. Mosaicism is much rarer at less than 2% and often these patients are less severely affected than those with trisomy. Congenital cardiac anomalies are present in approximately 40–60% of patients with Down Syndrome. Foetal echocardiography can help with early recognition of Down Syndrome, and it plays an important role in detection of structural and functional anomalies in the post-natal period, especially if cardiac surgery is to be performed. Although there are very few studies that have investigated the occurrence risk estimates with Down Syndrome in second- and third-degree relatives, there does not appear to be an increased risk.

2.31   E – No known family history is found in approximately 30% of cases

Haemophilia A and B (Christmas disease) is caused by deficiencies in factor VIII and IX, respectively. In approximately 70% of haemophilia cases, there is a known family history and therefore in 30% of cases, a family history is not known; hence E is the correct response. Haemophilia A is more common than haemophilia B (1 in 5000 compared to 1 in 30,000 male births, respectively).

Ristocetin cofactor can be added to platelet-rich plasma in order to measure ristocetin-induced platelet aggregation. This can be used as an *in vitro* test of functional von Willebrand factor, which can be deficient or defected in von Willebrand disease (the most common inherited bleeding disorder). There are three types of this disease, and the ristocetin assay is useful in distinguishing between the multiple variants of type 2 von Willebrand disease.

Haemophilia is an X-linked recessive condition where males are affected more frequently than females since they only have one X chromosome which contains the gene mutation. Hence fathers cannot pass this gene mutation to their sons. Penetrance is the proportion of individuals who have the trait genotype who also show the trait phenotype. When a genotype is known but a phenotype is not observable, i.e., an individual has a condition but shows no symptoms, the trait shows incomplete penetrance. Haemophilia shows complete penetrance, as does red-green colour blindness and Huntington's disease. Examples of conditions which show incomplete penetrance include von Willebrand disease and osteogenesis imperfecta.

2.32 $B - \dfrac{1}{150}$

The probability that the unaffected brother is a carrier is $\dfrac{2}{3}$. The probability that his partner is a carrier equals the frequency of carriers in the general population, i.e., 2pq in the Hardy-Weinberg distribution, where $q^2 = \dfrac{1}{25000} \therefore q = \dfrac{1}{50} \therefore 2pq = 2 \times \dfrac{49}{50} \times \dfrac{1}{50}$ $= 0.0392 \approx \dfrac{1}{25}$. The probability that two carrier parents will have an affected child is $\dfrac{1}{4}$. Therefore, the probability that the brother (of a sister with cystic fibrosis) and his partner will have an affected child with cystic fibrosis is $\dfrac{2}{3} \times \dfrac{1}{25} \times \dfrac{1}{4} = \dfrac{1}{150}$.

2.33   C – Children under 16 do not have capacity to make decisions about testing

Mature minors who understand the test and what it involves may give valid consent. It cannot be assumed that all children under the age of 16 lack capacity simply on the grounds of age. Each individual case must be considered on its merits. If parental guardians refuse to consent to testing for a child who is unable to consent, in certain jurisdictions this would be referred to the court for consideration of testing in the child's best interests; hence C is the correct response. All other options are valid.

2.34 *A – Down's syndrome*

In the UK, a 5-day old baby will have a heel prick test to test for nine rare conditions. These include sickle cell anaemia, cystic fibrosis, congenital hypothyroidism, and six inherited metabolic diseases – phenylketonuria, medium-chain acyl-CoA dehydrogenase deficiency, maple syrup urine disease, isovaleric acidaemia, glutaric aciduria type 1 and homocystinuria; hence A is the correct response. Down's syndrome is offered to women at 11–14 weeks gestation, but if later in pregnancy, it can be offered at 14–20 weeks. Diagnostic tests include chorionic villus sampling and amniocentesis. Screening is not routinely offered for Down's syndrome in the post-natal period, as clinical suspicion of the typical features would often prompt clinicians to karyotype the baby's chromosomes.

2.35 *C – Tuberous sclerosis*

Tuberous sclerosis is an autosomal dominant, neurocutaneous syndrome characterised by multiple skin lesions, such as hypomelanotic macules (ash leaf spots) and angiofibromas, shagreen patches on the trunk, multiple café-au-lait spots, ungual fibromas and confetti-like skin macules (pathognomonic of the disease); hence C is the correct response. Stickler syndrome or hereditary arthro-ophthalmopathy is an autosomal dominant condition of collagen types II or XI and characterised by ophthalmic abnormalities (high myopia, retinal degeneration often leading to detachment), craniofacial abnormalities (retrognathia, cleft palate, bifid uvula), hearing loss and skeletal abnormalities (joint laxity, degenerative arthropathy). Multiple endocrine neoplasia type I is an autosomal dominant disorder characterised by parathyroid adenomas, anterior pituitary adenomas and pancreatic neuroendocrine tumours. Neurofibromatosis type II is an autosomal dominant disorder characterised by bilateral acoustic neuromas, café-au-lait spots and cutaneous neurofibromas (often seen less than in type I). Piebaldism (partial albinism) is an autosomal dominant disorder characterised by discrete patches of leukoderma (absence of melanocytes) of skin and hair resulting in a white forelock.

2.36 *B – Beckwith-Wiedemann syndrome*

Beckwith-Wiedemann syndrome is an overgrowth syndrome caused by abnormal gene transcription in an imprinting domain on chromosome 11. It is characterised by macrosomia, macroglossia, neonatal gigantism and exomphalos. There is also an increased risk of tumours such as Wilms tumour, neuroblastoma and hepatoblastoma; hence B is the correct response. Acromegaly is usually caused by a pituitary growth hormone-secreting adenoma which leads to excessive production of growth hormone and insulin-like growth factor-1 (IGF-1). It can lead to pituitary gigantism in children. Hurler syndrome is a mucopolysaccharidoses which can present with early inguinal hernias, and later features including hepatosplenomegaly, macroglossia, coarse facial features, short stature and enlarged head circumference. Amyloidosis is a heterogenous group of disorders characterised by extracellular deposition of insoluble fibrils in various tissues of the body which eventually leads to organ failure, if not treated. Symptoms can include congestive cardiac failure, nephrotic syndrome, renal failure, orthostatic hypotension, macroglossia, and sensory and motor neuropathy. McCune-Albright syndrome, or polyostotic fibrous dysplasia, is characterised by endocrine abnormalities, such as precocious puberty, thyrotoxicosis, pituitary gigantism, Cushing's syndrome and café-au-lait skin patches.

2.37 *D – Zollinger-Ellison syndrome*

Zollinger-Ellison syndrome is caused by a neuroendocrine tumour (gastrinoma) that secretes gastrin, leading to gastric acid hypersecretion. Typically, this can cause peptic ulcers and severe oesophageal reflux disease. It is not a ciliopathy; hence D is the correct response. All other disorders listed are ciliopathies. Kartagener's syndrome, part of the primary ciliary dyskinesia family and referred to as immotile cilia syndrome, is an autosomal recessive disorder characterised by recurrent respiratory infections which lead to bronchiectasis, chronic sinusitis, and situs inversus. Infertility can result due to asthenozoospermia (poorly motile sperm). Retinitis pigmentosa is a progressive, degeneration of the retina which affects rod photoreceptors and can lead to night blindness and visual field defects. It can be inherited as an autosomal dominant, autosomal recessive or X-linked trait. Initially, this condition may not be thought of as a ciliopathy, but in fact multiple gene mutations have been studied which encode ciliary transport proteins, such as *TULP1* (Tubby-like protein 1), *USH2A* (Usherin) and *C2ORF71* (cilia localised protein). Similarly, polycystic kidney disease may not be thought of as a ciliopathy. However, single gene defects transmitted as either autosomal dominant or recessive traits can result in dysfunctional receptor-channel proteins in apical cilia membranes, hindering cilia function. In autosomal dominant conditions, defects in *PKD1* and *PKD2* can lead to cyst formation because of dysfunctional polycystin-1 and -2, and hence ciliary dysfunction. In autosomal recessive conditions, gene defects in *PKHD1* lead to dysfunctional fibrocystin/polyductin protein which is important in maintaining the structural integrity of cilia. Ellis-van Creveld syndrome, or chondroectodermal dysplasia, is an autosomal recessive disorder characterised by short limbs, dental anomalies, postaxial polydactyly, hypertelorism and cardiac defects. Gene mutations in *EVC1* and *EVC2* leads to disruption of intracellular proteins in primary cilia, and subsequently impaired cell signal transduction. Interestingly, there is an increased incidence in the Amish community.

2.38 A – Leber's hereditary optic neuropathy

Leber's hereditary optic neuropathy is a maternally inherited disease which results from three-point mutations in the mitochondrial genome. As a result, aerobic metabolism is hindered which subsequently affects highly ATP-dependent tissues such as the retina, optic nerve and extraocular muscles. Hence typically, it affects young adult males who present with acute or subacute bilateral loss of central vision. This visual loss can be accompanied by headaches, ocular discomfort and visual disturbances that occur with exercise and heat (Uhthoff's phenomenon). There are no trinucleotide-repeat mutations; hence A is the correct response. Fragile X syndrome is caused by CGG repeats in the *FMR1* gene, Friedrich ataxia is caused by GAA repeats in the *FXN* gene, myotonic dystrophy is caused by CTG repeats in the *DMPK* gene and Kennedy disease is caused by CAG repeats in the *AR* gene.

2.39 D – Leptotene

Prophase I can be divided into five stages: (1) *leptotene* – chromosomes condense and become clearly visible, two sister chromatids are closely aligned but not distinguishable; hence D is the correct response; (2) *zygotene* – homologous chromosomes align and pair (synapsis) via the synaptonemal complex along the entire length of the chromosome; (3) *pachytene* – further coiling and condensing of homologous chromosomes pairs (known as a bivalent), bivalent chromosomes undergo chromatid exchange in a process called crossing over or recombination; (4) *diplotene* – homologous chromosomes now begin to separate but remain attached at points where crossing over has occurred (chiasmata); and (5) *diakinesis* – homologous chromosomes continue to separate until they become maximally condensed.

2.40 B – Klinefelter syndrome

Klinefelter syndrome, or 47,XXY, is caused by an additional X chromosome in men, as can be seen in the figure; hence B is the correct response. Jacobs syndrome, or 47,XYY, is caused by an additional Y chromosome in men. Triple X syndrome, or 47,XXX, is caused by an additional X chromosome in women. Patau syndrome, or trisomy 13, is caused by an additional chromosome 13 in cells of the body, whereby there are three copies instead of the usual two. Edwards syndrome, or trisomy 18, is caused by an additional chromosome 18 in cells of the body.

2.41 E – Cri-du-chat syndrome

Cri-du-chat syndrome ('cry of the cat') results from a deletion on the short arm of chromosome 5; hence it can also be referred to as 5p minus syndrome. It is characterised by a high-pitched cat-like cry, microcephaly, micrognathia, hypertelorism, epicanthic folds, and significant intellectual disability. It is not a single gene defect disorder; hence E is the correct response. All other options are examples of single gene defect disorders. Marfan syndrome is caused by mutations in the gene encoding fibrillin-1. Cystic fibrosis is caused by mutation in the gene encoding cystic fibrosis transmembrane regulator. Huntingdon disease is caused by gene mutation associated with CAG trinucleotide repeats which encode the huntingtin protein. Myotonic dystrophy is caused by unstable CTG trinucleotide repeats in the gene which encodes a serine/threonine protein kinase.

2.42 C – McArdle disease – tyrosinase

McArdle disease is a glycogen storage disorder of skeletal muscles characterised by deficiency or absence of the enzyme glycogen phosphorylase (or myophosphorylase); hence C is the correct response. Glucose-6-phosphatase is an important enzyme in gluconeogenesis and glycogenolysis. Deficiency leads to Von Gierke disease, another glycogen storage disease (type I). All other options are correctly matched. Tay-Sachs disease is a neurodegenerative, lysosomal storage disorder caused by deficiency in hexosaminidase A which results in excessive accumulation of gangliosides in the brain. Niemann-Pick disease, another lysosomal storage disorder is caused by deficiency of acid sphingomyelinase which plays a role in sphingomyelin hydrolysis. Subsequently, this results in excessive accumulation of unesterified cholesterol and sphingomyelin throughout the viscera and brain. Cori disease, also known as Forbes disease, is another glycogen storage disease (type III) which is caused by mutations in a gene that encodes a debranching enzyme, namely amylo-1,6-glucosidase, and 4-α-glucanotransferase which are important in glycogen hydrolysis. Zellweger syndrome results from dysfunctional peroxisome biogenesis, often because of peroxisomal enzyme deficiencies, such as straight-chain acyl-CoA oxidase and α-methylacyl-CoA racemase. Peroxisomes are the site of beta oxidation of lipids and bile acid synthesis. Therefore, abnormal or absence peroxisomes can lead to cholestasis, paucity of bile ducts and hepatic fibrosis, in addition to craniofacial anomalies and glomerulocystic kidney disease.

2.43 A – DR3 – Rheumatoid arthritis

The human leukocyte antigen (HLA) system or major histocompatibility complex (MHC), located on the short arm of chromosome 6, plays an important role in the immune system. It is divided into three main sub-regions:

1. *class I* molecules are present on all nucleated cells and platelets, the heavy chain is encoded by genes at HLA A, B and C loci (classical molecules), some genes encode non-classical MHC molecules (A–E, -G, -H, -J, -K, -L), T cells that express CD8 molecules react with class I MHC (cytotoxic T cells).
2. *class II* molecules are expressed on antigen presenting cells (macrophages, dendritic cells, monocytes, B lymphocytes, Langerhans cells), the class II region encodes HLA-DR, -DQ and -DP, T cells reactive to class II molecules express CD4 (helper T cells).
3. *class III* molecules are less polymorphic and contain over 50 genes that encode several inflammatory mediators, such as complement components, heat shock proteins and the tumour-necrosis factor (TNF) family.

Various disorders linked to specific HLA alleles are shown in the table below. HLA-DR3 is not associated with rheumatoid arthritis (however, DR4 is); hence A is the correct response. All other options are correctly matched.

Disease	HLA
Rheumatoid arthritis	DR1, DR4, DR5
Ankylosing spondylitis, psoriatic arthritis, reactive arthritis	B27
Multiple sclerosis	B7, B16, DR2, DRB1
Narcolepsy	DQ1, DQ6, DR2
Type 1 diabetes mellitus	B18, DR3, DR4, DR5, DQ2, DQ8
Graves' disease	DR3, B8
Coeliac disease	DR4, DQ2, DQ8
Myasthenia gravis	B8, DR1, DR3
Systemic lupus erythematosus	DR2, DR3
Haemochromatosis	A3
Goodpasture syndrome	DQ2, DR2, DR15
Lymphoid leukaemia	B35
Addison's disease	B8, DR3, DR4
Antiphospholipid syndrome	DR5

2.44 *C – Factor V Leiden*

Factor V Leiden refers to an abnormal factor V protein resulting from a point mutation in exon 10 of the factor V gene where there is a G-to-A transition at nucleotide 1691 or 1746 (depending on start position). This results in arginine to glutamine substitution at either amino acid 506 or 534 of the protein. Historically, this has been known as R506Q, R534Q, 1691G→A or 1746G→A. Subsequently, activated protein C (which normally inactivates factor V, preventing fibrin formation and further clotting) does not inactivate factor V, so clotting remains active for longer, facilitating overproduction of thrombin, fibrin and clot formation; hence C is the correct response. Inherited protein C deficiency is caused by mutation in the *PROC* gene which leads to a faulty or absent protein C protein. Acquired protein C deficiency can be caused by large thrombi, disseminated intravascular coagulation, liver disease, sepsis and vitamin K deficiency (since protein C is a vitamin K-dependent plasma zymogen). Protein S serves as a cofactor for activated protein C, hence clinical presentation of both deficiencies is indistinguishable. Inherited protein S deficiency can be caused by mutation in the *PROS1* gene. Antithrombin III inactivates thrombin and various clotting factors (IX, X, XI and XII). Antithrombin deficiency is rare and the most thrombogenic of the inherited thrombophilias. Inherited antithrombin deficiency increases the risk of thrombotic events, whereas acquired does not. Multiple single point and gene mutations in the *SERPINC1* gene are responsible for many cases of inherited antithrombin deficiency. It can also be inherited in an autosomal dominant manner. Prothrombin G20210A is a polymorphism in the prothrombin (factor II) gene which leads to a hypercoagulable state. A single substitution of A for G at nucleotide 20210 results in lower prothrombin degradation; increasing circulating plasma levels of prothrombin which increases venous thromboembolism risk.

2.45 *C – CG*

Gene expression often correlates negatively with DNA methylation. Methyltransferases modify cytosine to 5-methylcytosine which occurs when cytosine is adjacent to guanine in the promoter region. These are known as CpG islands (where the p represents the linking phosphate), and when methylated they prevent transcription and decrease gene expression; hence C is the correct response. Hypermethylation can also lead to histone methylation and acetylation which can disrupt gene transcription and expression. Methylation of CpG islands are important epigenetic biomarkers as they have been shown to play a role in X-inactivation, genomic imprinting, gene silencing and cancer genetics.

2.46   *D – Antisense oligonucleotides*

Antisense oligonucleotides are short, single-stranded deoxyribonucleotides that can hybridize an RNA target in a sequence-specific manner, and subsequently modify, reduce or promote protein expression. Similar to small interfering RNA (siRNA), these molecules are capable of silencing gene expression and have great therapeutic potential. Clinically, these molecules are enzymatically unstable and are often inefficiently or inadequately delivered into cells, hence delivery vehicles are usually required; hence D is the correct response. All other options are suitable gene delivery modalities. Virus-mediated transduction using retroviruses (oncoretroviruses, lentiviruses) or adenoviruses can be used in gene therapy but convey a significant risk for insertional mutagenesis. Non-viral vectors such as naked-DNA (usually plasmids) and liposomes are less immunogenic and can be easily transfected into cells. The limitation of these non-viral modalities is inefficient DNA transfer.

2.47   *E – Melanoma affects women and men equally*

Melanoma is a malignant skin tumour that arises from uncontrolled proliferation of melanocytes. Melanoma affects women and men differently (not equally); hence E is the correct response. Adolescent and young adult women are more susceptible to melanoma than men, possibly as a result of these groups visiting indoor tanning studios. Men aged over 40 have a higher incidence of melanoma than in women. People who live closer to the equator are at a higher incidence of melanoma due to the higher degree of sun exposure. People who live at higher altitude are also at increased risk.

2.48   *B – Epistasis*

Epistasis, meaning 'standing upon', is the antagonistic interaction between non-allelic genes that influences a phenotype. It occurs when two or more genes contribute to the same phenotype, whereby one gene can mask or modify the phenotype of a second gene; hence B is the correct response. Epigenetics is the study of how behaviours and the environment can cause changes in gene activity without altering DNA sequences. Eugenics is the selection of desired heritable characteristics to improve specific species and future generations. Ecogenetics is the study of how genetics and the environment interact together. Epialleles are epigenetic variants within a genomic region in individuals within a population that are stably transmitted between generations.

2.49   *C – Lyonization*

Lyonization is the inactivation of one of the X-chromosomes in females. It occurs early in embryonic development, where one of the two X chromosomes is randomly inactivated, and it ensures that females (and males) have a functional X chromosome in each body cell; hence C is the correct response. Methylation is the process by which methyl groups are added to molecules. In DNA methylation, the epigenetic mechanism involves transferring a methyl group onto the C5 position of cytosine. This can often regulate gene expression. Hemizygosity is the presence of only one single copy of an allele, gene or chromosome in a diploid organism, such as the X chromosome in males. Segregation, in the genetic sense, is the random process by which each gamete receives only one form of the gene in gamete formation. Recombination or crossing over is the process of genetic exchange between chromatids when homologous pairs are close together.

2.50   *A – There is a 50% chance that babies will be of equal sex in dizygotic twin pregnancy*

Dizygotic twins (fraternal) result from fertilisation of two ova by two sperm and are always dichorionic and diamniotic (ca. two-thirds of twin pregnancies). Monozygotic twins (identical) originate from a single ovum that has been fertilised by a single sperm (ca. one-third of twin pregnancies). Approximately 70% of monozygotic twins are monochorionic and diamniotic and approximately 30% are dichorionic and diamniotic. Monozygotic twins share 100% of their genes, whereas dizygotic twins share on average 50%. There is a 50% chance that dizygotic twins will be of equal or opposite sex; hence A is the correct response. In monozygotic twins, gender is always the same. The chance that an uncle of an affected individual is a carrier for an autosomal recessive disorder is 1 in 2 (not 1 in 4). In autosomal dominant disorders, a penetrance of 0.55 means that 55% (not 45%) of heterozygotes will manifest the condition. Bayesian analysis plays an important role in the assessment of genetic risk. It allows calculation of the overall probability of an event or outcome (disease or carrier) based on ancestral information <u>and/or</u> genetic test results. Posterior probability is the final probability of an event occurring after considering ancestral (prior probability) and new information, i.e., it is the probability of event A occurring given that event B has occurred. It can be calculated by using Bayes' theorem to update prior probability, which is based on ancestral or anterior information.

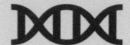

CHAPTER 3
Immunology

The deviation of man from the state in which he was originally placed by Nature seems to have proved to him a prolific source of diseases.

Edward Jenner

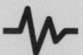

3.1 Which of the following regarding immunity is **not** correct?
A Neutrophils are cells of acute inflammation
B Mast cells participate in immediate-type hypersensitivity reactions
C Eosinophils have receptors for IgE
D Activation of C5a of the complement pathway leads to neutrophil chemotaxis
E T-helper 1 (Th1) cells are thought to be involved in the development of allergic disease

3.2 Which of the following are involved in Type IV hypersensitivity reactions?
A Graft-versus-host disease
B Asthma
C Transfusion reactions
D Viral hepatitis
E Graves' disease

3.3 Which of the following statements is correct in acute inflammation?
A Macrophages and lymphocytes predominate
B Increased vascular permeability and vasodilatation occur
C Granulomas are a common feature
D Healing by fibrosis and angiogenesis predominate
E Usually results in tissue destruction which occurs via necrosis

3.4 Which of the following gene clusters does **not** directly contribute to antigen binding?
A V_L
B V_H
C C_L
D D
E J

3.5 Which immunoglobulin is mainly involved in opsonisation?
A IgM
B IgG
C IgA
D IgD
E IgE

3.6 Which of the following best describes the processes underpinning type III hypersensitive reactions?
A IgE-mediated degranulation of mast cells
B Macrophage and T-cell accumulation
C IgM and IgG immune complexes deposited in tissues
D IgG directed against cell surface antigen mediates cell destruction
E T-cell sensitisation and T_H1 cytokine release

3.7 Activation of which of the following complement components results in both opsonisation and stimulation of phagocytosis?
A C3a
B C3b
C C4b
D C5a
E C5b

3.8 Which of the following would result from parasitic infections?
A ↑basophils   ↓IgM
B ↑eosinophils   ↑IgE
C ↓eosinophils   ↑IgM
D ↓basophils   ↑IgE
E ↓eosinophils   ↓IgE

3.9 Which of the following is a component of MHC Class I molecules?
A Interferon-γ
B β₂-microglobulin
C Tumour necrosis factor-beta
D HLA-DR
E Complement C3

3.10 Which of the following statements regarding immunoglobulin structure is correct?
A The light chain is found in the constant Fc region
B There are always two interchain (heavy) disulphide bonds
C The light chain determines immunoglobulin isotype
D Complement binding regions are found on the heavy chain only
E The N-terminus is located in the Fc region

3.11 Which of the following regarding T-cell receptors is **not** correct?
A It is a heterodimeric membrane protein
B Those with γδ chains are found on approximately 95% of human T lymphocytes
C αβ receptors recognise peptides presented by major histocompatibility complex molecules
D Antigens bind to variable domains
E They have a similar structure to the Fab portions of immunoglobulins

3.12 Which of the following regarding the major histocompatibility complex is correct?
A HLA is found on chromosome 17 in humans
B Class I molecules consist of an α and a β chain
C Class II molecules are expressed on neutrophils and hepatocytes
D Class I involves CD4 recognition
E Cytosolic peptides are associated with class I molecules

3.13 Which of the following regarding macrophages is correct?
A M1 macrophages are anti-inflammatory
B M2 macrophages are tumoricidal
C M1 activation is associated with graft rejection
D M2 activation is associated with immunoregulation
E Polarisation states of M1 and M2 macrophages are not interchangeable

3.14 Which of the following cytokines is **not** secreted by macrophages?
A TGF-β
B IL-8
C TNF
D IL-2
E IL-10

3.15 Which of the following conditions results in immune paresis where lymphoplasmacytoid cells produce monoclonal IgM?
A Multiple myeloma
B Waldenström's macroglobulinaemia
C Cryoglobulinaemia
D Monoclonal gammopathy of undetermined significance
E Amyloidosis

3.16 Which of the following proteins is correctly matched to the region found in protein electrophoresis?
A Haptoglobin – α1 region
B Transferrin – β2 region
C C3 – β1 region
D Immunoglobulins – γ region
E Albumin – α2 region

3.17 Which of the following immunoglobulins is the heaviest by mass?
  A IgG
  B IgA
  C IgM
  D IgE
  E IgD

3.18 Which of the following cytokines has an important role in neutrophil chemotaxis?
  A IL-5
  B IL-6
  C IL-8
  D GM-CSF
  E IFNγ

3.19 Which of the following proteinases is key to the lectin pathway?
  A Serine
  B Cysteine
  C Asparagine
  D Glutamine
  E Histidine

3.20 Which of the following conditions is **not** an example of a type II hypersensitivity reaction?
  A Haemolytic anaemia
  B Idiopathic thrombocytopenic purpura
  C Glomerulonephritis
  D Myasthenia gravis
  E Erythroblastosis fetalis

3.21 Which of the following regarding helper T cells is correct?
  A Th1 cells produce IL-5 and IL-13
  B Th2 cells produce IFN-γ and TNF-β
  C Th1 cells are associated with disease downregulation
  D Th2 cells stimulate T-cell proliferation
  E Th17 cells produce IL-21 and kill extracellular bacteria

3.22 Which of the following is **not** a component of cellular exudate formation?
  A Neutrophil margination
  B Leucocyte adhesion
  C Amoeboid movement of leucocytes
  D Persistent vasoconstriction
  E Diapedesis

3.23 Which of the following regarding the kinin system is correct?
  A Kallikrein converts kininogen into bradykinin
  B Neutrophils release Hageman factor
  C Prekallikrein is converted into kallikrein using activated factor X
  D Kallikrein converts plasmin into plasminogen
  E Kininogens activate pain receptors

3.24 Which of the following human immunoglobulins has the shortest half-life?
  A IgG
  B IgM
  C IgD
  D IgE
  E IgA

3.25 Which of the following cells is **not** a polymorphonuclear leucocyte?
   A Mast
   B Basophil
   C Macrophage
   D Eosinophil
   E Neutrophil

3.26 Which of the following terms best describes a small molecule that elicits an immune response only when conjugated to a larger molecule?
   A Epitope
   B Isotype
   C Allergen
   D Hapten
   E Opsonin

3.27 Which of the following is **not** correct regarding superantigens?
   A Stimulate T-lymphocytes via interaction with the T cell antigen receptor
   B Predominantly bacterial in origin
   C Bind MHC class II molecules
   D Predominantly processed intracellularly
   E Stimulate CD4 cells

3.28 Which of the following immunoglobulins is predominant in colostrum?
   A IgA
   B IgD
   C IgE
   D IgG
   E IgM

3.29 Which of the following is correct regarding IgD?
   A It is pentameric
   B It is present as a B cell receptor
   C It crosses the placenta
   D It has 4 antigen binding sites
   E It is composed of 2 α heavy chains and 2 light chains

3.30 Concentrations of immunoglobulins specific for a microbe that had previously infected a patient were analysed. The levels of IgM were extremely high but there were no detectable levels of IgG, IgA or IgE. Which of the following terms best describes why this patient was susceptible to recurrent infections with this microbe?
   A Class switching
   B Alloimmunity
   C Avidity
   D Single-nucleotide polymorphism
   E Somatic hypermutation

3.31 Which of the following cells produce the mediators perforin and granzymes?
   A CD4+ T lymphocytes
   B CD8+ T lymphocytes
   C B lymphocytes
   D Plasma cells
   E Eosinophils

3.32 Which of the following is correct regarding B-lymphocytes?
   A They are divided into three categories – B1, B2 and B3
   B They occur outside lymph nodes
   C They lack surface antigens
   D They are involved in cell-mediated immunity
   E They do not produce lymphokines

3.33 Which of the following regarding systemic effects of inflammation is **not** correct?
   A Phagocytosis stimulates release of endogenous pyrogens
   B Systemic lymph node enlargement is rare
   C Splenomegaly may be found in malaria
   D Anaemia can be present
   E Weight loss is common in extensive chronic inflammation

3.34 Which of the following is **not** a granulomatous disease?
   A Syphilis
   B Brucellosis
   C Sarcoidosis
   D Mycetoma
   E Pars planitis

3.35 Which of the following regarding X-linked agammaglobulinaemia is correct?
   A It has a prevalence of 1 in 100,000
   B All immunoglobulins except IgG are very low
   C B cells are often absent
   D T cells are dysfunctional
   E Btk protein is present

3.36 Which of the following self-antigens and associated autoimmune diseases are **not** matched correctly?
   A Acetylcholine – myasthenia gravis
   B Beta-2 glycoprotein I – Factor V Leiden
   C Platelets – thrombocytopenic purpura
   D Pyruvate dehydrogenase – primary biliary cirrhosis
   E Topoisomerase I – diffuse scleroderma

3.37 Which of the following regarding secondary immunodeficiency is **not** correct?
   A Hypogammaglobulinaemia is common in chronic bacterial sepsis
   B Albumin levels can be reduced in acute bacterial sepsis
   C Lymphopenia is common in chronic bacterial sepsis
   D Phagocytosis is normal or low in acute bacterial sepsis
   E T cell function may be markedly impaired in chronic bacterial sepsis

3.38 Which of the following is measured by the radioallergosorbent test (RAST)?
   A IgE concentration
   B IgG concentration
   C IgM concentration
   D Antigen concentration
   E Percentage of agglutination

3.39 Which of the following cells is **not** assigned to the mononuclear phagocyte system?
   A Monocytes
   B Kupffer cells
   C Pleural macrophages
   D Epithelioid cells
   E Endothelial cells

3.40 Which of the following would indicate a previous but not current infection?
   A IgD positive, IgM negative
   B IgD negative, IgM negative
   C IgG negative, IgM positive
   D IgG positive, IgM negative
   E IgG positive, IgM positive

3.41 Which of the following regarding immunology of thyroid disease is **not** correct?
  A In Grave's disease, CD4⁺ T-cell infiltration of the thyroid is predominant
  B Postpartum thyroiditis is associated with HLA-DR5
  C In de Quervain's thyroiditis, antibodies against thyroglobulin are present in low titres, and can be undetectable
  D In primary hypothyroidism, elevated levels of antibodies to thyroid peroxidase are detected
  E In Hashimoto's thyroiditis, there is increased antigen expression of MHC class I on thyroid cells

3.42 Which of the following antibodies would **not** help in the diagnosis of type I diabetes mellitus?
  A Glutamic acid decarboxylase (GAD)
  B Insulinoma-associated protein 2 (IA2)
  C Zinc transporter (ZnT8)
  D Islet cell
  E MuSK

3.43 Which of the following conditions would anti-glial nuclear (AGNA) and P/Q- type voltage-gated calcium channel antibodies (P/Q-VGCC) be present?
  A Lambert-Eaton myasthenic syndrome
  B Guillain-Barré syndrome
  C Encephalitis
  D Optic neuritis
  E Myasthenia gravis

3.44 Which of the following antibodies is **not** correctly matched to the associated disease?
  A anti-Jo-1 – polymyositis
  B anti-cardiolipin – antiphospholipid syndrome
  C anti-GM1 – multifocal motor polyneuropathy
  D anti-Hu – paraneoplastic syndromes
  E anti-La – bullous pemphigoid

3.45 Which of the following regarding autoimmunity is correct?
  A IgE anti-ACh-receptor antibodies are detected in ~90% of patients with myasthenia gravis
  B Intrinsic factor antibodies have a higher sensitivity than gastric parietal cell antibodies in patients with pernicious anaemia
  C Haptoglobin levels are decreased in autoimmune haemolytic anaemia
  D Over 70% of patients with Felty's syndrome are ANCA negative
  E Mitochondrial antibodies are rarely found in primary biliary cirrhosis

3.46 Which of the following cells become tumorigenic in myeloma?
  A Neutrophil
  B Plasma
  C Basophil
  D T lymphocyte
  E Macrophage

3.47 Which of the following is characterised by the presence of Reed-Sternberg cells?
  A Chronic myeloid leukaemia
  B Chronic lymphocytic leukaemia
  C Non-Hodgkin's lymphoma
  D Hodgkin's lymphoma
  E Multiple myeloma

3.48 Which of the following is **not** a recognised cause of angioedema?
  A ACE deficiency
  B C2-hydroxylase inhibitor deficiency
  C SLE
  D Ramipril
  E Simvastatin

3.49   Which of the following conditions results in athymia in children?

    A   Cushing's syndrome

    B   Conn's syndrome

    C   Acromegaly

    D   Gigantism

    E   DiGeorge syndrome

3.50   Which of the following is the correct definition of a prion?

    A   Chemoattractant proteins that stimulate migration and activation of leucocytes

    B   Small antibacterial proteins produced by neutrophils

    C   Serum proteins involved in inflammation, phagocytosis and cell lysis

    D   Infectious circular RNA molecules that lack a protein coat

    E   Abnormally folded, protease-resistant isoform of an endogenous host protein

Answers

3.1 *E – T-helper 1 (Th1) cells are thought to be involved in the development of allergic disease*

T-helper 2 (Th2) (not Th1) cells are involved in activation and/or recruitment of IgE antibody producing B cells, eosinophils and mast cells; hence E is the correct response. Th2 cells secrete several cytokines, namely interleukins (IL-4, IL-5, IL-6, IL-9, IL-10 and IL-13), and they regulate eosinophil and B cell-mediated responses. Th1 cells provide protection against intracellular pathogens evoking cell-mediated immunity and phagocyte-dependent inflammation. They secrete interferon-γ (INFγ), IL-2 and tumour necrosis factor-β (TNFβ). Th1 cells are involved in the pathogenesis of certain autoimmune disorders, recurrent abortions, and renal allograft rejection, whereas Th2 are responsible for various atopic disorders.

3.2 *A – Graft-versus-host disease*

Type I, II and III hypersensitivity reactions are caused by antibodies. Type IV reactions are caused by T-lymphocytes. Broadly speaking, Type I reactions are immediate and mediated by IgE antibodies, Type II reactions are cytotoxic and antibody-mediated, typically IgM or IgG, type III reactions are immune-complex mediated, and type IV reactions are cell-mediated or delayed. Examples of type I reactions include anaphylaxis, asthma and various food allergies. Examples of type II reactions include autoimmune haemolytic anaemia, immune thrombocytopaenia, Goodpasture's syndrome, myasthenia gravis, Graves' disease, bullous pemphigoid, pemphigus vulgaris, transfusion reactions and pernicious anaemia. Examples of type III reactions include systemic lupus erythematosus, serum sickness, small-vessel vasculitis, extrinsic allergic alveolitis, chronic viral hepatitis and post-streptococcal glomerulonephritis. Examples of type IV reactions include contact dermatitis, the Mantoux test used to detect tuberculosis, organ transplant and chronic graft rejections, graft versus host disease, multiple sclerosis, type I diabetes mellitus and delayed drug reactions (erythema multiforme, Steven-Johnson syndrome, lichenoid drug eruptions); hence A is the correct response.

3.3 *B – Increased vascular permeability and vasodilation occur*

In the early stages of acute inflammation, there is active hyperaemia with blood vessel vasodilatation, blow flow is reduced due to increase vascular permeability, blood viscosity increases, and cellular exudate is formed; hence B is the correct response. Neutrophil polymorphs are the most abundant cells in acute inflammation, whereas macrophages and lymphocytes are the most abundant in chronic inflammation. Granulomas are aggregates of epithelioid histiocytes and are a common feature of chronic inflammation (not acute inflammation). Inflammatory cells release pro-inflammatory cytokines which recruit T-lymphocytes which exacerbate the inflammatory response. Subsequently endothelial cells promote angiogenesis. Fibrosis results when most of the chronic inflammatory cell infiltrate has subsided; hence is a common feature of chronic inflammation (not acute inflammation). Acute inflammation usually resolves quickly (and not by excessive necrosis causing tissue destruction), and causes can include microbial infections, physical and chemical agents, hypersensitivity reactions and tissue necrosis (usually because of ischaemic infarction). Acute inflammation which does not resolve can lead to excessive necrosis which often results in fibrosis, excessive exudate which can lead to suppuration and abscess formation, or chronic inflammation.

3.4 *C – C_L*

The basic unit of immunoglobulins consists of two heavy and two light chains. Light chains can be either κ or λ, and both have a constant domain (C_L) and variable domain (V_L). Heavy chains can be one of five isotypes: IgA, IgD, IgE, IgG and IgM. Immunoglobulins have three functional components: two fragment antigen binding (Fab) regions and the fragment crystalline (Fc) region, where the two are linked by a hinge region. The hypervariable region of the Fab is composed of loops of variable heavy (V_H) and light (V_L) domains. The heavy chain consists of V_H, and three constant domains C_H1, C_H2 and C_H3. The Fab region is formed by pairing of the V_L and C_L of the light chains with the V_H and C_H1 of the heavy chains. The V_L region is further subdivided into D and J genes. The Fc constant region contains C_H2 and C_H3 domains which interact with one another. The C_L region does not directly contribute to antigen binding; hence C is the correct response.

3.5 *B – IgG*

Opsonisation is the process of coating antigens with substances such as antibodies or complement so that they can be more easily engulfed by phagocytes. Phagocytes have receptors for the Fc region of IgG (FcγRIII) and for the C3b fragment of complement. IgG and C3b are key opsonins that facilitate phagocytosis; hence B is the correct response. Neutrophils and macrophages have specific surface receptors for the Fc region of IgG and C3b and can phagocytose IgG-coated antigens. Complement activation by antibody binding via the classical pathway, or by direct binding to microbial cell walls via the alternative or lectin pathways generate bound C3-derived fragments on phagocytic cells.

3.6 C – IgM and IgG immune complexes deposited in tissues

In type III hypersensitivity reactions, immune complexes composed of antigen-antibody aggregates form in tissues and lead to an abnormal immune response; hence C is the correct response. IgE-mediated degranulation of mast cells is a type I hypersensitivity response. Macrophage and T-cell accumulation is a type IV hypersensitivity response. IgG (and IgM) directed against cell surface antigen mediating cell destruction is a type II hypersensitivity response. T-cell sensitisation and T_H1 cytokine release is a type IV hypersensitivity response.

3.7 B – C3b

The complement system is composed of plasma proteins that interact in order to opsonise pathogens, marking them for destruction by phagocytes, and inducing multiple inflammatory processes that help combat infection. The complement pathway can be triggered by (1) the classical pathway, where the first protein complex, C1q binds directly to the pathogen surface or to antibody-antigen complexes; (2) the alternative pathway, where activated complement components spontaneously bind directly to the pathogen surface without the need for complement components, C1, C2 or C4; and (3) the mannose-binding lectin pathway, where mannose-binding lectin binds avidly to mannose-containing carbohydrates on pathogen surfaces. Mannose-binding lectin has a similar structure to C1q and activates complement through mannose-binding serine proteinase, i.e., via the classical pathway without the need for antibody. All three pathways converge to form C3 convertase which cleaves complement C3 into C3a and C3b. C3b plays an important role in opsonisation and removal of immune of complexes; hence B is the correct response. C3b also binds the C3 convertase to form C5 convertase, which form C5a and C5b. Multiple polymerisation reactions ensue where terminal complement components (C5–C9) interact to form a membrane attack complex which results in cell lysis. C4a is generated by the cleavage of C4 in the classical pathway, and not by the action of C3 convertase. C3a, C4a and C5a are important peptide mediators of inflammation and have roles in cell recruitment. On an extra note, IgM and IgG activate the classical pathway, but IgA, IgD and IgE do not.

3.8 B – ↑eosinophils ↑IgE

Eosinophils are granulocytes associated with asthma, allergic disease, and parasite and helminth infections. Eosinophils have FcεR receptors for IgE and upon antigen binding, toxic metabolites are released from eosinophil granules. Elevated eosinophil count (eosinophilia) and raised IgE result from parasitic infections; hence B is the correct response.

3.9 B – β₂-microglobulin

Major histocompatibility complex (MHC) antigens are cell surface glycoproteins which have two classes: class I (subdivided into A, B and C) antigens are expressed by most nucleated cells and composed of a heavy alpha chain and a smaller chain called β_2-microglobulin, and class II (with multiple loci such as HLA-DP, HLA-DQ and HLA-DR) antigens are found on B-lymphocytes, activated T cells, dendritic cells, and macrophages; hence B is the correct response. Other cells such as astrocytes express MHC class II only when exposed to the cytokine interferon-γ (IFN-γ), which then participate in antigen presentation.

3.10 D – Complement binding regions are found on the heavy chain only

Complement binding regions are found on the heavy chain, specifically in the C_H2 region of the Fc region; hence D is the correct response. The light chain is found in the Fab region (not the Fc region). In humans, the number of interchain (heavy) disulphide bonds varies between immunoglobulins: IgA has 2, IgD has 1, IgE has 2, and IgM has 3. IgG has four subtypes, all of which have a different number: IgG1 has 2, IgG2 has 4, IgG3 has 11 and IgG4 has 2. The heavy chain (not light chain) determines immunoglobulin isotype, which differs in sequence and number of constant regions, hinge structure and the number of binding sites. The N-terminus is located in the Fab region (not the Fc region).

3.11 B – Those with γδ chains are found on approximately 95% of human T lymphocytes

T lymphocytes recognise antigens by one of two types of T-cell receptors: α/β receptors, which are heterodimers of alpha and beta chains, or γ/δ receptors, which are heterodimers of gamma and delta chains. In adults, the α/β receptors are more abundant, whereas ca. 10% of epithelial structures contain γ/δ receptors; hence B is the correct response. All other options are factually correct.

3.12 E – Cytosolic peptides are associated with class I molecules

Cytosolic peptides are associated with class I molecules; hence E is the correct response. HLA is found on chromosome 6 (not 17) in humans. Class II (not class I) molecules consist of an α and a β chain. Class I molecules originate from a single heavy α-chain. Class I (not class II) molecules are expressed on most nucleated cells, including neutrophils and hepatocytes. Class II (not class I) involves CD4 recognition. Class I recognition involves CD8.

3.13 D – M2 activation is associated with immunoregulation

Macrophages can change phenotype and function upon polarisation by the microenvironment. Thus, diversity and plasticity are hallmarks of macrophages. Depending on the activation state of the macrophage, they can be divided into two interchangeable types: M1 (classically activated macrophage) and M2 (alternatively activated macrophage). M1 macrophages are pro-inflammatory and can be polarised by lipopolysaccharide with or without T_H1 cytokines, such as IFNγ which can differentiate macrophages into M1 macrophages. M1 macrophages secrete pro-inflammatory cytokines, such as IL-1β, IL-6, IL-12, IL-23 and TNFα, and have a positive effect on the immune response. M2 macrophages are anti-inflammatory and immunoregulatory, and are polarised by T_H2 cytokines, such as IL-4 and IL-13, and produce anti-inflammatory cytokines, such as arginase-I, IL-10 and TGF-β. They play an important role in wound healing and tissue repair; hence D is the correct response. M1 macrophages are tumoricidal. M2 macrophages are associated with graft rejection, where they can often accumulate, promote interstitial fibrosis and contribute to graft failure.

3.14 D – IL-2

Upon exposure to an inflammatory stimulus, macrophages secrete pro-inflammatory cytokines such as TNFα, IL-1, IL-6, IL-8, IL-12, IL-18, IL-23 and IL-27. Many other cells also produce these cytokines, namely fibroblasts, endothelial cells and activated lymphocytes. Macrophages also produce anti-inflammatory cytokines which are important regulators of inflammation, often acting as inhibitors or antagonists. They include IL-4, L-10, IL-13 and TGF-β. They are produced by macrophages, and many suppress the production of pro-inflammatory cytokines. IL-2 is produced primarily by helper T cells and is known to have immunoregulatory and immunostimulatory functions. It can promote CD8 and natural killer cell cytotoxic activity. Smaller quantities of IL-2 can also be released from eosinophils and B cells, but not macrophages; hence D is the correct response.

3.15 B – Waldenström's macroglobulinaemia

Waldenström's macroglobulinaemia is a rare B cell neoplasm, specifically a lymphoplasmacytoid lymphoma involving B lymphocytes, plasmacytoid lymphocytes and plasma cells, characterised by accumulation of monoclonal IgM paraprotein. This often results in hyperviscosity. Median age is the 7th decade and there is a male predominance; hence B is the correct response. Multiple myeloma is a malignant neoplasm of plasma cells in bone marrow which produce monoclonal IgG, IgA, IgE or IgD paraproteins. Excess light chains can also be produced in the urine, as either κ or λ chains, and known as Bence-Jones proteins. Cryoglobulinaemia refers to the presence of serum proteins that precipitate at temperatures below 37°C and redissolve on rewarming. Most cryoglobulins are IgG or IgM, and rarely IgA or free light chains. There are three types: *type I* are single monoclonal immunoglobulins linked to a B cell lymphoproliferative disorder, such as myeloma or lymphoma, *type II* are polyclonal immunoglobulins IgG linked with monoclonal IgM with rheumatoid factor activity, such as myeloma, lymphoma, connective tissue diseases and hepatitis C infection, and *type III* are polyclonal immunoglobulins IgG linked with polyclonal IgM with rheumatoid factor activity, such as in connective tissue disorders and infections. Type II and III are also known as *mixed cryoglobulinaemias*. Interestingly, over 80% of patients with hepatitis C develop cryoglobulinaemia vasculitis. Monoclonal gammopathy of undetermined significance (MGUS) is a premalignant clonal plasma cell proliferative disorder characterised by the presence of low serum paraprotein (<3 g/dL), bone marrow with <10% monoclonal plasma cells, and the absence of end-organ damage related to the lymphoproliferative process. Amyloidosis is a multisystem disease characterised by extracellular deposition of insoluble protein fibrils, and over 20 different proteins are known to form amyloid structures. Common amyloid proteins include that found in the human brain, amyloid-β which is associated with Alzheimer's disease, dialysis-associated amyloid caused by polymerisation of β2-microglobulin, amyloid-associated prion disease such as Creutzfeldt-Jakob and inherited amyloidosis, caused by mutations that lead to dysfunctional proteins (such as cystatin C, lysozyme and transthyretin).

3.16 D – Immunoglobulins – γ region

Protein electrophoresis separates proteins according to charge and size using an electric field. Albumin is the most abundant protein in serum and forms a single distinct band closest to the anode. γ-globulins form a diffuse band closest to the cathode. The other four bands are the α_1–, α_2–, β_1– and β_2-globulins. Various proteins found within these zones are highlighted below; hence D is the correct response.

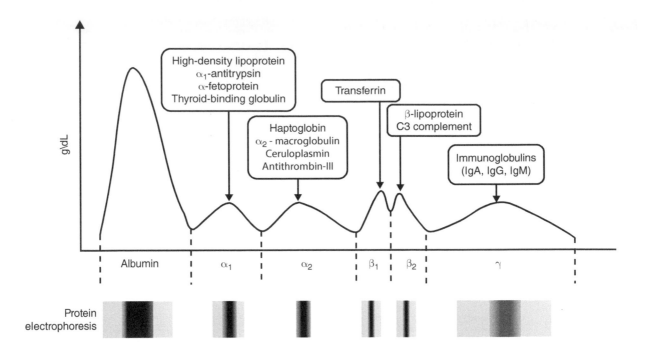

3.17 *C – IgM*

IgM is ~900 kDa, and is the heaviest immunoglobulin; hence C is the correct response. IgG is ~150 kDa, IgA is ~380 kDa, IgE is ~200 kDa and IgD is ~185 kDa.

3.18 *C – IL-8*

IL-8 is a chemoattractant cytokine which targets, attracts and activates neutrophils in inflammatory regions. It is a chemokine that is important in cell proliferation, tissue remodelling and angiogenesis; hence C is the correct response. IL-5 acts as an eosinophil stimulating factor, in addition to inducing isotype switching in B-cells. IL-6 is a pro-inflammatory cytokine which stimulates acute phase proteins such as CRP, in addition to playing a role in differentiation of T- and B-cells, and haematopoiesis. GM-CSF activates mature neutrophils and macrophages and induces production of pro-inflammatory cytokines. IFNγ activates macrophages, endothelial cells, and natural killer cells, and inhibits production of IgE.

3.19 *A – Serine*

The lectin pathway is part of the innate immune system. It activates the complement system using pattern recognition proteins – mannose-binding lectin (MBL), collectin-11, ficolin-1, ficolin-2 and ficolin-3, instead of immunoglobulins to target activation (as seen in the classical pathway of complement activation). Each of these proteins complex with MBL-associated serine proteinases (MASPs); hence A is the correct response. MBL is structurally related to C1q and activates complement via MASP, which are structurally and functionally similar to C1r and C1s of the classical pathway.

3.20 *C – Glomerulonephritis*

Acute post-streptococcal glomerulonephritis results from a streptococcal throat or skin infection, usually 10–14 days later. IgG and C3 immune complexes are deposited in the glomerular basement membrane, an example of a type III hypersensitivity reaction; hence C is the correct response. All other options are examples of type II hypersensitivity reactions.

3.21 *E – Th17 cells produce IL-22 and kill extracellular bacteria*

Th cells express CD4 protein on their surface which recognise foreign antigens complexed with MHC class II molecules on antigen presenting cells. Th17 cells are a subset of T-helper cells that produce different cytokines to Th1 and Th2. In fact, the cytokines IL-4 and IFNγ that are released from Th1/Th2 cells are known to suppress Th17 differentiation. Th17 cells mediate immune responses against extracellular bacteria and fungi. They are also known to mediate some autoimmune responses. Th17 cells produce IL-17, IL-21, IL-22, and IL-23; hence E is the correct response. Th1 cells mediate immune responses against intracellular pathogens. Th1 produce IL-2, IL-3, TNF-β and IFNγ. IFNγ is important in activating cytotoxic T cells, natural killer cells and macrophages to increase their microbicidal activity. Th2 cells mediate host defence against extracellular parasites such as helminths. Th2 cells produce IL-4, IL-5, IL-6, IL-9, IL-10, IL-13 and IL-25. These cells are involved in the development of allergic diseases.

3.22 *D – Persistent vasoconstriction*

Acute inflammation is an immediate, innate immune response to tissue injury. It has five main features: rubor (redness), dolor (pain), calor (heat), tumour (swelling) and loss of function. Initially, there is transient (not persistent) arteriolar vasoconstriction to control blood loss, followed by persistent vasodilation which provides blood to surrounding tissues; hence D is the correct response. Cellular exudate is formed due to increased permeability of blood vessels because of histamine release from mast cells at the site of injury. Neutrophils are abundant during the acute phase and undergo a regulated sequence of events involving margination, rolling, adhesion and migration. Neutrophils undergo chemotaxis whereby they are chemoattracted to the site of injury, transmigrating through capillary walls in an amoeboid manner, i.e., changing shape to fit through small pores. This process is known as diapedesis.

3.23 *A – Kallikrein converts kininogen into bradykinin*

The kallikrein-kinin system is an important cascade in inflammation, blood pressure regulation, cell proliferation, pain, and vasodilation. Kinins are released from either the plasma or by tissues. In plasma, activated factor XII (Hageman factor) and plasmin convert prekallikrein into kallikrein. This stimulates the conversion of kininogens to kinins, such as bradykinin. Bradykinin is a potent vasodilator, which stimulates endothelial nitric oxide synthesis and increases vascular permeability; hence A is the correct response. Factor XII is synthesised by hepatocytes in the liver (not neutrophils). Prekallikrein is converted into kallikrein using activated factor XII (not factor X). Plasmin activates conversion of prekallikrein into kallikrein (not kallikrein converts plasmin into plasminogen). Kinins (not kininogens), especially bradykinin, can induce pain via the activation of kinin receptors, B1 and B2.

3.24 *D – IgE*

IgE has the shortest half-life at ~2 days; hence D is the correct response. Total IgG has the longest half-life between 20 and 26 days, depending on the subclass. IgM has a half-life between 5 and 10 days. IgD has the second shortest half-life at ~3 days. IgA has a half-life at ~6 days.

3.25 *C – Macrophage*

Polymorphonuclear leucocytes are the most abundant circulating white blood cell with a multilobed nucleus and granule-containing cytoplasm. They are granulocytes which include basophils, neutrophils, eosinophils and mast cells. In contrast, monocytes, macrophages and lymphocytes are agranulocytes; hence C is the correct response.

3.26 *D – Hapten*

Hapten (from the Greek word meaning 'to hold') are small molecular structures that can complementarily bind to antibodies but are too small to be complete antigens and so need to be coupled to larger, more immune invoking carrier proteins; hence D is the correct response. An epitope is a region of a molecule, often an antigen and a protein, which generate an antigenic response and allow antibody binding. Isotypes are macromolecules that share common features, such as immunoglobulins – IgA, IgD, IgE, IgG and IgM, which are classed according to the heavy chain they contain – α, δ, ε, γ and μ, respectively. Allergens are foreign molecules that cause an abnormal immunological response involving IgE. Opsonins are molecules that facilitate recognition and binding of microorganisms to enhance phagocytosis.

3.27 *D – Predominantly processed intracellularly*

Superantigens are proteins derived exogenously from bacteria, viruses and mycoplasma or expressed endogenously in an organism that can activate T-cells, B-cells, and natural killer cells. They are powerful immunomodulators that simultaneously bind to T-cell receptors on CD4 T-cells and MHC class II molecules on antigen-presenting cells which leads to an overactive immune response, and often a profound release of cytokines. They are processed extracellularly which circumvents intracellular processing to trigger activation of T-cells; hence D is the correct response.

3.28 *A – IgA*

IgA is secreted locally in tears, saliva, mucus and colostrum; hence A is the correct response. IgD is a membrane immunoglobulin found on the surface of B-cells where it functions as a receptor for an antigen and is often co-expressed with IgM. It can be found in low quantities throughout life in salivary, lacrimal, pancreatic and cerebrospinal fluids. IgE is produced by plasma cells located in lymph nodes, or at the sites of allergic reactions. It is tightly bound to the surface of mast cells and basophils through the IgE FcεRI receptor. IgG is the only immunoglobin that can cross the placenta to provide immune protection to a foetus. It plays a central role in the humoral immune response. It is the most abundant immunoglobulin in the extracellular fluid and plasma. IgM is the first antibody produced after initial antigen exposure and is found at a low concentration in human serum and interstitium, later being replaced by IgG. It is also the first immunoglobulin found in the foetus. It is the only isotype besides IgG that binds and activates complement.

3.29 *B – It is present as a B cell receptor*

The δ heavy chain of IgD is present on the surface of B-cells where it functions as a receptor for an antigen, or as a soluble form in plasma; hence B is the correct response. Similar to IgE and IgG, IgD is monomeric (not pentameric). IgM is pentameric and IgA is dimeric. Only IgG crosses the placenta. Similar to IgE and IgG, it has 2 antigen binding sites (not 4). IgA has 4 and IgM has 10 binding sites. IgD is composed of two heavy (2δ) and two light chains (not α chains).

3.30 *A – Class switching*

Immunoglobulin class switching, also known as isotype switching or class-switch recombination, is a mechanism by which activated B-cells change the class of antibody being produced, i.e., IgM is changed to IgA, IgG or IgE. The constant region of the heavy chain (C_H) is changed, but the variable region does not change, hence class switching does not affect antigen specificity. Switch regions are found within the constant regions and when two switch regions upstream of a constant region undergo switch recombination, the preceding constant regions are excised; hence A is the correct response. Alloimmunity is the process by which an immune response is invoked against antigens from members of the same species, i.e., in graft rejection. Avidity refers to the strength of the interaction between the antigen-binding site on an immunoglobulin and the antigen. Single-nucleotide polymorphisms are variations in bases of DNA between organisms and are the largest source of sequence variation in humans. Somatic hypermutation is a process by which immunoglobulins increase their affinity in an immune response, i.e., the immune system adapts to the foreign material. Somatic hypermutation and class switching are both important events observed in B-cells. Whereas somatic hypermutations introduce nucleotide variations in the heavy and light chain genes, class-switching exchanges the C_H region for other downstream C_H exons.

3.31 *B – CD8+ T lymphocytes*

Perforin is a pore-forming glycoprotein, which as the name suggests, perforates target cell membranes to facilitate the entry of granzymes – serine proteases released from lytic granules. This leads to apoptosis. Granules that store perforin and granzymes are found in cytotoxic CD8+ T lymphocytes; hence B is the correct response. CD4+ cells can kill other cells, but they do not contain granules that store perforin or granzymes. B lymphocytes and plasma cells do not make or store perforins. Interestingly, some studies have highlighted that granzymes are secreted by B lymphocytes when recognising viral antigens during acute phase viral disease and when induced by cytokines. Eosinophils do not contain perforin or granzymes.

3.32 *B – They occur outside lymph nodes*

B-lymphocytes are found in primary lymphoid tissues, such as the bone marrow and Peyer's patches of the ileum, and in secondary lymphoid tissues, such as the tonsils, spleen and lymph nodes; hence B is the correct response. They are divided into two categories – B1 and B2 (not three), which are distinguished by the expression of antigens on the cell surface. B1 cells do not display a strong memory response, whereas B2 cells do. B1 cells do not require cognate T-cell interactions for differentiation into plasma cells, whereas B2 cells do. B1 cells show little somatic hypermutation, whereas B2 cells do and hence produce high-affinity immunoglobulins. They are involved in the humoral immune response (not cell-mediated) whereby immunoglobulins are produced by B-cells which cause destruction of extracellular microorganisms. Lymphokines are cytokines produced predominantly by T-lymphocytes (and macrophages) in an endocrine or paracrine manner, and by B-lymphocytes in an autocrine manner.

3.33 *B – Systemic lymph node enlargement is rare*

Lymphatic vessels undergo profound enlargement at the site of inflammation where they become leakier. They are critical in an inflammatory response as they help drain excess extravasated fluid that has arisen from leaky blood vessels. Systemic lymph node enlargement is common in systemic acute or chronic infections, autoimmune conditions and malignant disease; hence B is the correct response. All other options are factually correct.

3.34 *E – Pars planitis*

The ciliary body is the site of aqueous humour production and located between the iris and choroid of the eye. The anterior portion is known as the pars plicata, and the posterior portion is known as the pars plana (or orbicularis ciliaris). Pars planitis is inflammation of the pars plana which can lead to blurred vision, floaters and even progressive vision loss. It is an idiopathic chronic uveitis which predominantly affects children and adolescents. The exact underlying cause is unknown, but one hypothesis is that it is an autoimmune condition. It is not a granulomatous disease; hence E is the correct response. All other options are examples of granulomatous diseases. Tertiary syphilis shows necrotising granulomatous inflammation. Brucella infection can cause suppurative granulomas (brucellomas). Sarcoidosis is a multisystem granulomatous disease, most commonly affecting the lungs and lymphatics. Mycetoma is a chronic subcutaneous infection caused by bacteria or fungi which results in granulomatous tissue.

3.35 *C – B cells are often absent*

X-linked agammaglobulinaemia or Bruton's disease is an X-linked recessive condition caused by mutations of the *btk* gene located at Xq21.3-22. This gene encodes a tyrosine kinase which is involved in B-cell maturation. The condition usually presents early in male children with a family history, who experience recurrent lung and ear infections. B cells are often absent (or very low); hence C is the correct response. It has an incidence of 1 in 100,000 and a prevalence of 1 in 10,000. All immunoglobulins are absent or low. T cells function normally. The btk protein is absent.

3.36 *B – Beta-2 glycoprotein I – Factor V Leiden*

Beta-2 glycoprotein I and other anticoagulant proteins (lupus, cardiolipin) are associated with antiphospholipid syndrome (not Factor V Leiden); hence B is the correct response. All other options are matched correctly.

3.37 *A – Hypogammaglobulinaemia is common in chronic bacterial sepsis*

Secondary causes of immunodeficiency are far more common than primary causes. Hypergammaglobulinaemia is common in chronic bacterial sepsis, whereas hypogammaglobulinaemia is common in acute bacterial sepsis; hence A is the correct response. Hypogammaglobulinaemia can also result from renal protein loss as seen in nephrotic syndrome, and via the gut as seen in protein-losing enteropathy.

3.38 *A – IgE concentration*

Radioallergosorbent testing or RAST is a method employed in allergy testing that detects specific IgE antibodies against a known allergen, such as peanuts, pollen, house dust mite, cat or dog dander, latex, venom, and certain drugs. The test is not a marker of the reaction severity that the patient has experienced, nor does it predict if a subsequent reaction will occur in the future. Total IgE measurements are of <u>no</u> value in allergy testing; hence A is the correct response.

3.39 *E – Endothelial cells*

The mononuclear phagocyte system involves non-specific phagocytosis of foreign agents, in addition to processing and presentation of specific antigens to T-cells by antigen-presenting cells. It consists of myeloid cells such as monocytes, macrophages, dendritic cells, Kupffer cells in the liver, alveolar and pleural macrophages in the lungs, red pulp macrophages in the spleen, osteoclasts in bone, Hofbauer cells in placenta, and epithelioid cells in granulomas. Endothelial cells are not members of the mononuclear phagocyte system; hence E is the correct response.

3.40 *D – IgG positive, IgM negative*

IgM antibodies are produced upon initial antigen exposure providing short-term immunity. They increase over weeks and decline as IgG begins to be produced. IgG antibodies are the most abundant in the blood and form the basis of long-term immunity against microorganisms. Upon exposure to the same antigen, IgG antibodies are produced more rapidly and vigorously as they bind with higher affinity to the antigen. These antibodies rise for a few weeks and then decline and stabilise. The figure below shows primary and secondary antibody responses. IgD is not routinely measured. Hence D is the correct response.

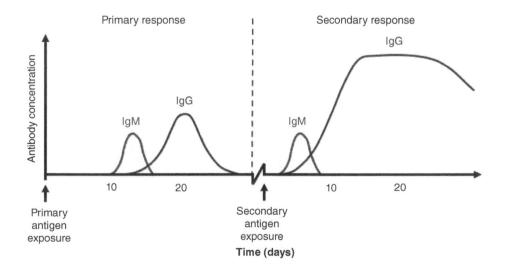

3.41 *E – In Hashimoto's thyroiditis, there is increased antigen expression of MHC class I on thyroid cells*

Hashimoto's thyroiditis is the most common cause for hypothyroidism. It is more common in women of late-middle age who present usually with a goitre. Anti-thyroid peroxidase (TPO) is present in very high titres (far greater than in Grave's disease). There are an increased number of helper and cytotoxic T-cells, and there is increase antigen expression of MHC class II (not class I) on lymphocytes and thyroid cells; hence E is the correct response.

3.42 *E – MuSK*

MuSK (muscle-specific tyrosine kinase) is a tyrosine kinase receptor found at the neuromuscular junction. MuSK activation leads to downstream signal transduction and pre- and post-synaptic differentiation whereby acetylcholine receptors begin to cluster in the synapse. Defects in MuSK signalling can lead to myasthenia gravis; hence E is the correct response. Autoantibodies associated with type I diabetes include GAD, IA2, ZnT8, islet cell, insulin, glucose transporter (GLUT-2), heat-shock protein 65, and carboxy-peptidase H.

3.43 *A – Lambert-Eaton myasthenic syndrome*

Lambert-Eaton myasthenic syndrome is a neuromuscular junction disorder which may present as a primary autoimmune disorder or as a paraneoplastic syndrome. Over 50% of cases are associated with small cell lung cancer. Over 80% of cases demonstrate antibodies against the P/Q subtype of voltage-gated calcium channels on pre-synaptic neurones. Anti-glial nuclear antibody is a specific marker for Lambert-Eaton associated with small cell lung cancer. A small number of patients may also have antibodies to synaptotagmin, a synaptic vesicle protein that senses calcium in neurotransmission; hence A is the correct response.

3.44 *E – anti-La – bullous pemphigoid*

Antibodies to La (and Ro) are found mainly in primary Sjögren's syndrome, being present in over 60%. Anti-La is also found in ca. 15% of patients with systemic lupus erythematosus; hence E is the correct response. Autoantibodies are directed against the basement membrane in bullous pemphigoid, which is hallmarked by the production of autoantibodies against two keratinocyte hemidesmosomal anchoring proteins, BP180 and BP230.

3.45 *C – Haptoglobin levels are decreased in autoimmune haemolytic anaemia*

Serum haptoglobins are decreased due to haemolysis in autoimmune haemolytic anaemia; hence C is the correct response. IgG (not IgE) anti-ACh-receptor antibodies are detected in ~90% of patients. Intrinsic factor antibodies have higher specificity but lower sensitivity than gastric parietal cell antibodies. Over 70% of patients with Felty's syndrome are ANCA positive (mostly anti-lactoferrin), and nearly all are rheumatoid factor positive. Mitochondrial antibodies are found in over 95% of patients with primary biliary cirrhosis.

3.46 *B- Plasma*

Myeloma is a tumour of plasma cells which leads to clonal expansion; hence B is the correct response.

3.47 *D – Hodgkin's lymphoma*

Hodgkin's lymphoma is characterised by the presence of Reed-Sternberg cells; hence D is the correct response. These are multinucleated cells with prominent eosinophilic nuclei that surround an abundant slightly basophilic cytoplasm.

3.48 *C – C2-hydroxylase inhibitor deficiency*

Angioedema is an urticarial-like, deep subcutaneous swelling caused by increased vascular permeability. Any part of the body can be involved, in particular the mucosa and submucosa of the respiratory and gastrointestinal tract. Hereditary and acquired C1-esterase inhibitor deficiency (not C3-hydroxylase inhibitor deficiency) are known to cause angioedema; hence C is the correct response. Drugs, such as ACE inhibitors, angiotensin-II receptor blockers, NSAIDs, statins and proton-pump inhibitors are also common causes of angioedema. ACE inhibitors are thought to inhibit angiotensin I-converting enzyme (kininase II), which breaks down bradykinin, as well as converting angiotensin I to angiotensin II. Angioedema can also be idiopathic.

3.49 *E – DiGeorge syndrome*

DiGeorge syndrome is a primary immunodeficiency caused by microdeletion on chromosome 22q11.2 in over 90% of patients. Most babies have a small thymus which results in low T-cell number and less than 1% are completely athymic; hence E is the correct response. In addition, babies can have cardiac abnormalities such as truncus arteriosus, interrupted aortic arch or tetralogy of Fallot, facial dysmorphia, such as hypertelorism, micrognathia or low-set ears, feeding problems, neurobehavioural problems, hypoparathyroidism and hypocalcaemia.

3.50 *E – Abnormally folded, protease-resistant isoform of an endogenous host protein*

Amyloids are aggregated fibrillary tangles with regular β-sheet repetitions that run perpendicular to the fibril axis. They have been linked to numerous neurodegenerative diseases, such as Alzheimer's disease, Parkinson's disease and Creutzfeldt-Jakob disease. Prions (the shortened version of proteinaceous infectious particles) are thought to be a subclass of amyloids that are infectious, abnormally folded, and protease-resistant isoforms of an endogenous host prion protein (PrP). Aggregations of these isoforms form highly structured amyloid fibres, which accumulate into plaques; hence E is the correct response. Prions lack genes and consist only of protein. They are responsible for some transmissible and inherited spongiform encephalopathies, such as bovine spongiform encephalopathy in cattle, scrapie in sheep, and Creutzfeldt-Jakob disease, kuru and Gerstmann-Sträussler-Scheinker syndrome in humans. Chemoattract proteins that stimulate migration and activation of leucocytes are chemokines. Small antibacterial proteins produced by neutrophils are defensins. Serum proteins involved in inflammation, phagocytosis and cell lysis are complement (C3a and C5a; C3b; and C5b-9, respectively). Infectious circular RNA molecules that lack a protein coat are viroids.

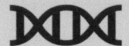

CHAPTER 4
Pharmacology

Any fool can know. The point is to understand.
Albert Einstein

4.1 Which of the following is the correct definition of bioavailability?
  A The biological effects of a drug on the body
  B The effects the body has on a drug over time
  C The effects of genetic variability on a drug
  D The proportion of unchanged drug that reaches the systemic circulation following any route of administration
  E The proportion of drug lost during absorption

4.2 Which of the following phases of drug development involves large numbers of patients and randomized controlled trials?
  A Pre-clinical
  B Phase I
  C Phase II
  D Phase III
  E Phase IV

4.3 Which of the following is a phase II metabolic reaction?
  A Oxidation
  B Reduction
  C Hydrolysis
  D Glucuronidation
  E Alcohol dehydrogenation

4.4 Which of the following regarding cytochrome P_{450} is **not** correct?
  A Enzymes are most highly expressed in the liver
  B Metabolic drug modification includes oxidation and hydrolysis
  C Phenytoin is a P_{450} enzyme-inducing drug
  D It is largely located within the nucleus of the cell
  E Grapefruit juice increases the concentration of metabolised drugs

4.5 Which of the following routes of administration is the most suitable for administering an antidote to a patient with a drug overdose?
  A Oral
  B Intravenous
  C Intramuscular
  D Subcutaneous
  E Transdermal

4.6 Which of the following antibiotics inhibit DNA gyrase?
  A Ciprofloxacin
  B Nitrofurantoin
  C Vancomycin
  D Chloramphenicol
  E Lymecycline

4.7 Which of the following is an osmotic laxative?
  A Senna
  B Docusate
  C Lactulose
  D Bisacodyl
  E Sodium picosulfate

4.8 Which of the following drugs are contraindicated in patients with renal artery stenosis?
  A Atenolol
  B Ramipril
  C Furosemide
  D Bendroflumethiazide
  E Diltiazem

4.9 Which of the following chemotherapy drugs is a dihydrofolate reductase inhibitor?

A 5-fluorouracil
B Cisplatin
C Methotrexate
D Vincristine
E Imatinib

4.10 Which of the following drugs does deferoxamine reverse?

A Morphine
B Iron
C Lorazepam
D Rocuronium
E Aspirin

4.11 Which of the following increases gastric emptying by relaxing the pyloric sphincter?

A Metoclopramide
B Prochlorperazine
C Cyclizine
D Ondansetron
E Haloperidol

4.12 Which of the following is **not** a risk factor for digoxin toxicity?

A Hypokalaemia
B Hypomagnesemia
C Hypocalcaemia
D Hypothyroidism
E Hypovolaemia

4.13 Which of the following does **not** cause hyperkalaemia?

A Ramipril
B Burns
C Renal tubular acidosis
D Spironolactone
E Conn's syndrome

4.14 Which of the following drugs does **not** contain a beta lactam?

A Ertapenem
B Piperacillin
C Cefuroxime
D Vancomycin
E Aztreonam

4.15 Which of the following long-term adverse effects of drugs is **not** correct?

A Thiazide diuretics – gout
B Corticosteroids – osteoporosis
C Anticonvulsants – megaloblastic anaemia
D Amiodarone – pulmonary fibrosis
E Hydralazine – insomnia

4.16 Which of the following is **not** a muscarinic antagonist?

A Atropine
B Hyoscine
C Tiotropium
D Solifenacin
E Rocuronium

4.17   Which of the following is the correct effect of hormones on blood glucose?
A   Insulin – increased gluconeogenesis
B   Adrenaline – decreased glycogenolysis
C   Glucagon – increased glycogenolysis
D   Growth hormone – decreased gluconeogenesis
E   Glucocorticoids – increased glucose uptake

4.18   Which of the following functional groups confers the most acidity?
A   Aniline
B   Amidine
C   Guanidine
D   Carboxyl
E   Phenol

4.19   Which of the following characteristics of β_2 adrenoceptors is **not** correct?
A   Dilate bronchi
B   Relax bladder detrusor
C   Contract urethral sphincter
D   Relax ciliary muscles
E   Increase force of contraction of the heart

4.20   Which of the following drugs is only a selective α_1 antagonist?
A   Labetalol
B   Doxazosin
C   Timolol
D   Terbutaline
E   Mirtazapine

4.21   Which of the following regarding coagulation is **not** correct?
A   Heparin inhibits coagulation by activating antithrombin III
B   Vitamin K antagonists interfere with post-translational amination of glutamic acid
C   Fondaparinux increases the action of antithrombin III on factor Xa
D   Sensitivity to protamine occurs in some patients with fish allergies
E   Clopidogrel inhibits platelet responses to adenosine diphosphate

4.22   Which of the following actions of 5-hydroxytryptamine is correct?
A   Decreased gastrointestinal motility
B   Relaxation of smooth muscle of the uterus
C   Platelet aggregation
D   Inhibition of peripheral nociceptive nerve endings
E   Vasodilatation does not occur

4.23   Which of the following regarding mediators of inflammation is **not** correct?
A   Histamine causes cardiac stimulation by acting on H_2 receptors
B   Prostaglandin D_2 acts on thromboxane receptors which mediates bronchoconstriction
C   Arachidonate is metabolised by cyclo-oxygenase to prostanoids
D   Leukotriene B_4 is found in inflammatory exudates
E   Bradykinin causes decreased vascular permeability

4.24   Which of the following drugs is **not** a cytokine inhibitor?
A   Cyclophosphamide
B   Etanercept
C   Anakinra
D   Rituximab
E   Tofacitinib

4.25 Which of the following regarding theophylline is correct?
A It blocks acetylcholine receptors
B It decreases intracellular cyclic AMP
C It is a pentylxanthine
D It is a phosphodiesterase inhibitor
E It can only be given orally

4.26 Which of the following oral corticosteroids is the longest acting?
A Prednisolone
B Hydrocortisone
C Methylprednisolone
D Triamcinolone
E Dexamethasone

4.27 Which of the following is a progestogen-only pill?
A Ethinylestradiol
B Norethisterone
C Ergometrine
D Mifepristone
E Clomiphene

4.28 Which of the following is a contraindication in the use of risedronate?
A Hyponatraemia
B Hypokalaemia
C Hypoglycaemia
D Hypocalcaemia
E Hypophosphataemia

4.29 Which of the following is an inhibitory neurotransmitter?
A Acetylcholine
B Dopamine
C GABA
D Glutamate
E Epinephrine

4.30 Which two amino acids must bind to NMDA receptors for activation?
A Glycine and glutamate
B Glycine and aspartate
C Glutamine and methionine
D Asparagine and glutamate
E Lysine and aspartate

4.31 Which of the following regarding adenosine receptors is correct?
A A_1, A_2 and A_3 receptors are tyrosine kinases
B A_1 receptors produce vasoconstriction in coronary vessels
C Stimulation of platelet aggregation occurs via A_2 receptors
D Stimulation of neurotransmitter release at synapses occurs via A_1 receptors
E A_3 receptors on mast cells release mediators which contributes to bronchoconstriction

4.32 Which of the following regarding neurotransmitters is correct?
A NMDA receptors are aspartate receptors
B Flumazenil is a $GABA_A$ receptor antagonist
C Baclofen inhibits $GABA_B$ receptors by decreasing post-synaptic Ca^{2+} influx
D Dopamine D1 receptors are linked to inhibition of adenylate cyclase
E Botulinum toxin prevents GABA release from neurones

4.33   Which of the following regarding opioid receptors is correct?
A   Pure agonists have high affinity for δ receptors
B   Partial agonists cause dysphoria rather than euphoria
C   Only μ receptors are G-protein mediated
D   Antagonists have low affinity for κ receptors
E   σ receptors are responsible for most of the analgesic effects of opioids

4.34   Which of the following regarding cholinergic transmission is **not** correct?
A   Five molecular subtypes of muscarinic receptors are known
B   Acetylcholine release occurs by calcium ion-mediated exocytosis
C   Botulinum toxin inhibits acetylcholine release
D   Suxamethonium can lead to malignant hypothermia
E   Neostigmine acts on neuromuscular junctions

4.35   Which of the following is **not** a serotonin-norepinephrine reuptake inhibitor (SNRI)?
A   Duloxetine
B   Venlafaxine
C   Trazodone
D   Dosulepin
E   Tramadol

4.36   Which of the following drugs used to treat open-angle glaucoma is a carbonic anhydrase inhibitor?
A   Brimonidine
B   Acetazolamide
C   Latanoprost
D   Timolol
E   Pilocarpine

4.37   Which of the following antiepileptic drugs may exacerbate seizures in people with myoclonic and atonic seizures?
A   Carbamazepine
B   Lamotrigine
C   Levetiracetam
D   Sodium valproate
E   Clobazam

4.38   Which of the following drugs is **not** known to cause gum hypertrophy?
A   Phenytoin
B   Verapamil
C   Cyclosporin
D   Irbesartan
E   Sodium valproate

4.39   Which of the following regarding ACE inhibitors is **not** correct?
A   Increase levels of bradykinin
B   Increase vasodilation of vascular smooth muscle
C   Decrease preload and afterload
D   Decrease the secretion of aldosterone
E   Increase retention of sodium and water

4.40   Which of the following regarding platelet aggregation inhibitors and their drug interactions is **not** correct?
A   Dual use of aspirin and ketorolac can lead to increased bleeding
B   Clopidogrel and ranitidine have a strong drug interaction
C   Ticagrelor and itraconazole should be avoided
D   Dipyridamole increases exposure to adenosine and should be avoided
E   Tirofiban and fluoxetine can lead to increased bleeding

4.41 Which of the following is **not** the correct mechanism of action for drugs used in the treatment of diabetes?
  A Gliclazide blocks ATP-sensitive potassium ion channels which results in depolarization
  B Metformin reduces hepatic gluconeogenesis
  C Sitagliptin is an active dipeptidyl peptidase-4 (DPP-4) inhibitor
  D Pioglitazone stimulates peroxisome proliferator-activated receptor- γ (PPAR$_\gamma$) receptors
  E Empagliflozin increases urinary glucose excretion by inhibiting sodium-glucose linked transporter 1 (SGLT1)

4.42 Which of the following regarding nitric oxide is correct?
  A Nitric oxide synthase isoenzymes are all trimers
  B Aspartate is important in nitric oxide biosynthesis
  C Sodium-calmodulin activates nitric oxide synthase
  D High concentrations of nitric oxide can cause methaemoglobinaemia
  E Nitric oxide biosynthesis is increased in patients with hypercholesterolaemia

4.43 Which of the following regarding antibiotics is **not** correct?
  A Tetracyclines are bacteriostatic
  B Sulfonamides cross the placenta and blood-brain barrier
  C Clavulanic acid is a β-lactamase inhibitor
  D Clindamycin has no activity against anaerobes
  E Vancomycin is bactericidal

4.44 Which of the following antifungal drugs is only used in topical therapy?
  A Miconazole
  B Itraconazole
  C Fluconazole
  D Voriconazole
  E Ketoconazole

4.45 Which of the following drugs is known to cause oligohydramnios?
  A Warfarin
  B Prednisolone
  C Ramipril
  D Tetracycline
  E Gentamicin

4.46 Which of the following anti-cancer drugs induces cytotoxicity through inhibition of microtubule formation?
  A Cisplatin
  B Cytarabine
  C Anastrozole
  D Paclitaxel
  E Bleomycin

4.47 Which of the following regarding drugs used in the haemopoietic system is **not** correct?
  A Folic acid contains a pteridine ring and glutamic acid
  B Vitamin B$_{12}$ helps convert homocysteine to methionine
  C Hypoxia-inducible factor-2 (HIF-2) induces erythropoietin production in juxtatubular cells
  D Tetracycline is an iron-chelating agent
  E Fe^{2+} is converted to Fe^{3+} for absorption in the gastrointestinal tract

4.48 Which of the following regarding general anaesthetic drugs is correct?
  A Ketamine produces negligible anaesthetic effects
  B Propofol can cause profound vasoconstriction
  C Nitrous oxide can cause malignant hyperthermia
  D Sevoflurane is contraindicated in patients with liver disease
  E Etomidate can cause adrenocortical suppression

4.49   Which of the following regarding drugs that affect kidney function is correct?

    A   Furosemide increases excretion of uric acid

    B   Bendroflumethiazide increases Ca^{2+} excretion

    C   Eplerenone inhibits distal Na^+ retention and K^+ secretion

    D   Ethanol stimulates ADH secretion

    E   Amiloride leads to an increase in Na^+ reabsorption in the collecting duct

4.50   Which of the following regarding antimicrobial drugs is correct?

    A   Penicillin V is a broad spectrum antibacterial

    B   Ceftriaxone is a first-generation cephalosporin

    C   Teicoplanin is not administered per os

    D   Metronidazole is the treatment of choice for giardiasis

    E   Atovaquone with proguanil is used to treat amoebiasis

Answers

4.1 *D – The proportion of unchanged drug that reaches the systemic circulation following any route of administration*

Bioavailability is the proportion (or fraction) of unchanged drug that reaches the systemic circulation following any route of administration; hence D is the correct response. In addition, it is the rate at which this occurs. It is measured by determining the plasma drug concentration versus time curves and calculated from the area under these curves. It is important to remember that bioavailability is not a characteristic of the drug preparation alone, and factors such as enzyme activity within the GI tract, pH and GI motility all play a role. Intravenous formulations have 100% bioavailability, while other routes have less than 100% bioavailability.

4.2 *D – Phase III*

Pre-clinical studies aim to link drug discovery in a laboratory to the initiation of clinical trials in humans. Phase I trials are performed on small groups of people (20–80) and aim to assess safety, tolerability and pharmacokinetic properties. Phase II trials are performed on larger group of people (100–300) and aim to assess efficacy. Phase III trials are double-blind randomized controlled trials, often multicentred and performed on much larger groups of people (1000–3000); hence D is the correct response. These trials are costly and time consuming. They aim to confirm effectiveness, monitor side effects, and compare the new drug with a standard/similar treatment. These trials also aim to assess pharmacoeconomics of a new drug. At the end of Phase III trials, the drug is submitted to the relevant regulatory body for licencing such as the FDA in the US, and the MHRA in the UK. Upon approval, the drug is made available to the public via Phase IV trials which aim to detect longer-term adverse effects.

4.3 *D – Glucuronidation*

Biotransformation is predominantly a hepatic metabolic process which alters the chemical structure of exogenous and endogenous substances aiding in excretion. There are three phases which can occur sequentially or simultaneously. Phase I involves biotransformation of molecules to less lipophilic, more water-soluble active metabolites. Examples include oxidation with cytochrome P450, reduction and hydrolysis. Alcohol dehydrogenation is an oxidation reaction. For example, blue cheese is often high in tyramine, and if it is not oxidized to inactive *p*-hydroxyphenylacetic acid by the enzyme monoamine oxidase, tyramine builds up in synaptic vesicles which can lead to a hypertensive crisis. It is for this reason that patients taking monoamine oxidase inhibitors such as phenelzine for depression should not consume large quantities of blue cheese (or any food/drink containing high levels of tyramine). Phase II reactions yield a large polar metabolite by conjugation with hydrophilic groups that form water-soluble, pharmacologically inactive compounds that can be excreted in urine. Examples include glucuronidation (hence D is the correct response), methylation, acetylation, sulfation and conjugation with an endogenous ligand (e.g., glutathione, glycine, sulfate, acetate). Phase III reactions involve further metabolism, hepatocellular efflux and biliary excretion. Recognised membrane transporters involved in these reactions include the ATP-binding cassette (ABC) and soluble carrier (SLC) transporters.

4.4 *D – It is largely located within the nucleus of the cell*

Cytochrome P450 are a family of haem-containing monooxygenases that catalyse oxidative reactions, and in its reduced state, binds carbon monoxide to give a complex that absorbs light at a maximum absorption of 450 nm. These enzymes use molecular oxygen and NADPH as cofactors to add oxygen to amino acids in a regio- and stereoselective manner. They are found extensively in the liver, and certain subfamilies can also be found in enterocytes. They are expressed as membrane bound proteins found predominantly in the endoplasmic reticulum (not the nucleus) of the liver; hence D is the correct response.

4.5 *B – Intravenous*

Intravenous injection is the fastest and most certain of drug administration with 100% of the dose entering the systemic circulation. By definition, bioavailability is 100%; hence B is the correct response. Oral administration is the most common and a drug's plasma concentration following oral administration is determined by its bioavailability and the rate by which it is metabolised by the liver and excreted by the kidneys. Hence bioavailability is widely varied due to the extent of absorption in the small intestine and first-pass elimination by the liver. Intramuscular and subcutaneous injections produce a faster effect than oral administration, but absorption can be less predictable depending on the site of injection and regional blood flow. Transdermal methods often produce a prolonged steady-state drug delivery via skin absorption and avoid pre-systemic metabolism, such as the first-pass effect. Similarly, avoidance of the first-pass effect is seen with sublingual and rectal routes of administration.

4.6 *A – Ciprofloxacin*

Ciprofloxacin belongs to the quinolones and inhibit bacterial DNA synthesis by inhibiting DNA gyrase as well as topoisomerase IV; hence A is the correct response. DNA gyrase is an important enzyme in DNA replication as it is responsible for maintaining the helical shape. It is particularly effective against Gram-negative bacteria, such as *Escherichia coli, Pseudomonas aeruginosa, Haemophilus influenzae* and *Klebsiella pneumoniae*. The mechanism of action of nitrofurantoin is complex. Essentially, nitrofurantoin is reduced by bacterial flavoproteins to reactive intermediates which inactivate ribosomal proteins and hence alter a wide range of essential, metabolic processes such as DNA, RNA and protein synthesis. It has activity against both Gram-positive bacteria such as *Staphylococcus saprophyticus, Staphylococcus aureus*, and coagulase-negative staphylococci; and Gram-negative bacteria such as *Escherichia coli*. It has no activity against *Pseudomonas* species. Vancomycin is a glycopeptide active against Gram-positive bacteria which inhibits cell wall synthesis. Chloramphenicol is a naturally-occurring bacteriostatic antibiotic that contains nitrobenzene. It inhibits protein synthesis by competing with messenger RNA for ribosomal binding and prevents chain elongation by inhibiting peptidyl transferase. Lymecycline belongs to the tetracyclines which have bacteriostatic activity against many Gram-positive and Gram-negative bacteria. It inhibits protein synthesis by blocking aminoacyl-tRNA attachment to the ribosome.

4.7 C – Lactulose

There are a variety of laxatives available, and they all have different modes of action. Osmotic laxatives such as lactulose increase the water content in the large bowel by increasing inflow of fluid and electrolytes; hence C is the correct response. They can act as stool softeners and help stimulate contraction of the colon. Stimulant laxatives such as the anthraquinone senna, bisacodyl and sodium picosulfate help stimulate colonic motility and intestinal secretion but can often cause abdominal cramp. Docusate (also called dioctyl sodium sulphosuccinate) is a stimulant laxative thought to decrease surface tension and stimulate intestinal fluid secretion which increases penetration into faecal matter, thereby softening the stool.

4.8 B – Ramipril

Renin is released from the renal cortex in response to reduced renal arterial pressure, sympathetic neural activity and sodium concentration in the distal tubule. Renin acts on angiotensinogen to yield angiotensin I. Ramipril is an angiotensin-converting enzyme (ACE) inhibitor which inhibits conversion of angiotensin I to angiotensin II. Angiotensin is a vasoconstrictor which stimulates renal hypertension and aldosterone synthesis. Ramipril causes vasodilation and reduces aldosterone synthesis, in addition to increasing concentrations of other vasodilating agents such as prostaglandins and kinins. In renal artery stenosis, or secondary hyperaldosteronism, patients are hypertensive due to excess renin and angiotensin II production. There is narrowing of the renal artery (or arteries) which leads to reduced renal perfusion pressure at the distal side of the stenosis; hence B is the correct response. ACE inhibitors are an absolute contraindication in patients with renal artery stenosis. Aetiology is either by atherosclerotic reno-vascular disease or fibromuscular dysplasia.

4.9 C – Methotrexate

Methotrexate is structurally similar to folic acid. Folic acid is converted to folinic acid by dihydrofolate reductase, the receptor for the antineoplastic drug methotrexate. Methotrexate is an antimetabolite which inhibits dihydrofolate reductase, hence preventing synthesis of purines and pyrimidines needed for nucleic acid synthesis; hence C is the correct response. 5-fluoruracil acts by blocking thymidylate synthase, an enzyme essential for pyrimidine synthesis. Cisplatin exerts a cytotoxic effect by forming intra- and interstrand crosslinks which inhibit DNA synthesis. Vincristine (and vinblastine) is a vinca alkaloid, derived from the periwinkle plant *Vinca rosea*, which inhibits tubulin polymerisation and leads to disruption in the assembly of microtubules, especially during metaphase of mitosis. Imatinib is a tyrosine kinase inhibitor which prevents phosphorylation by ATP of the Bcr-Abl oncoprotein and used in the treatment of chronic myeloid leukaemia.

4.10 B – Iron

Deferoxamine is a potent iron-chelating agent which chelates free iron (non-transferrin bound), iron which exists between transferrin and ferritin, ferritin, and haemosiderin. The bound complex is then excreted via the urine or bile; hence B is the correct response. Morphine excess and overdose can be reversed by naloxone, an opioid-receptor antagonist. Lorazepam is a benzodiazepine which, in excess, can be reversed by flumazenil, a competitive benzodiazepine-receptor antagonist. Rocuronium is a non-depolarising skeletal muscle relaxant used in endotracheal intubation, which can be reversed by anticholinesterases such as neostigmine or sugammadex, a modified gamma cyclodextrin. There is no antidote to aspirin overdose/excess, and management is directed towards preventing further absorption and promoting elimination. Due to the weakly acidic nature of aspirin, sodium bicarbonate can be administered which causes an alkalosis and helps neutralise serum acidosis.

4.11 A – Metoclopramide

All options are examples of antiemetics. Metoclopramide is a central D_2-receptor antagonist (as is domperidone), and peripheral 5-HT_3-receptor antagonist and 5-HT_4-receptor agonist. It stimulates oesophageal, gastric and pyloric motor activity. It increases lower oesophageal sphincter tone while relaxing the pyloric sphincter, stimulates gastric contractions and enhances gastric emptying. In this regard, it acts as a prokinetic agent as it selectively stimulates gut motor function; hence A is the correct response. All other options do not increase gastric emptying by relaxing the pyloric sphincter, and they are not prokinetic agents. Prochlorperazine is a phenothiazine which acts as a D_2-receptor antagonist. It produces vagal blockade in the GI tract. Cyclizine is a piperazine which acts as a H_1-receptor antagonist. Ondansetron is a selective 5-HT$_3$-receptor antagonist which acts centrally in the vomiting centre and chemoreceptor trigger zone, and peripherally, by blocking receptors on intestinal vagal and spinal afferent nerves. Haloperidol is a butyrophenone which acts as a D_2-receptor antagonist and a first-generation antipsychotic.

4.12 A – Hypocalcaemia

Digoxin is a cardiac glycoside that increases the force of myocardial contraction and reduces conductivity within the AV node. It is indicated for treatment of chronic heart failure and persistent atrial fibrillation. Hypocalcaemia is not a risk factor for digoxin toxicity; hence C is the correct response. However, hypercalcaemia is. All other options are known risk factors for digoxin toxicity, as is increasing age (>55 years), decreased renal clearance and polypharmacy. Common drugs which alter digoxin levels include diltiazem, verapamil, amiodarone, ketoconazole, itraconazole, spironolactone, erythromycin and clarithromycin.

4.13 E – Conn's syndrome

Conn's syndrome, or primary hyperaldosteronism, is the most common cause of secondary hypertension. It is caused by aldosterone-producing adenomas, bilateral idiopathic adrenal hyperplasia, aldosterone-secreting adrenal carcinomas (rare) and familial hyperaldosteronism. Increasing aldosterone levels causes renal sodium reabsorption and water retention, with potassium loss. This results in plasma volume expansion, hypertension and hypokalaemia (in addition to hypernatraemia and metabolic alkalosis); hence E is the correct response. All other options cause hyperkalaemia.

4.14 D – Vancomycin

All options are examples of antibiotics. Vancomycin is a glycopeptide antibiotic that inhibits bacterial cell wall synthesis and alters cell membrane permeability. It is bactericidal and only effective against Gram-positive bacteria. It is the drug of choice for staphylococcal and streptococcal infections, and in patients who are allergic to penicillins and cephalosporins. It is a branched, tricyclic and glycosylated peptide which does not contain a beta lactam; hence D is the correct response. All other antibiotics contain a beta lactam ring.

4.15 E – Hydralazine – insomnia

Hydralazine is a direct vasodilator used to treat essential hypertension. It is not a first-line agent since it stimulates the sympathetic nervous system. It can also be used to rapidly reduce blood pressure in hypertensive emergencies when administered intravenously. The most common adverse effects which have been reported when using hydralazine include headaches, hypotension, flushing, dizziness, angina, myalgia, palpitations, tachycardia, nausea and vomiting. Insomnia is not a recognised adverse effect of hydralazine; hence E is the correct response. All other options are recognised adverse effects of the drugs listed.

4.16 E – Rocuronium

Rocuronium is an aminosteroid, non-depolarising neuromuscular blocker used as a muscle relaxant in anaesthetics. It is fast-acting and reversible. It competitively binds to nicotinic cholinergic receptors at the motor endplate of neurones. It is not a muscarinic antagonist; hence E is the correct response. All other options are examples of muscarinic antagonists.

4.17 C – Glucagon – increased glycogenolysis

The following table summarises the effect of hormones on blood glucose; hence C is the correct response.

Hormone	Main action	Main effect
Insulin	↑ glucose uptake ↑ glycogen synthesis ↓ glycogenolysis ↓ gluconeogenesis	↓ blood glucose
Glucagon	↑ glycogenolysis ↑ gluconeogenesis	↑ blood glucose
Adrenaline (epinephrine)	↑ glycogenolysis	
Growth hormone	↓ glucose uptake ↑ gluconeogenesis	
Glucocorticoids	↑ gluconeogenesis ↓ glucose uptake	

4.18 *D – Carboxyl*

The charge state of compounds, in particular drugs, under varying pH conditions greatly affect absorption, distribution, metabolism, excretion and toxicity. The acid–base character of drugs affects potency, selectivity and solubility, and has significant impact on pharmacokinetics. It is important to remember that pK_a and pK_b values quoted in the literature tell us very little about whether the drug behaves more as an acid or a base. The only sure way of knowing this is to learn the functional groups that confer acidity or basicity. Common acidic groups include carboxylates, phenols, sulfonamides, hydroxamates, and acidic amides and imides. The lower the pK_a value, the stronger the acid. Phenols have a pK_a of ca. 10 and are thus significantly less acidic than carboxylic acids; hence D is the correct response.

Common basic groups include heterocyclic nitrogen atoms, aliphatic amines, amidines, anilines, guanidines and basic amides. Remember not all nitrogen-containing compounds are basic. In fact, amides contain nitrogen and are neutral, and many drugs that contain nitrogen atoms are acidic. This is due to the availability of the lone pair of electrons on the nitrogen, and often, when unavailable for reaction with protons, they are so weakly basic that they behave as acids.

4.19 *C – Contract urethral sphincter*

Alpha and beta adrenoceptors are activated by the catecholamines adrenaline and noradrenaline. Adrenaline has a much higher affinity for beta receptors than noradrenaline, whereas noradrenaline has a much higher affinity for alpha receptors. Alpha receptors lead to smooth muscle contraction whereas beta receptors lead to smooth muscle relaxation. Beta adrenoceptors consist of 7 G-protein coupled transmembrane receptor proteins, of which there are three subtypes: β_1, β_2 and β_3.

β_1 receptors are known to play a critical role in mediating the inotropic effects of the heart – increased heart rate, stroke volume, cardiac output and blood pressure, and cause renin release from juxtaglomerular cells of the kidney which increase blood pressure.

β_2 receptors regulate aspects of airway function, such as mediating mast cell release and airway smooth muscle tone – smooth muscle relaxation and bronchodilation, detrusor muscle relaxation – urinary retention and decreased urination, uterine relaxation, vascular smooth muscle relaxation and vasodilation, ciliary muscle relaxation and increase production of aqueous humor, increase insulin release from the pancreas and lead to gluconeogenesis and glycogenolysis in the liver.

β_3 receptors are by far the least studied isotype and are found in various tissues including the myocardium, brain, adipose tissue, retina, kidneys and bladder. Studies have found that activated receptors can lead to lipolysis in adipose tissue, and detrusor muscle relaxation.

Activation of α_1 receptors (not β_2) lead to urethral sphincter contraction; hence C is the correct response.

4.20 *B – Doxazosin*

Doxazosin is a long acting selective α_1 adrenoceptor antagonist used in the management of benign prostatic hyperplasia to relieve symptoms of urinary obstruction, and hypertension; hence B is the correct response. Labetalol is used in cases where mixed adrenergic antagonism is desirable since it acts as a competitive antagonist at α_1 and β adrenoceptors. Timolol is a non-selective β-adrenoceptor antagonist that prevents action of catecholamines. It is applied topically to the eyes as it lowers intraocular pressure by blocking ciliary body receptors which reduce the rate at which aqueous humor is produced. Terbutaline is a selective β_2-adrenoceptor agonist, but it also has low affinity for β_1-adrenoceptors. It is used in the management of reversible airways obstruction, and in premature labour, since it relaxes uterine smooth muscle and reduce uterine contractility. Mirtazapine is a noradrenergic and serotonergic antidepressant that also has α_2 antagonism.

4.21 *B – Vitamin K antagonists interfere with post-translational amination of glutamic acid*

Vitamin K antagonists, such as the anticoagulant warfarin, inhibits the vitamin K epoxide reductase complex 1, which is an essential enzyme for vitamin K activation and required for the production of functionally active, γ-carboxylated coagulation proteins (factors II, VII, IX and X) and anticoagulant proteins (protein C and protein S). Oral anticoagulant drugs act indirectly on the carboxylation (not amination) of glutamic acid of vitamin K-dependent proteins in the liver; hence B is the correct response.

4.22 *C – Platelet aggregation*

5-hydroxytryptamine, or serotonin (interestingly named because the substance released from a blood clot into the serum acted as a vasoconstrictor, i.e., added tone), is a neurotransmitter synthesised from 5-hydroxytryptophan, and in the pineal gland, acts as a precursor of melatonin. Over 90% of serotonin is found in enterochromaffin cells of the GI tract. In the blood, it is found in platelets and leads to platelet aggregation by activating 5-HT_2 receptors; hence C is the correct response. Serotonin leads to stimulation of gastrointestinal smooth muscle, increasing tone and motility. It also stimulates uterine smooth muscle contractions in pregnant women. Similar to histamine, serotonin is a potent stimulant of peripheral nociceptive nerve endings. It is a powerful vasoconstrictor; however, in cardiac and skeletal muscle, it acts as a vasodilator. Clinically, carcinoid tumours release excess serotonin which is metabolised by monoamine oxidase to 5-hydroxyindolacetic acid (5-HIAA). It is for this reason that a 24-hour urine collection of 5-HIAA is used as a diagnostic test for carcinoid tumours.

4.23 *E – Bradykinin causes decreased vascular permeability*

Kinins are potent vasodilators formed when serine proteases (kallikreins) act on protein substrates (kininogens). Bradykinin is released from high-molecular-weight kininogen by plasma kallikrein. Kinins cause arteriolar dilation in vascular beds, likely as a result of nitric oxide release or the vasodilatory effect of prostaglandins. Interestingly in contrast, kinins cause venoconstriction, likely due to smooth muscle stimulation in veins or as a result of prostaglandins which cause the veins to contract. Kinins increase flow in capillary beds and vascular permeability; hence E is the correct response.

4.24 *A – Cyclophosphamide*

Cyclophosphamide is an alkylating cytotoxic drug that belongs to the class of nitrogen mustard agents that binds to DNA and disrupts replication. It is used to treat various leukaemias and lymphomas, and autoimmune diseases such as systemic lupus erythematosus and multiple sclerosis; hence A is the correct response. All other options are cytokine inhibitors. Etanercept is a biologic tumour necrosis factor (TNF) inhibitor used in the treatment of ankylosing spondylitis, rheumatoid arthritis, psoriatic arthritis and juvenile idiopathic arthritis. Anakinra is a biologic interleukin-1 receptor antagonist which has anti-inflammatory and immunomodulatory actions, and is used in the treatment of rheumatoid arthritis, Still's disease and cryopyrin-associated period syndromes (autosomal dominant genetic autoinflammatory syndromes). Rituximab is an anti-CD20 monoclonal antibody used in the treatment of non-Hodgkin's lymphoma, chronic lymphocytic leukaemia, rheumatoid arthritis, pemphigus vulgaris, microscopic polyangiitis and granulomatosis with polyangiitis. Tofacitinib is a Janus-associated tyrosine kinase (JAK) inhibitor, specifically a potent JAK1 and JAK3 inhibitor (but less active against JAK2) used in the treatment of rheumatoid arthritis, psoriatic arthritis, ulcerative colitis and ankylosing spondylitis. It has been shown to suppress cytokine signalling by inhibiting signal transducer and activator of transcription (STAT) transcription factors.

4.25 *D – It is phosphodiesterase inhibitor*

Theophylline is a phosphodiesterase inhibitor and an inducer of catecholamine release; hence D is the correct response. It is a potent inhibitor of adenosine (not acetylcholine) receptors. Adenosine causes airway narrowing. It prevents intracellular breakdown of cAMP, resulting in increased intracellular cAMP which reduces smooth muscle tone and dilation of the airways. It is a methylxanthine related to caffeine, not a pentylxanthine. It can be administered orally or intravenously. Theophylline is used in the treatment of asthma and COPD.

4.26 *E – Dexamethasone*

Dexamethasone (and betamethasone) are the longest acting oral corticosteroids (when using hydrocortisone as a standard); hence D is the correct response. Prednisolone, methylprednisolone and triamcinolone are intermediate acting. Hydrocortisone and cortisone are short acting.

4.27 *B – Norethisterone*

Progestogen-only pills (POP), as the name suggests, contain only progestogen, unlike the combined pill which contains an oestrogen and a progestogen. POPs include norethisterone and levonorgestrel; hence B is the correct response. Longer acting progestogen-only contraceptives are also available which can be given intramuscularly, such as medroxyprogesterone, and the subcutaneous implant of levonorgestrel. The oestrogen in most combined second-generation pills is ethinylestradiol. Ergometrine is a myometrial stimulant (oxytocic) that contracts the uterus and can be used to treat postpartum haemorrhage. Mifepristone is a partial agonist at progesterone receptors, and in combination with a prostaglandin analogue, can be used as a medical alternative to surgical termination of early pregnancy. Clomiphene is an oestrogen antagonist that stimulates gonadotrophin release (and thereby LH and FSH) by inhibiting the negative feedback effects of endogenous oestrogen. It is used to stimulate ovulation in anovulatory infertility.

4.28 *D – Hypocalcaemia*

Risedronate is a bisphosphonate which resists enzymatic hydrolysis and deemed to be analogues of pyrophosphate. The main action is to block bone resorption by osteoclasts. Bisphosphonates have a high affinity for bone and are not metabolised. Contraindications include hypocalcaemia (hence D is the correct response); hypersensitivity to bisphosphonates, chronic kidney disease where the eGFR is less than 30 mL/minute/1.73 m^2, an inability to stand or sit upright for at least 30 minutes, oesophageal disorders (achalasia, strictures, Barrett's, previous bariatric surgery), and a history of atypical femur fractures or osteonecrosis of the jaw secondary to bisphosphonate.

4.29 *C – GABA*

GABA, or γ-aminobutyric acid, is the main inhibitory neurotransmitter in the brain, and it is scarce in peripheral tissues; hence C is the correct response. It is formed from glutamate by the action of glutamic acid decarboxylase. Glycine is also an inhibitory neurotransmitter mainly found in the spinal cord. Excitatory neurotransmitters include acetylcholine, dopamine and epinephrine. Glutamate and aspartate are excitatory amino acids in the CNS. Histamine has both excitatory and inhibitory effects.

4.30 *A – Glycine and glutamate*

N-methyl-D-aspartate (NMDA) receptors are a family of L-glutamate receptors that play an important role in learning and memory. They are tetrameric ion channels composed of various types of subunits. They are highly permeable to calcium cations but are readily blocked by magnesium cations. Activation of NMDA receptors requires glycine and glutamate, and both sites are distinct from each other; hence glycine acts as an allosteric modulator. Both sites must be occupied by glycine and glutamate for the channel to open; hence A is the correct response.

4.31 *E – A$_3$ receptors on mast cells release mediators which contributes to bronchoconstriction*

Adenosine receptors are 7-transmembrane receptors that mediate the central and peripheral actions of methylxanthines, theophylline and caffeine. There are four subtypes of receptors – A$_1$, A$_{2A}$, A$_{2B}$ and A$_3$ which exert their effects by coupling to different G proteins and, in turn, activate downstream signalling pathways via stimulation or inhibition of adenylate cyclase. All four receptors are members of the rhodopsin-like family of transmembrane receptors (not tyrosine kinases). A$_1$ receptors cause arteriolar vasoconstriction (in the kidneys) and A$_2$ receptors induce vasodilatation (including the coronary vessels). Inhibition (not stimulation) of platelet aggregation occurs via A$_2$ receptors. Inhibition (not stimulation) of neurotransmitter release at central and peripheral synapses occurs via A$_1$ receptors. A$_3$ receptors on mast cells release mediators which contributes to bronchoconstriction; hence E is the correct response.

4.32 *B – Flumazenil is a GABA$_A$ receptor antagonist*

Flumazenil, a water-soluble imidazodiazepine, is a competitive antagonist or inverse agonist at the benzodiazepine binding site on GABA$_A$ receptors; hence B is the correct response. NMDA receptors are glutamate (not aspartate)-activated calcium ionophores. Baclofen is a selective GABA$_B$ receptor agonist used for muscle spasms and spasticity. Baclofen has both pre-synaptic and post-synaptic actions. In pre-synaptic neurones, GABA$_B$ receptors modulate neurotransmitter release by inhibiting Ca^{2+} influx, while post-synaptic GABA$_B$ receptors couple mainly to K$^+$ channels. There are two types of dopamine receptors which have been further subdivided. D$_1$ and D$_5$ receptors stimulate adenylate cyclase and activate protein kinase A. D$_2$, D$_3$ and D$_4$ receptors inhibit calcium channels and adenylate cyclase. In general, activation of D$_2$ receptors opposes the effects of D$_1$ receptor activation. Botulinum toxin acts selectively to prevent glycine (not GABA) release from inhibitory neurons in the spinal cord.

4.33 *B – Partial agonists cause dysphoria rather than euphoria*

Partial agonists combine a degree of agonism and antagonism on different receptors. Buprenorphine is a partial agonist at the μ receptor, but also a weak κ receptor antagonist and δ receptor agonist. Euphoria is mediated by μ receptors, whereas activation of κ receptors produce dysphoria; hence B is the correct response. Pure agonists have high affinity for μ receptors (and low affinity for δ and κ receptors). All opioid receptors are G-protein-coupled receptors. Antagonists, such as naloxone and naltrexone, block the effects of opiates. They have a high affinity for μ receptors (and in general, κ receptors). Although not a true opioid receptor, σ receptors account for the dysphoric effects such as anxiety and hallucinations. The μ receptors are responsible for most of the analgesic effects.

4.34 *D – Suxamethonium can lead to malignant hypothermia*

Suxamethonium, or succinylcholine (succinic acid with a choline molecule attached at each carboxyl group), is the only depolarising neuromuscular blocking agent which acts as a muscle relaxant. It is an analogue of acetylcholine, and it acts as an agonist at nicotinic cholinergic receptors on the post-synaptic membrane. It is rapid acting and continues to be used in rapid-sequence inductions and in the treatment of laryngospasms. However, its use in anaesthetics is declining as a result of the numerous side effects due to its depolarising role. These include arrhythmias, bradycardia, hyperkalaemia, muscle pains and malignant hyperthermia (not hypothermia); hence D is the correct response.

4.35 *C – Trazodone*

Trazodone is used in the treatment of major depression and is in the serotonin-antagonist-and-reuptake-inhibitor class (not norepinephrine); hence C is the correct response. There are three SNRIs currently available: duloxetine, venlafaxine and desvenlafaxine. They inhibit both serotonin and norepinephrine reuptake. These can be used in the treatment of major depression and neuropathic pain. Duloxetine is also efficacious for generalised anxiety disorder. Dosulepin is a thio-derivative of amitriptyline and a tricyclic antidepressant. It inhibits reuptake of serotonin, norepinephrine and dopamine. Tramadol, although a weak opioid, is similar in structure to venlafaxine, and similarly, plays an inhibitor role on serotonin and norepinephrine reuptake. Interestingly, weak opioids such as tramadol (and codeine) require cytochrome P450 2D6 for conversion to an active opioid agonist, and many antidepressants are CYP2D6 inhibitors. Clinically, this is important since combined use may lead to reduced analgesic effects.

4.36 B – Acetazolamide

Acetazolamide is a carbonic anhydrase (an enzyme that catalyses the formation of carbonic acid from water and carbon dioxide) inhibitor; hence B is the correct response. It is used primarily for the treatment of open-angle glaucoma (and acute mountain sickness). It was introduced in the early 50s as a diuretic since it increases urinary sodium excretion, blocks bicarbonate absorption in the proximal tubule and increases H^+ in the plasma, hence alkaline urine and metabolic acidosis. It is now seldom used as a diuretic. Brimonidine is a highly selective α_2-adrenergic agonist which lowers IOP by inhibiting adenyl cyclase, reduces aqueous humor synthesis and increases outflow. Latanoprost is a prostaglandin $F_{2\alpha}$ analogue used to reduce IOP by increasing outflow of aqueous humor through the uveoscleral pathway. Timolol is a non-selective β-adrenoceptor antagonist that lowers IOP by reducing the production rate of aqueous humor. Pilocarpine is a cholinergic muscarinic agonist that contracts the ciliary muscle, increasing outflow of aqueous humor and reducing IOP.

4.37 A – Carbamazepine

Antiepileptic drugs that may exacerbate seizures in people with myoclonic and atonic seizures include carbamazepine, gabapentin, oxcarbazepine, pregabalin, tiagabine and vigabatrin; hence A is the correct response. Phenytoin can exacerbate myoclonic seizures. All other options can be used to help prevent myoclonic seizures. Tonic and atonic seizures are treated with sodium valproate, lamotrigine, clobazam, topiramate and rufinamide. Interestingly, a ketogenic diet can also be recommended as an add-on treatment under supervision of a dietician.

4.38 D – Irbesartan

Drugs are the most common reason behind gum hypertrophy. It is a side effect seen in patients taking anticonvulsants such as phenytoin, sodium valproate, phenobarbitone, vigabatrin and ethosuximide, immunosuppressants such as cyclosporin, tacrolimus and sirolimus, and calcium channel blockers, such as nifedipine, amlodipine, verapamil and diltiazem. Irbesartan is an angiotensin-II receptor antagonist used to treat hypertension and is not known to cause gum hypertrophy; hence D is the correct response.

4.39 E – Increase retention of sodium and water

ACE inhibitors decrease angiotensin II production and therefore decreases aldosterone secretion. Aldosterone is responsible for sodium and water retention; therefore, ACE inhibitors cause vasodilation and sodium and water loss (not retention); hence E is the correct response. ACE inhibitors can decrease systemic venous tone which reduces preload, but they also decrease peripheral vascular resistance and ventricular afterload. ACE is also an enzyme that degrades bradykinin; therefore ACE inhibitors increase bradykinin levels.

4.40 B – Clopidogrel and ranitidine have a strong drug interaction

Clopidogrel is a prodrug that is metabolised to its active form by carboxylesterase-1. The active form is a platelet inhibitor that prevents platelet aggregation. There are no known interactions between clopidogrel and ranitidine; hence B is the correct response. However, omeprazole, a proton-pump inhibitor, competitively inhibits the CYP2C19 isoenzyme which is known to metabolise clopidogrel to its active form, and therefore reducing the ability of clopidogrel to inhibit platelet aggregation. Therefore, these drugs are generally not recommended but lansoprazole can be used at the lowest effective dose as an alternative when patients have dyspepsia or when dual antiplatelets are used (which can increase the risk of gastrointestinal bleeding).

4.41 E – Empagliflozin increases urinary glucose excretion by inhibiting sodium-glucose linked transporter 1 (SGLT1)

Empagliflozin is a selective inhibitor of sodium-glucose linked transporter 2 (SGLT2) which reduces hyperglycaemia in patients with type 2 diabetes by decreasing renal glucose reabsorption and increasing urinary glucose excretion; hence E is the correct response.

4.42 D – High concentrations of nitric oxide can cause methaemoglobinaemia

Methaemoglobinaemia is caused by oxidation of the iron in haemoglobin from the ferrous state (Fe^{2+}) to the ferric state (Fe^{3+}). Nitric oxide acts as an oxidising agent since it rapidly reacts with reduced oxyhaemoglobin; hence D is the correct response. Nitric oxide synthases (NOSs) are enzymes that oxidise arginine to citrulline, generating nitric oxide (which can be reduced to N_2O and N_2). NOSs are functional as homodimers (not trimers) and there are three NOS isoforms – neuronal NOS (nNOS), endothelial (eNOS) and inducible (iNOS). All three isoforms are found in the kidney. Arginine (not aspartate) is important in nitric oxide biosynthesis. Calcium-calmodulin (not sodium) activates nitric oxide synthase. It has been proposed that this complex acts as a molecular switch, inducing a conformational change in NOS that facilitates electron flow. Since NO is synthesised in functionally intact endothelium, hypercholesterolaemia and atherosclerosis impair endothelial function, hence reduce eNOS activity (not increase it).

4.43   D – Clindamycin has no activity against anaerobes

Clindamycin is a lincosamide, bacteriostatic antibiotic which is active against several aerobic Gram-positive cocci (staphylococci and streptococci, but not enterococci) and a variety of anaerobes (*Bacteroides* spp and *Clostridium perfringens*). It is not active against aerobic and facultatively anaerobic Gram-negative bacilli; hence D is the correct response.

4.44   A – Miconazole

All drugs listed are members of the azoles which are known to inhibit lanosterol 14α-demethylase, an important enzyme in ergosterol biosynthesis. Ergosterol is an integral part of the fungal cell membrane. Depending on the number of nitrogen atoms in the five-membered azole ring, azoles can be classified as imidazoles or triazoles. Imidazoles contain two nitrogen atoms in the ring and include miconazole, ketoconazole and clotrimazole. Miconazole and clotrimazole are only used in topical therapy; hence A is the correct response. Although ketoconazole is more commonly used to topically treat fungal skin infections and seborrhoeic dermatitis, it can also be administered orally in the treatment of endogenous Cushing's syndrome. It acts as a potent inhibitor of cortisol and aldosterone synthesis by inhibiting 17α-hydroxylase activity, thereby inhibiting steroidogenesis and decreasing levels of glucocorticoids. Triazoles contain three nitrogen atoms in the ring and include itraconazole, fluconazole and voriconazole.

4.45   C – Ramipril

Oligohydramnios is defined as decreased amniotic fluid volume of less than 500 ml, or an amniotic fluid index (AFI) of less than 5 cm. It typically presents in the third trimester with genitourinary abnormalities such as bladder outlet obstruction, dysplastic kidneys and renal agenesis. There are many causes such as foetal – chromosomal and congenital factors, intrauterine growth restriction, and premature rupture of membranes; placental – abruption and twin-twin transfusion syndrome in monochorionic twins; maternal – dehydration, hypertension, pre-eclampsia, diabetes, uteroplacental insufficiency and hypoxia; idiopathic and drug-induced – indomethacin and ACE inhibitors, such as ramipril; hence C is the correct response. Similar to adult kidneys, ACE inhibitors block the conversion of angiotensin I to angiotensin II in the developing foetal kidneys. ACE inhibitors are contraindicated after the first trimester.

4.46   D – Paclitaxel

Paclitaxel, or taxol, is extracted from the pacific yew tree, *Taxus baccata*. It is an antimicrotubule that promotes assembly of microtubules, stabilising them and preventing depolymerisation. As a result of this stabilisation, normal reorganisation of the microtubules is inhibited and cytotoxicity ensues; hence D is the correct response. This contrasts with the vinca alkaloids, such as vinblastine and vincristine (obtained from the Madagascan periwinkle plant) which induce microtubule disassembly. Cisplatin intercalates into DNA causing inter- and intrastand crosslinks that arrest the cell cycle and induce apoptosis. Cytarabine is a pyrimidine analogue which competes with cytidine to intercalate within DNA, thus ceasing DNA replication. Anastrozole is an aromatase (oestrogen synthase) inhibitor which suppresses oestrogen levels and is indicated in the treatment of hormone-receptive breast cancer in postmenopausal women. Bleomycin is a glycopeptide antibiotic used as a cytotoxic antineoplastic agent. It oxidatively damages DNA by binding to metal ions forming metallobleomycin complexes and reactive oxygen species. These cause DNA strand breaks which then produce free base propenals known to cause cell cycle arrest.

4.47   E – Fe^{2+} is converted to Fe^{3+} for absorption in the gastrointestinal tract

Dietary iron is absorbed by enterocytes of the duodenum by the divalent metal transporter-1 in the ferrous state (Fe^{2+}) which is reduced from the ferric state (Fe^{3+}) by duodenal cytochrome B. Transferrin-bound iron is taken up by the transferrin-receptor-1 which is internalised into endosomes via endocytosis, released and reduced to Fe^{2+}; hence E is the correct response.

4.48   E – Etomidate can cause adrenocortical suppression

Etomidate is an ultrashort-acting, non-barbiturate hypnotic anaesthetic agent, which is only administered intravenously, has no analgesic effects and is often used due to its favourable haemodynamic profile (ideal for shocked, hypovolaemic patients, or those with significant cardiovascular disease). Although its pharmacokinetics are favourable, it has limited use for continuous infusions due to endocrine side effects. It causes a dose-dependent inhibition of 11β-hydroxylase, an enzyme responsible for converting 11-deoxycortisol to cortisol which results in adrenocortical suppression; hence E is the correct response. Ketamine is a water and lipid-soluble NMDA antagonist which differs from most other intravenous anaesthetics since it produces profound analgesia. It is unique at induction as it produces a dissociative anaesthetic state characterised by analgesia and amnesia, despite the patients' eyes remaining open. Propofol is a potent hypnotic commonly used for induction and maintenance of anaesthesia. It activates $GABA_A$ receptors and inhibits NMDA receptors. It decreases cerebral blood flow, intracranial pressure, and systemic blood pressure as a result of profound vasodilation (not vasoconstriction). Hence it is relatively contraindicated in haemodynamically unstable patients. Nitrous oxide does not cause malignant hyperthermia. Inhaled, volatile halogenated anaesthetic agents such as isoflurane, sevoflurane and desflurane, commonly used in induction and/or maintenance of anaesthesia (in oxygen/oxygen-enriched air, or nitrous oxide-oxygen environments) can cause malignant hyperthermia. Sevoflurane (or any halogenated anaesthetic) is not contraindicated in hepatic impairment, but it can cause hepatotoxicity in patients previously sensitised to them. In addition, halogenated anaesthetic agents should be used with caution in patients with renal impairment (risk of nephrotoxicity from either inorganic fluoride ions or the haloalkene degradation product).

4.49 C – Eplerenone inhibits distal Na+ retention and K+ secretion

Eplerenone (and spironolactone) is a potassium-sparing diuretic and aldosterone antagonist. It binds to receptors on the distal convoluted tubule and collecting duct to increase sodium, water and calcium excretion and decrease potassium loss. Therefore, inhibiting the activity of the Na^+/K^+-ATPase pump reducing Na^+ reabsorption and K^+ excretion (increasing K^+ in the blood); hence C is the correct response. Furosemide is a loop diuretic which reduces uric acid excretion due to increased uric acid reabsorption in the proximal tubule. Bendroflumethiazide is a thiazide diuretic which lowers calcium excretion and increases serum calcium levels. Ethanol inhibits the secretion of ADH causing a water diuresis (like a transient diabetes insipidus). Amiloride is a potassium-sparing diuretic which inhibits sodium reabsorption in the distal convoluted tubules and collecting ducts, leading to sodium and water loss.

4.50 D – Metronidazole is the treatment of choice for giardiasis

Metronidazole is the treatment of choice for giardiasis, a diarrhoeal disease caused by a parasite and often associated with recent foreign travel, particularly South Asia; hence D is the correct response. Tinidazole is at least equally effective as metronidazole and can be administered as a single oral dose. Penicillin V (phenoxymethylpenicillin) is a narrow spectrum antibacterial (not broad spectrum). Narrow spectrum antibiotics are active against a narrow or selected group of bacterial types, while broad spectrum antibiotics are effective against a broader number. Broad spectrum antibiotics are mainly used when the infecting bacteria is unknown. Ceftriaxone is a third-generation (not first) cephalosporin, as are cefotaxime, cefixime and ceftazidime. First-generation cephalosporins include cefalexin, cefadroxil and cefazolin. Second-generation cephalosporins include cefaclor and cefuroxime. Fifth-generation cephalosporins are now available, which include ceftaroline fosamil, ceftobiprole and ceftolozane with a β-lactamase inhibitor such as tazobactam. Teicoplanin is a glycopeptide antibiotic which has bactericidal activity against aerobic and anaerobic Gram-positive bacteria. It can be administered per os (by mouth), intravenously, intramuscularly and intraperitoneally. On the other hand, vancomycin, another glycopeptide antibiotic, is not administered intramuscularly. Atovaquone with proguanil is used both in the treatment and chemoprophylaxis of falciparum malaria (not amoebiasis). Metronidazole followed by the anti-protozoal drug diloxanide is used to treat confirmed cases of amoebiasis or amoebic dysentery.

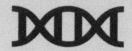

CHAPTER 5

Histology and Histopathology

Learn to see microscopically.
Rudolf Virchow

Single Best Answers for Medical Students: Basic Science, First Edition. Stuart Kyle.
© 2024 John Wiley & Sons Ltd. Published 2024 by John Wiley & Sons Ltd.

Histology

5.1 Which of the following is correct regarding epithelium?
A Pseudostratified epithelium has all cells in contact with the underlying extracellular matrix
B Nuclei of columnar epithelial cells are basal and arranged randomly
C Cuboidal epithelium is a characteristic cell lining the endometrium
D Holocrine secretion is common in cells lining the pancreas
E Bullous pemphigoid results from autoantibodies directed against proteins in occluding junctions of epithelial cells

5.2 Which of the following is **not** a component of the basement membrane?
A Type IV collagen
B Heparan sulphate
C Fibronectin
D Fibrillin
E Laminin

5.3 Which of the following contain Paneth cells?
A Stomach
B Liver
C Small intestine
D Pancreas
E Testes

5.4 Which of the following structure–tissue matches are correct?
A Epididymis – pseudostratified cuboidal epithelium
B Vas deferens – stratified squamous epithelium
C Epiglottis – ciliated pseudostratified columnar epithelium
D Anal canal – cuboidal epithelium
E Trachea – ciliated stratified squamous epithelium

5.5 Which of the following cells' main function is to produce acid?
A Sertoli
B Merkel
C Oxyphil
D Parietal
E Mesangial

5.6 Which of the following regarding the female reproductive system is correct?
A The development of primary follicles is dependent on luteinizing hormone
B The primary oocyte arrests in the dictyate stage of prophase II
C Secondary follicles contain liquor folliculi which fill spaces between granulosa cells
D Simple columnar epithelium is found in the ovarian medulla
E Ciliated peg cells facilitate capacitation of spermatozoa

Questions 5.7 to 5.9 relate to the following histological section.

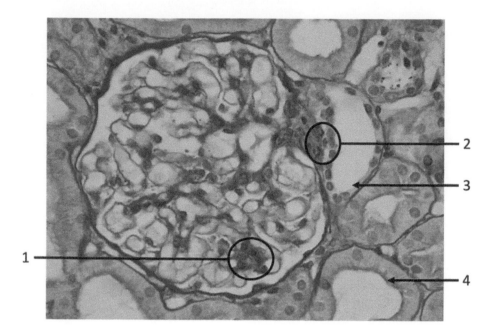

5.7 Which of the following cells is located in region labelled 1?
  A Transitional epithelial
  B Microvillus epithelial
  C Goblet
  D Mesangial
  E Lacis

5.8 Which of the following is **not** correct regarding region labelled 2?
  A Cells detect changes in luminal sodium chloride concentration
  B Renal blood flow and glomerular filtration rate are controlled
  C Renin is release by juxtaglomerular cells
  D Adenosine binds to afferent arterioles and causes vasoconstriction
  E Hypotension results in renin release causing vasodilation of efferent arterioles

5.9 Which of the following regarding labels 3 and 4 is correct?
  A Cells lining both 3 and 4 are mainly columnar
  B Brush borders are greater in number at 3 than 4
  C More urine is filtered at 3 than 4
  D Aldosterone causes 3 to reabsorb sodium ions
  E Only ~40% of filtered glucose and amino acids are reabsorbed at 4

5.10 Which of the following is correct regarding histology of the liver?
  A Canals of Hering are lined by simple cuboidal epithelium
  B Spaces of Dissé separate bile canaliculi from hepatocytes
  C Kupffer cells contain few lysosomes
  D Endothelial cells are tightly packed with little intercellular space
  E Stellate cells store and regulate transport of vitamin K

Questions 5.11 to 5.13 relate to the following histological sections of the liver. Reticulin fibres stain black in Y.

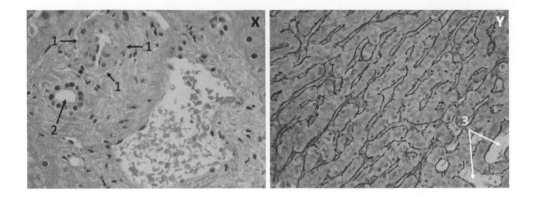

5.11 Which of the following corresponds to the structure enclosed within label 1?
  A Kupffer cell
  B Hepatocyte
  C Portal vein
  D Hepatic artery
  E Central vein

5.12 Which of the following epithelium lines structure labelled 2?
  A Simple cuboidal
  B Pseudostratified squamous
  C Simple squamous
  D Stratified cuboidal
  E Stratified columnar

5.13 Which of the following corresponds to label 3?
  A Canaliculi
  B Bile ductules
  C Sinusoids
  D Hepatic acini
  E Adipose tissue

Questions 5.14 to 5.15 relate to the following histological section of the tongue.

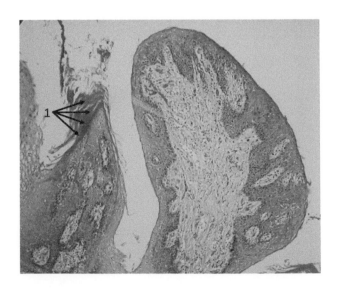

5.14 Which of the following types of papillae are observed in this section?
   A Circumvallate and filiform
   B Filiform and foliate
   C Fungiform and filiform
   D Circumvallate and fungiform
   E Foliate and fungiform

5.15 Which of the following corresponds to label 1?
   A Lamina propria
   B Serous glands of von Ebner
   C Taste buds
   D Keratin
   E Skeletal muscle

5.16 Which of the following epithelium lines the lingual surface of epiglottis?
   A Keratinised stratified squamous
   B Non-keratinised stratified squamous
   C Stratified columnar
   D Simple columnar
   E Pseudostratified ciliated columnar

Questions 5.17a to 5.17e relate to the following histological section.

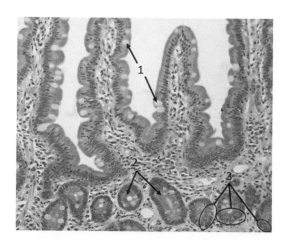

5.17a Which of the following organs is this histological section taken from?
   A Stomach
   B Large intestine
   C Small intestine
   D Oesophagus
   E Pancreas

5.17b Which of the following cells corresponds to label 1?
   A Enterocytes
   B Enteroendocrine cells
   C Paneth cells
   D Tuft cells
   E Goblet cells

5.17c Which of the following is **not** correct regarding label 2?
   A Stem cells are abundant
   B Simple columnar epithelium is present
   C A central lacteal is present
   D There are higher rates of mitotic divisions
   E There is a high concentration of lysozyme

5.17d Which of the following cells correspond to label 3?
   A Enterocytes
   B Enteroendocrine cells
   C Paneth cells
   D Tuft cells
   E Goblet cells

5.17e Which of the following lies immediately beneath label 3?
   A Muscularis mucosae
   B Plicae circularis
   C Peyer's patch
   D Brunner's glands
   E Lamina propria

5.18 Which of the following is correct regarding the skin?
   A Keratinocytes are constantly produced in the stratum corneum
   B Melanocytes are located in the hypodermis
   C Eccrine glands are essential for thermoregulation
   D Rete ridges are dermal downgrowths which extend into hypodermis
   E Meissner corpuscles found within dermal papillae are sensitive to deep vibration and pressure

Questions 5.19 to 5.21 relate to the following histological section.

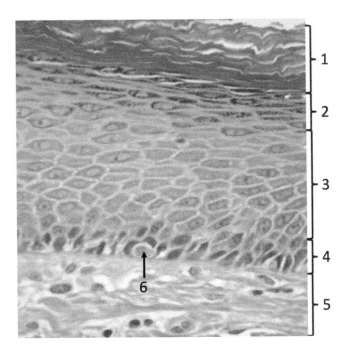

5.19 Which of the following (A–E) match labels (1–4)?

	1	2	3	4
A	Stratum corneum	Stratum granulosum	Stratum basale	Stratum spinosum
B	Stratum corneum	Stratum spinosum	Stratum granulosum	Stratum basale
C	Stratum spinosum	Stratum corneum	Stratum granulosum	Stratum basale
D	Stratum corneum	Stratum granulosum	Stratum spinosum	Stratum basale
E	Stratum granulosum	Stratum corneum	Stratum basale	Stratum spinosum

5.20 Which of the following layers contain the highest proportion of connective tissue?
   A 1
   B 2
   C 3
   D 4
   E 5

5.21 Which of the following corresponds to label 6?
   A Fibroblast
   B Neutrophil
   C Melanocyte
   D Langerhans
   E Keratinocyte

5.22 Which of the following regarding the following histological section is **not** correct?

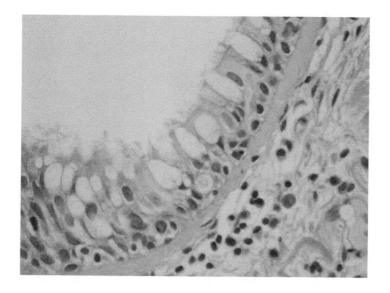

   A Pseudostratified cuboidal epithelium is evident
   B Cilia are present
   C Basement membrane lies above the lamina propria
   D This is typical of respiratory mucosa
   E Mucus-secreting cells are abundant

Questions 5.23 and 5.24 relate to the following histological section.

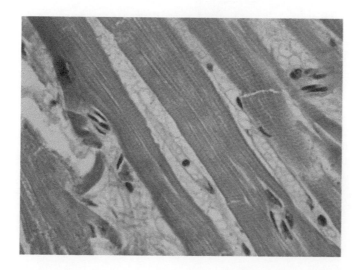

5.23   Which of the following muscle types is highlighted in this section?
   A   Transverse section of cardiac muscle
   B   Longitudinal section of cardiac muscle
   C   Transverse section of skeletal muscle
   D   Longitudinal section of skeletal muscle
   E   Smooth muscle

5.24   Which of the following regarding this type of tissue is correct?
   A   This tissue is under voluntary control of the somatic nervous system
   B   Thick and thin filaments are not organised into sarcomeres
   C   Intercalated discs are present
   D   Multiple nuclei are located near the sarcolemma
   E   Auerbach's plexus is found in this tissue

5.25   Which of the following is correct regarding muscle?
   A   In the sarcomere, the I and A bands represent areas where actin and myosin do not overlap
   B   All types of muscle tissue have a sarcomere
   C   With age, lipofuscin often builds up in skeletal muscle
   D   Multinucleated cells with peripherally situated nuclei is a feature of skeletal muscle
   E   In cardiac muscle, intercalated discs occur at the M line of the sarcomere

5.26   Which of the following regarding the histology of bone is correct?
   A   Osteoblasts lie in Howship's lacunae
   B   Osteoclasts are uninucleated
   C   Trabecular bone is composed of osteons
   D   Osteocytes produce bone matrix
   E   Haversian canals run longitudinally in osteons

5.27   Regarding histology of bone, which of the following (A–E) corresponds to lacunae?

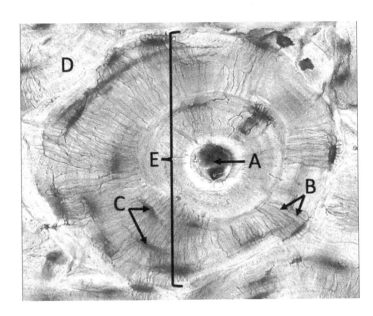

5.28   Which of the following regarding histology of the colon and anus is **not** correct?
   A   Myenteric plexus is located in the muscularis externa
   B   Meissner's plexus is located in the submucosa
   C   There are no plicae circularis in the colon
   D   Three longitudinal bands of smooth muscle form taeniae coli
   E   The anal canal is composed of keratinised simple columnar epithelium

5.29 Which of the following is a non-ciliated, non-mucous secreting cell found in the bronchioles?
  A Bushy
  B Clara (Club)
  C Foveolar
  D Oxyphil
  E Chromaffin

5.30 Which of the following zones of the adrenal gland predominantly secretes glucocorticoids?
  A Capsule
  B Zona glomerulosa
  C Zona reticularis
  D Zona fasciculata
  E Medulla

5.31 Which of the following is **not** found in olfactory mucosa?
  A Glands of Bowman
  B Olfactory cell
  C Sustentacular cell
  D Basal cell
  E Stereocilia

5.32 Which of the following glands is the following histological section most likely taken from?

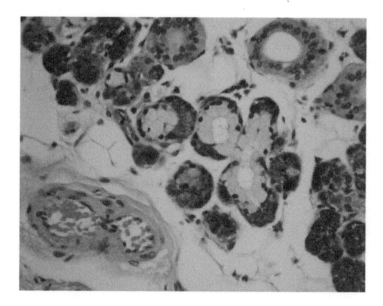

  A Submandibular
  B Parotid
  C Brunner
  D Pancreas
  E Lacrimal

5.33 Which of the following transitions occur at the gastro-oesophageal junction?
  A Simple columnar to non-keratinised stratified columnar epithelium
  B Stratified cuboidal to simple columnar epithelium
  C Non-keratinised stratified squamous to simple columnar epithelium
  D Keratinised stratified squamous to simple columnar epithelium
  E Pseudostratified columnar to simple cuboidal epithelium

Questions 5.34 and 5.35 relate to the following histological section of the spleen.

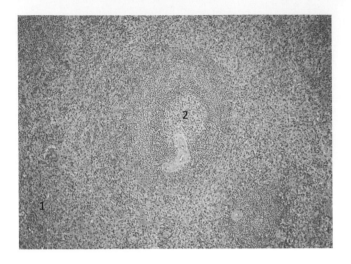

5.34   Which of the following is **not** evident in this histological section?
   A   Arteriole
   B   Red pulp
   C   Sinusoids
   D   White pulp
   E   Capsule

5.35   Which of the following is correct regarding labels 1 and 2?
   A   Follicular dendritic cells predominate in region 1
   B   Small, immature lymphocytes are common in region 1
   C   Cords of Billroth are found in region 2
   D   Antibody production is rich in region 2
   E   Periarteriolar lymphoid sheaths are equally abundant in regions 1 and 2

5.36   Which of the following contain glands of Littré and lacunae of Morgagni?
   A   Penile urethra
   B   Prostatic urethra
   C   Seminal vesicles
   D   Epididymis
   E   Ductus deferens

5.37   Which of the following organs of the female reproductive system is the following histological section most likely taken from?

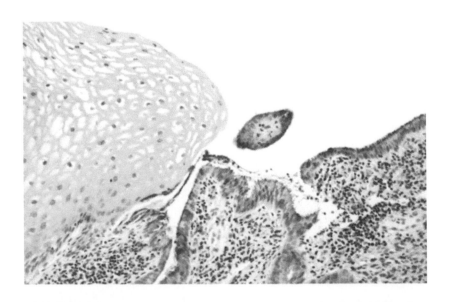

A Uterus
B Fallopian tube
C Ovary
D Cervix
E Vagina

5.38 Which of the following parts of the eye contains zonular fibres and is lined by simple cuboidal epithelium?
A Cornea
B Iris
C Lens
D Retina
E Conjunctiva

5.39 Which of the following (A–E) corresponds to a monocyte?

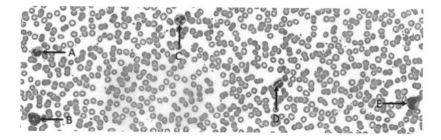

5.40 Which of the following is correct regarding blood cells?

A Erythrocytes contain no other proteins other than haemoglobin
B Neutrophils are agranular
C Eosinophils contain basophilic granules
D Monocytes often have a reniform nucleus
E Basophils have highly specific membrane receptors for IgG

Histopathology

5.41 A 28-year-old female presents with abdominal bloating, fatigue and iron-deficiency anaemia. She underwent an endoscopy and duodenal biopsies were taken. The histology from a normal duodenal biopsy is shown in A. The histology from the duodenal biopsy taken from this 28-year-old is shown in B, and the histology from the duodenal biopsy after the patient was partially treated is shown in C. Which of the following is the most likely diagnosis?

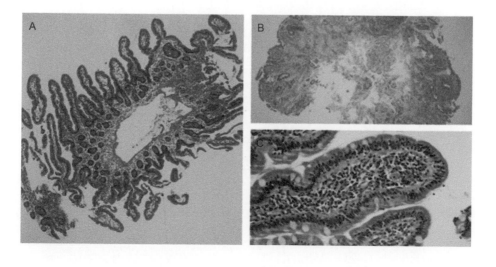

A Duodenal ulcer
B Crohn's disease
C Duodenal adenocarcinoma
D Coeliac disease
E Irritable bowel syndrome

5.42 A 42-year-old male smoker presents with chronic heartburn for over 10 years which has now become drug-resistant. He is obese and has been taking over-the-counter ibuprofen for lower back pain for several years. He underwent an endoscopy and biopsies were taken. A section of oesophagus is shown below. Which of the following is the most likely diagnosis?

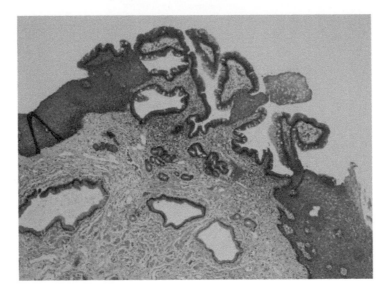

A Gastro-oesophageal reflux disease
B Oesophagitis
C Gastritis
D Oesophageal adenocarcinoma
E Barrett's oesophagus

5.43a A 31-year-old male presents with diarrhoea, weight loss, fatigue and spasmodic abdominal pain. He undergoes a colonoscopy and excisional biopsy. A section of bowel is shown below. Which of the following is the most likely diagnosis?

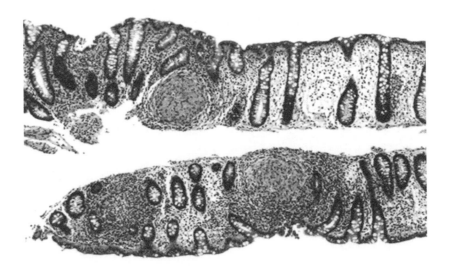

A Ulcerative colitis
B Crohn's disease
C Coeliac disease
D Giardiasis
E Colon carcinoma

5.43b Subsequently, the patient was initially treated, but this was stopped due to increasing dyspnoea. A chest radiograph and CT thorax was arranged, and he underwent bronchoscopy. A Ziehl-Neelsen stain was performed as shown below. Which of the following is the most likely diagnosis?

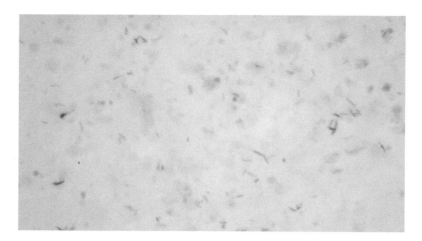

A Tuberculosis
B Aspergillosis
C Sarcoidosis
D Pneumonitis
E Pneumoconiosis

5.44 A 27-year-old female presents with heartburn, acid reflux, halitosis and epigastric pain. She underwent a gastroscopy and excisional biopsy. A section of stomach is shown below. She was diagnosed with chronic gastritis. Which of the following is the most likely cause?

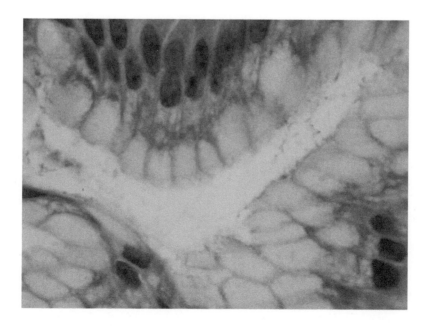

A Drug induced
B Autoimmune
C Dietary
D *Helicobacter pylori*
E Bile reflux

5.45 A 68-year-old undergoes excision of a skin lesion from his cheek. The histology is shown below. Which of the following is **not** a precursor to this neoplasm?

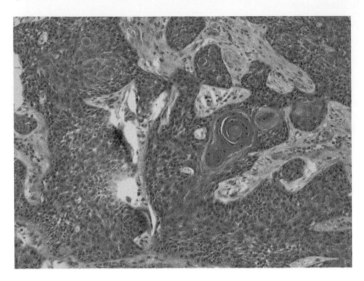

A Bowen's disease
B Seborrhoeic keratosis
C Keratoacanthoma
D Discoid lupus erythematosus
E Actinic keratosis

5.46 A 64-year-old smoker presents with chronic dyspnoea, wheeze, and a cough worse in the morning and night. Multiple treatment failures and worsening symptoms resulted in bronchoscopy-guided bronchial epithelium sampling. The histology is shown below. Which of the following is the most likely diagnosis?

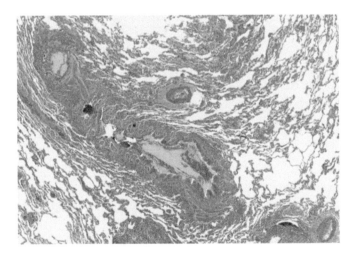

A Chronic obstructive pulmonary disease
B Bronchiectasis
C Asthma
D Idiopathic pulmonary fibrosis
E Eosinophilic pneumonia

5.47 A 39-year-old female barrister presents with persistent fatigue, malaise, and right upper quadrant discomfort. She has a BMI of 26 kg/m², drinks 24 units of alcohol per week and smokes 15 cigarettes per week. She drinks more alcohol at weekends. On examination, she has hepatomegaly. Blood tests reveal a mildly raised ALT only. An ultrasound reveals hyperechogenicity. Despite lifestyle measures, her symptoms remained, and a liver biopsy was performed. The histology is shown below. Which of the following is the most likely diagnosis?

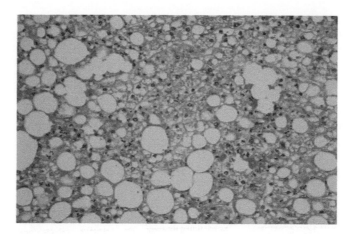

A Autoimmune hepatitis
B Cirrhosis
C Non-alcoholic fatty liver disease
D Acute steatohepatitis
E Chronic steatohepatitis

5.48 A 69-year-old male presents with a red-looking patch of crusty skin on his lower leg (A). It measures 7 mm in diameter, is irregular and slightly ulcerated, and has slowly enlarged over years. A skin biopsy was performed, and the histology is shown below (B). Which of the following is the most likely diagnosis?

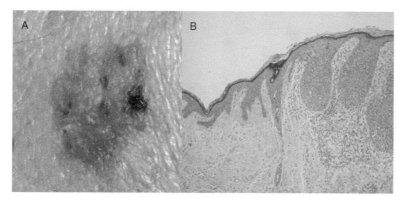

A Amelanotic melanoma
B Squamous cell carcinoma *in situ*
C Squamous cell carcinoma
D Basal cell carcinoma
E Actinic keratosis

5.49 A 62-year-old non-diabetic man presents with persistent fatigue, dyspnoea, weight loss and peripheral oedema. His blood pressure has been well controlled with medication, but more recently it has been 90/55 mmHg. Blood biochemistry showed serum creatinine was 740 μmol/L (baseline 98 μmol/L) and serum albumin was 24 g/L (baseline 36 g/L). Urine analysis revealed proteinuria (9 g in 24 hours). An ultrasound showed bilateral atrophic kidneys with increased echogenicity and cortical thinning. A core biopsy was performed and histology, as shown below, showed extensive reddish orange Congophilic deposits in the mesangium and surrounding interstitium under normal light (A), and apple-green birefringence under polarised light (B). Which of the following is the most likely diagnosis?

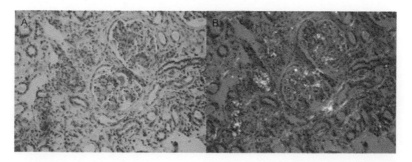

    A Nephrotic syndrome
    B Multiple myeloma
    C Glomerulonephritis
    D Sarcoidosis
    E Amyloidosis

5.50 A 71-year-old obese lady presents with polyarthritic firm joint swellings which continue to discharge. She has been having difficulty walking and opening tins in the kitchen. Joint fluid was sent for microscopy, culture, and crystal analysis. Under polarised light, the following photomicrograph was obtained. Which of the following is the most likely diagnosis?

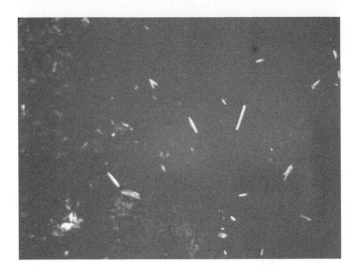

    A Rheumatoid arthritis
    B Pseudogout
    C Gout
    D Septic arthritis
    E Oxalate arthropathy

Answers

Histology

5.1 *A – Pseudostratified epithelium has all cells in contact with the underlying extracellular matrix*

Pseudostratified epithelium consists of more than one type of epithelium of different size and shape. Epithelial cells appear to be arranged in layers, and all cells are in contact with an underlying basement membrane and extracellular matrix. The term *pseudostratified* relates to the fact that the cells do not fully penetrate the epithelium and only some reach the surface; hence A is the correct response. The nuclei of columnar epithelial cells are basal but are not arranged randomly. They are centrally placed in an ordered layer. The endometrium consists of simple columnar epithelium (not cuboidal). Glands of pancreatic acini and ducts show merocrine secretion (not holocrine).

Exocrine glands release secretions via three mechanisms: (1) merocrine secretions (most common) exit the cell via exocytosis and no cell damage occurs; an example is eccrine sweat glands; (2) apocrine secretions exit the cell via budding or pinching off the apical cytoplasm, breaking off into the duct and part of the cell membrane is lost; an example is the mammary gland; and (3) holocrine secretions exit the cell via complete rupturing of the cell membrane, releasing products into the duct; an example is the sebaceous glands.

Bullous pemphigoid results from autoantibodies directed against proteins in hemidesmosomes, specifically bullous pemphigoid antigens 1 and 2 (BPAG1 and BPAG2), and not occluding (tight) junctions of epithelial cells.

5.2 *D – Fibrillin*

Basement membranes are specialised sheets of extracellular matrix that lie between parenchymal cells and provide an adhesive substrate for cell attachment and migration. The basement membrane has five major components: type IV collagen, heparan sulphate, laminin, fibronectin and entactin; hence D is the correct response. Fibrillin is a cysteine-rich glycoprotein found in microfibrils of connective tissue, predominantly elastic tissue.

5.3 *C – Small intestine*

Paneth cells occur in all parts of the small intestine but are especially numerous in the lower third of the crypts of the ileum. They have basal nuclei and distinctive eosinophilic granules. They secrete defensins which function in the immune response; hence C is the correct response.

5.4 *C – Epiglottis – ciliated pseudostratified columnar epithelium*

The epiglottis has two surfaces: (1) the anterior or lingual surface is covered by non-keratinised stratified epithelium which is directly continuous with the posterior (dorsal) part of the tongue, and (2) the posterior surface, often referred to as the respiratory epithelium, is directed towards to the pharynx and larynx, and is covered in stratified squamous epithelium (upper half) and a transitional zone of stratified columnar to ciliated pseudostratified columnar epithelium (lower half); hence C is the correct response.

The epididymal duct is lined by pseudostratified columnar (not cuboidal) epithelium containing basal (stem) cells and principal columnar cells. The duct of the vas deferens is lined with pseudostratified columnar (not stratified squamous) epithelium containing basal cells and principal columnar cells. The anal canal marks the transition from simple columnar epithelium of the colon to stratified columnar epithelium, which then becomes non-keratinised stratified epithelium at the pectinate (dentate) line. There is no cuboidal epithelium lining the anal canal. The surface of the trachea (and bronchi) is lined with tall, ciliated columnar epithelium (not stratified squamous), intermixed with goblet and basal cells.

5.5 *D – Parietal*

Parietal cells, previously called oxyntic cells, from the Greek *oxyntos* meaning to 'make an acidic substance', are the functional units of the gastric acid secretory system of the stomach; hence D is the correct response. They predominate in the neck, isthmus and lower pit regions. Parietal cells also synthesise and secrete intrinsic factor which binds to vitamin B_{12}.

Sertoli cells are found in the seminiferous tubules and provide nutritional support for developing germ cells. They secrete various proteins and hormones, such as androgen-binding protein, inhibin and anti-Müllerian hormone. Merkel cells are epithelial neuroendocrine cells found in the basal layer of the epidermis and around hair follicles. They act as adapting mechanoreceptors. Oxyphil cells, or oncocytes, are interspersed between chief cells of the parathyroid gland and have a characteristic granular, eosinophilic cytoplasm with an abundance of closely packed mitochondria. Mesangial cells, together with surrounding matrix, make up the mesangium of the glomerulus and provide a scaffold for surrounding capillaries.

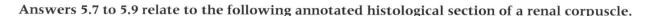

5.6 *C – Secondary follicles contain liquor folliculi which fill spaces between granulosa cells*

Secondary (antral) follicles have an oocyte surrounded by granulosa cells, which secrete hyaluronic acid, growth factors and steroid hormones. As spaces coalesce within the follicle, fluid accumulates (liquor folliculi) creating a single large antrum; hence C is the correct response. The development of primordial and primary follicles is dependent on cyclical secretion of follicle-stimulating hormone from the pituitary (not luteinizing hormone). The primary oocyte arrests in the dictyate stage of prophase I (not prophase II). The surface of the ovary is covered by epithelium, sometimes unhelpfully referred to as germinal epithelium, even though it does not contain germ cells. In fact, these cells are modified mesothelial cells which line the peritoneal cavity. The ovary consists of the outer cortex and inner medulla; both of which contain stromal cells. Embedded within the cortex are many follicles which contain oocytes surrounded by granulosa cells. Simple columnar epithelium is not found in the ovarian medulla. The oviduct epithelium consists of ciliated cells which help move the ovum towards the uterus, and non-ciliated cells (peg cells) which release nutrients, aid in maintenance of the spermatozoa and ovum, and capacitate spermatozoa.

Answers 5.7 to 5.9 relate to the following annotated histological section of a renal corpuscle.

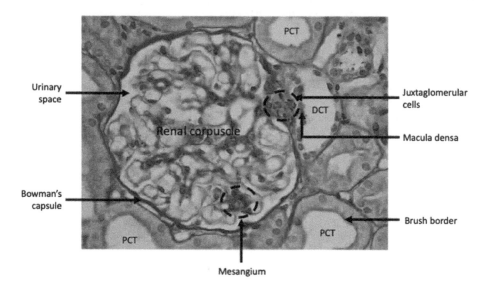

The renal corpuscle is found in the cortex of the kidney. It has a vascular pole where the afferent arteriole enters and the efferent arteriole exits, and a urinary pole where the proximal convoluted tubule (PCT) begins. Each corpuscle consists of the Bowman's capsule and the glomerulus. The distal convoluted tubule (DCT) can easily be distinguished from the PCT due to the absence of a brush border (although short microvilli can sometimes be evident), and a typically wider lumen compared to the PCT. The DCT also has far less cuboidal cells lining their epithelium. The juxtaglomerular apparatus is composed of three parts: the macula densa, granular cells and extraglomerular mesangial (lacis) cells.

5.7 *D – Mesangial*

Region labelled 1 corresponds to the mesangium, an area where the nuclei of endothelial cells and mesangial cells reside; hence D is the correct response. This region is often associated closer to the vascular pole of the glomerulus and are thought to play a role in maintaining the glomerular filtration membrane. Transitional and microvillus epithelium is not found within region labelled 1. Goblet cells are mucus-secreting cells commonly found in the intestinal mucosa and respiratory epithelium. Lacis cells are extraglomerular mesangial cells that are found between the glomerulus and macula densa of the DCT. They contain renin and play a role in autoregulation of blood flow to the kidney.

5.8 *E – Hypotension results in renin release causing vasodilation of efferent arterioles*

Region labelled 2 corresponds to the juxtaglomerular apparatus (JGA) or complex. The JGA is located near the vascular pole of the renal corpuscle and is the primary site of renin storage and release. A reduction in afferent arteriole pressure causes renin release from the cells of the JGA, whereas higher pressures inhibit renin release. The macula densa senses changes in sodium and chloride ions in the surrounding fluid, and a reduction of these ions stimulates renin release from the JGA. Conversely, high concentrations cause renin release to be inhibited. This is an important mechanism for blood pressure control since afferent arteriole hypotension causes a reduction in glomerular filtration which reduces sodium chloride concentration in the tubules. This leads to decreased ATP and adenosine release by the macula densa, causing afferent arteriole vasodilation which then increases glomerular filtration. This tubuloglomerular feedback mechanism does not involve the efferent arteriole; hence E is the correct response.

5.9   D – Aldosterone causes 3 to reabsorb sodium ions

Labels 3 and 4 correspond to the DCT and brush border of the PCT, respectively. Aldosterone acts on the principal cells of the DCT and collecting duct by increasing expression of sodium channels and sodium-potassium ATPase in cell membranes. Ultimately sodium ions are absorbed from the lumen, with water absorption (in the presence of ADH), causing increased serum osmolality. Translated clinically, antihypertensive medication which decrease aldosterone cause hyponatraemia, hyperkalaemia and hypovolaemia; hence D is the correct response. Cells lining both 3 and 4 are mainly cuboidal (not columnar). Brush borders are greater in 4 (PCT) than 3 (DCT). More urine is filtered at 4 (PCT) than 3 (DCT). Almost all glucose and amino acids are reabsorbed in the PCT (not ~40%).

5.10   A – Canals of Hering are lined by simple cuboidal epithelium

Canals of Hering are lined by simple cuboidal epithelium; hence A is the correct response. These are small ducts that drain bile canaliculi close to the periphery of liver lobules. Spaces of Dissé separate sinusoids (not canaliculi) from surrounding hepatocytes. Kupffer cells are macrophages of the liver characterised by abundant lysosomes and endocytic vesicles within the cytoplasm. Endothelial cells intersperse between sinusoids and Kupffer cells and are fenestrated (not tightly packed), which increases permeability. Stellate cells are found between sinusoids and hepatocytes in the space of Dissé where they store and regulate transport of vitamin A (not vitamin K).

5.11   D – Hepatic artery

The characteristically thick tunica media and narrow lumen corresponds with the hepatic artery; hence D is the correct response. The portal vein can also be seen in this section, shown in the bottom right, with its large lumen.

5.12   A – Simple cuboidal

Label 2 corresponds to the bile duct. It is lined by simple cuboidal to columnar epithelium and functions to drain bile from hepatocytes.

5.13   C – Sinusoids

Label 3 corresponds to sinusoids. Hepatic sinusoids are lined by specialised endothelial cells which provide a porous barrier for exchange between blood, hepatocytes and the perisinusoidal space (space of Disse). Additional cells housed within sinusoids are phagocytic Kupffer cells, hepatic stellate cells, which help in hepatic repair, and pit cells, which are natural killer cells of the liver. Surrounding sinusoids are liver plates which are composed of polygonal anastomosing hepatocytes. Bile canaliculi and adipose tissue may be present but have not been stained. CD10 is a useful immunohistochemical stain for antigens expressed on the canalicular membrane of hepatocytes. There are no bile ductules or hepatic acini evident in this section. Hepatic acini are the functional units of the liver. They are ovoid or elliptical areas of tissue with two adjacent terminal hepatic venules located on the long axis and two adjacent portal triads located on the short axis. They are divided into three zones based on the distance from the arterial blood supply, i.e., hepatocytes in zone 1 receive the greatest oxygen supply.

5.14   C – Fungiform and filiform

Fungiform (on the right) and filiform (on the left) papillae are observed in this section; hence C is the correct response. The tongue is covered by stratified squamous epithelium, thicker on the upper surface and thinner on the lower surface. Papillae are found in far greater numbers on the upper and lateral surface of the tongue compared to the lower surface. Fungiform, circumvallate and foliate contain taste buds and are responsible for gustatory perception.

Fungiform papillae, derived from the Latin for mushroom, are located on the anterior two thirds of the dorsal tongue, with a much higher number being distributed anteromedially. They are found all over the dorsal surface and house numerous taste buds among the epithelial cells of the papillae. Those found anteriorly detect sweet taste and those found along the lateral border detect salty taste. These papillae are non-keratinised but are highly vascular, and look red. The papillae are innervated by the facial nerve.

Filiform papillae, derived from the Latin for thread-like filum, appear conical and pointed with a thin sheet of keratin, particularly at the tip. They are the most numerous and found in large numbers on the anterior two-thirds of the dorsal surface of the tongue. They do not contain taste buds and serve as a mechanical, abrasive cleaner, transducing touch, temperature, and nociception. They run in rows parallel to the sulcus terminalis. They are innervated by the facial nerve.

Circumvallate papillae are the largest but least numerous (between 8 and 12) and form an inverted V at the posterior one-third of the dorsal surface of the tongue. They appear as flattened domes, of which the base becomes depressed below the dorsal surface. They are surrounded by a groove, which contain over 300 taste buds in the epithelium, and detect bitter tastes. These papillae are innervated by the glossopharyngeal nerve.

Foliate papillae (leaf-like) are located along both sides of the posterolateral margins of the tongue and consist of ridges. They are innervated by the glossopharyngeal and facial nerve. They are vestigial and rarely found in humans since they degenerate in childhood.

5.15 *D – Keratin*

Label 1 corresponds to keratin found on a filiform papilla; hence D is the correct response.

5.16 *B – Non-keratinised stratified squamous*

The epiglottis covers the entrance to the larynx and is attached to the hyoid bone. It consists of a central sheet of elastic cartilage and has an anterior (lingual) surface lined with non-keratinised stratified squamous epithelium which is continuous with the dorsal surface of the tongue, and a posterior surface which is lined by non-keratinised stratified squamous epithelium (upper half) and ciliated pseudostratified columnar epithelium (lower half). The lower half contains many seromucous glands; hence B is the correct response.

Answers 5.17a to 5.17e relate to the following annotated histological section of the small intestine.

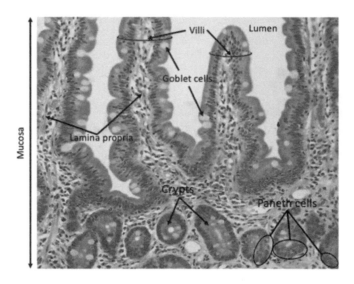

The duodenum is the most proximal section of the small intestine. The duodenal surface is composed of crescent-shaped folds known as plicae circularis, or valves of Kerckring. Proximally it is a continuation of the pylorus of the stomach and distally it continues with jejunum. It is approximately 12 inches in length (hence its name is derived from the Greek *dodekadaktulus* meaning 12 finger breadths) and is subdivided into four parts. The duodenal mucosa resembles that of the entire small intestine and is covered in villi. It consists of simple columnar epithelium, lamina propria composed on connective tissue and lamina muscularis, composed of smooth muscle. The crypts of Lieberkühn are present in the mucosa, located at the base of the villi. Brunner's glands are a characteristic feature of the submucosa of the first part (proximal) of the duodenum. These are mucus-secreting glands that contain bicarbonate which helps neutralise gastric acid. Additionally, numerous blood vessels and Meissner's plexus is present in the submucosa. The lamina muscularis consists of inner circular and outer longitudinal muscle, and an interjacent Auerbach's plexus.

The jejunum begins at the duodenojejunal flexure, where the ligamentum of Treitz attaches to the diaphragm. The mucosa is lined by simple columnar epithelium which contain enterocytes and goblet cells, together with crypts and villi which project into the lumen. The jejunum contains no Brunner's glands.

The ileum is the terminal part of the small intestine and is separated from the large intestine most distally by the ileocaecal valve. The mucosa consists of simple columnar epithelium with interspersed enterocytes and goblet cells. Histology of the ileum is very similar to the jejunum, except it contains Peyer's patches within the mucosa and submucosa. These are a collection of lymphoid tissues, and an important part of gut-associated lymphoid tissue (GALT). The lamina propria serosa covers the entire ileum and is composed of simple squamous epithelium and connective tissue.

5.17a *C – Small intestine*

5.17b *E – Goblet cells*

5.17c *C – A central lacteal is present*

Label 2 corresponds to the crypts of Lieberkühn. A central lacteal, an arteriole-capillary network, and nerves are found within the fat of the lamina propria of the villi (not the crypts); hence C is the correct response. Lacteals are an important lymphatic component of the villi that collect fluids, salts and proteins from the interstitium. Chylomicrons (triglyceride-loaded particles) made by enterocytes in the small intestine, undergo exocytosis and enter the lacteals. They are then transported to the cisterna chyli, into the thoracic duct and then the subclavian vein. Intestinal stem cells are abundant at the base of the crypts, which can ultimately differentiate into a variety of specialised cells, including enterocytes, Paneth, tuft, goblet and enteroendocrine cells. Higher rates of mitotic divisions occur at the base of the crypts, where stem cells are found. Paneth cells and crypts secrete lysozyme, an enzyme with potent antibacterial properties.

5.17d *C – Paneth cells*

Label 3 corresponds to Paneth cells; hence C is the correct response. These are specialised secretory cells found at the base of the crypts, and more abundant in the jejunum and ileum than the duodenum. Histologically, these have a bright red granular cytoplasm. The eosinophilic granules contain a variety of microbicidal proteins including lysozyme, α-defensin and phospholipase-A_2.

5.17e *A – Muscularis mucosae*

The typical histological pattern of the entire small intestine is mucosa, submucosa, muscularis and serosa. Crypts lie between the villi and the base (where Paneth cells are located) and extend into the lamina muscularis mucosae; hence A is the correct response. Plicae circulares are large circular folds found in the mucosa. Peyer's patches are found in the lamina propria of the mucosa and submucosa. Brunner's glands are found within the submucosa which lies beneath the lamina muscularis mucosae. The lamina propria lies beneath the lamina epithelialis, but above the lamina muscularis mucosae.

5.18 *C – Eccrine glands are essential for thermoregulation*

Eccrine glands produce sweat, and with cholinergic innervation, they serve a thermoregulatory role, maintaining body temperature; hence C is the correct response. Keratinocytes are constantly produced in the deepest layer of the epidermis, the stratum basale (not the stratum corneum). The stratum corneum is the outermost layer of the epidermis, made of dead cells which form a tough, water-repellent barrier. Melanocytes produce melanin and are found between cells of the stratum basale (not the hypodermis). The hypodermis is deep to the dermis and contains adipose lobules, hair follicles and blood vessels. Rete ridges are downgrowths, or downward ridge-like extensions of epidermis that project into dermis. They do not project into hypodermis. Meissner corpuscles are mechanoreceptors that mediate low-frequency vibrations and fine touch. Pacinian corpuscles are receptors located in deeper regions of the dermis that respond to deep pressure and high-frequency vibration.

Answers 5.19 to 5.21 relate to the following annotated histological section of the skin.

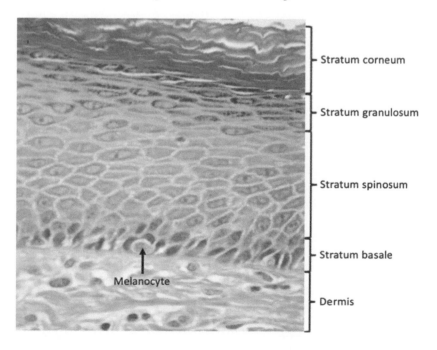

5.19 | D | Stratum corneum | Stratum granulosum | Stratum spinosum | Stratum basale |

5.20 E – 5

Label 5 corresponds to the dermis. This layer is located deep to the epidermis, sandwiched between this layer and the subcutaneous fat layer. It consists predominantly of a rich extracellular matrix of connective tissue, such as collagen (types I and III) and elastic fibres, nerve endings, vasculature, glands, and hair follicles; hence E is the correct response. Fibroblasts are abundant within this layer and help to maintain structure and function of the dermis by synthesising many extracellular matrix components. This layer functions to support and protect deeper anatomical structures, aids in thermoregulation and contain numerous mechanoreceptors (Pacinian and Meissner's corpuscles) which provide deep pressure and vibratory sensation.

5.21 C – Melanocyte

Label 6 corresponds to a melanocyte; hence C is the correct response. Melanocytes are melanin-producing cells of the skin (and eye) and are found along the stratum basale (label 4) and in hair follicles. Melanocytes contain numerous melanosomes, which are lysosome-related organelles that produce and store melanin. Melanocyte dendrites then translocate the melanosomes to neighbouring keratinocytes. Approximately 8–10% of epidermal cells are melanocytes and histologically, they have a small, dark, ovoid nucleus with a clear cytoplasm. They can often appear round, fusiform or oval. As seen in the histological section (label 6), they reside scantly along the dermo-epidermal junction, interspersed between keratinocytes, the most abundant cell in the epidermis. Fibroblasts are the main cell type of the dermis. Neutrophils are rare in normal skin but are common following tissue injury. Langerhans's cells are antigen-presenting cells found in the stratum spinosum. Keratinocytes are the predominant cell type of the entire epidermis but originate in the stratum basale.

5.22 A – Pseudostratified cuboidal epithelium is evident

This histological section (as shown labelled below) highlights the bronchial surface epithelium with tall, ciliated columnar cells interspersed with goblet cells (mucus-secreting cells), and basal cells (stem cells) which lie on the basement membrane. The basement membrane lies above the lamina propria. This epithelium is typically pseudostratified since the nuclei are located at different levels and not all the cells reach the lumen; hence A is the correct response. Histologically, these cells become simple columnar and then cuboidal at distal bronchi and smaller peripheral branches. Neuroendocrine cells are also evident on the basement membrane. These are small cells with characteristically dark-stained nuclei and a clear cytoplasm. They contain neuroendocrine granules and secrete hormones, such as serotonin.

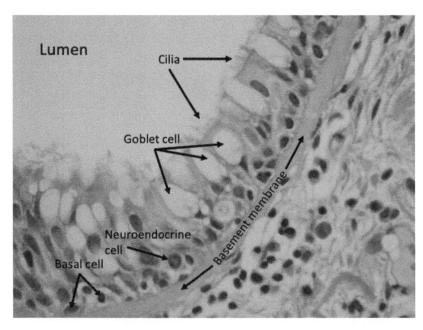

Answers 5.23 and 5.24 relate to the following histology of longitudinal and transverse sections of cardiac muscle.

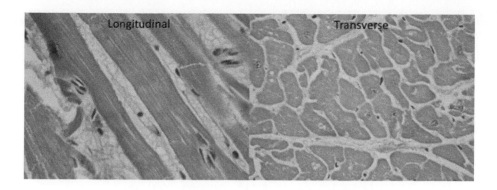

5.23 *B – Longitudinal section of cardiac muscle*

Cardiac muscle is striated, like skeletal muscle, but cardiac muscle cells are mononuclear, whereas skeletal muscle cells are multinucleated. In a longitudinal section of cardiac muscle, muscle fibres are extensively branched, cells are centrally placed with a single ovoid nucleus, and often a binucleated cell can be present. Interspersed between fibres is a fibrocollagenous septa containing an extensive capillary network; hence B is the correct response. Unique to cardiac muscle are intercalated discs which are the junctions of myocytes. When viewed in transverse section, cardiac muscle cells are irregularly shaped, and nuclei occupy the centre.

In contrast, skeletal muscle cells are more cylindrical and elongated where the nuclei are located peripherally, fusing to form a syncytia. In longitudinal section, distinct striated patterns are evident which correspond to the A and I bands of the myofibril. Nuclei will be located at the periphery. Similar to cardiac muscle, fibrocollagenous septa surround the cells which contains nerves and blood vessels.

Smooth muscle does not show the highly organised network of myosin and actin filaments seen in striated muscle. It lacks striations, consists of mononucleated cells and it is the main contractile cell found in the walls of the viscera and blood vessels. Cells have a small diameter, but their length can vary considerably depending upon on location.

5.24 *C – Intercalated discs are present*

Although not particularly evident in these images, intercalated discs are junctions between myocytes and often appear as dark, jagged transverse lines between cells in longitudinal section; hence C is the correct response. Cardiac and smooth muscle are both involuntary muscles, not under conscious control. Unlike skeletal muscle which is a voluntary muscle. Cardiac muscle, like skeletal muscle, shows an organised arrangement of thick and thin filaments, and where thin filaments have a central Z line which demarcate each sarcomere. Cardiac muscle, like smooth muscle, is mononucleated not multinucleated. Auerbach's plexus (myenteric) is a group of ganglia that run from the oesophagus to the rectum, innervating smooth muscle not cardiac muscle.

5.25 *D – Multinucleated cells with peripherally situated nuclei is a feature of skeletal muscle*

Skeletal muscle fibres are elongated, cylindrical cells with peripherally located nuclei (multinucleated); hence D is the correct response. The arrangement of filaments in a sarcomere can be seen in Question 1.25. The A and I bands represent the thick (myosin-containing) and thin (actin-containing) filaments, respectively. In the centre of the A band is a H zone which indicates where no thin (actin) filaments overlap the thick (myosin) filaments. The Z line/disc runs in the centre of the I band, and the M line runs down the centre of the H zone/band. Skeletal and cardiac muscle have sarcomeres, but smooth muscle does not, and this is evident by lack of visible striations when imaging the ultrastructure of smooth muscle. Smooth muscle does not show the highly organised system of contractile proteins as seen in striated muscle. Instead, proteins create a criss-cross lattice that insert into the cell membrane. In addition, actin filaments in smooth muscle do not contain troponin; hence the contraction mechanism is very different to that of striated muscle. Lipofuscin is an orange-brown granular material found within the cytoplasm and is commonly referred to as a 'wear-and-tear' pigment as it accumulates in older cells. Due to the long-lived nature of cardiac muscle cells, they often accumulate lipofuscin with advancing age (unlike skeletal muscle). In cardiac muscle, two myocytes meet at intercalated discs, located at the Z line, which demarcate each sarcomere (not the M line).

5.26 *E – Haversian canals run longitudinally in osteons*

Bone has a basic architecture composed of an outer compact (cortical) region or inner spongy (cancellous or trabecular) region. Compact bone is composed of many Haversian systems or osteons which appear round in transverse section and run longitudinally in the long axis. Osteons are cylindrical and contain a central Haversian canal which are surrounded by lamellae; hence E is the correct response. These canals are linked by perpendicular Volkmann's canals. Osteoprogenitor cells differentiate into osteoblasts, bone-forming cells which induce matrix mineralisation (osteoid). They then become osteocytes, mature bone cells which reside in lacunae. Osteoclasts, bone resorbing cells, erode and remove bone matrix, and reside in resorption cavities/bays/pits known as Howship's lacunae. Osteoclasts are large, multinucleated giant cells that derive from monocyte fusion. Compact bone is composed of osteons, not trabecular bone. Bone marrow occupies the spaces between the trabecular networks.

5.27 *C – Lacunae*

Concentric lamellae contain Howship's lacunae which are arranged around a vascular space known as the Haversian canal; hence C is the correct response, as shown below.

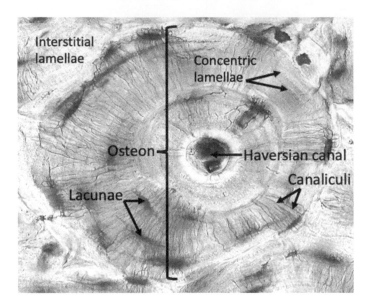

Haversian canals are connected to each other by perpendicular vascular spaces known as Volkmann's canals, as shown below.

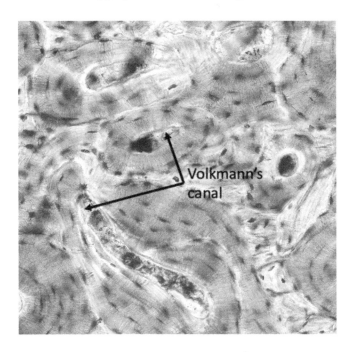

5.28 *E – The anal canal is composed of keratinised simple columnar epithelium*

The colon begins at the ileocaecal junction and terminates at the anorectal junction. It consists of the caecum, appendix, ascending, transverse and descending colon, sigmoid colon, and rectum. The colon is lined by simple columnar epithelium, like the small intestine, but they lack villi and contain larger crypts. There is an abundance of mucus-secreting goblet cells, far more than seen in the small intestine, which increase in number towards the distal rectum. The rectal mucosa is like the colon and lined with simple columnar epithelium. The anorectal junction, marked by the pectinate line, is a transition zone where simple columnar epithelium changes to stratified columnar epithelium and then non-keratinised stratified squamous epithelium; hence E is the correct response. Three longitudinal bands consisting of an inner circular muscle layer and an outer longitudinal layer form taeniae coli which run the entire length of the colon. Sacculated pouches between taeniae coli form haustra, and between these are semilunar or crescent-shaped folds called plicae semilunares. Plicae circularis are found in the small intestine.

5.29 B – Clara (Club)

Clara or Club cells are non-ciliated, non-mucous secreting cells of the bronchiolar epithelium. These dome-shaped cells provide secretory surfactants and proteins, such as surfactant proteins A, B and C, and Clara cell 10-kDa secretory protein (CCSP) to the extracellular fluid. They also serve as a pool of progenitor cells that help other cells of the epithelium with regeneration following injury, and, due to an abundance of cytochrome P450-dependent mixed function oxygenases, metabolise xenobiotic agents which helps in detoxification.

Bushy cells are found in the anteroventral cochlear nucleus, which lies between the cochlear nerve. They receive excitatory inputs from auditory nerve fibres of the cochlear nerve, specifically via synaptic terminals called endbulbs of Held. Foveolar cells are tall, columnar, mucin-secreting cells lining gastric pits of the gastric mucosa. Oxyphil cells are one of two main cell types of the parathyroid gland, the other being chief cells. They are larger than chief cells and have an abundant eosinophilic granular cytoplasm owing to the presence of numerous mitochondria. Little is known about the function of these cells, but interestingly they are rare before puberty and increase with age. However, they do not synthesise parathyroid hormone and appear to have no endocrine function. Chromaffin cells are neuroendocrine cells of the adrenal medulla which produce catecholamines, such as epinephrine and norepinephrine.

5.30 D – Zona fasciculata

The adrenal gland lies on the superior poles of the kidneys and consists of an outer cortex and inner medulla. The cortex has three distinct zones which are bound by the fibrous capsule externally, and the medulla internally. The outermost zona glomerulosa contain glomerulosa cells which contain aldosterone synthase, therefore synthesising and secreting mineralocorticoids, such as aldosterone and deoxycorticosterone. The middle zona fasciculata synthesises and secretes glucocorticoids, such as cortisol; hence D is the correct response. Interestingly, both the mineralocorticoid and glucocorticoid pathways are catalysed by the same enzymes, 21-hydroxylase and 11β-hydroxylase. However, in the mineralocorticoid pathway progesterone is the initial substrate, whereas in the glucocorticoid pathway it is 17α-hydroxyprogesterone. The innermost zona reticularis produces androgenic steroids (and a very small amount of glucocorticoids), specifically dihydroepiandrosterone (DHEA) and dihydroepiandrosterone sulphate. DHEA is converted to androstenedione by 3β-hydroxysteroid dehydrogenase, which is converted to testosterone by 17β-hydroxysteroid dehydrogenase. Testosterone is then converted to oestradiol by aromatase.

5.31 E – Stereocilia

The olfactory mucosa, which senses smell, is found in the roof of the nasal cavity, superior concha and extends down the nasal septum. It is lined with pseudostratified columnar epithelium composed of olfactory cells, sustentacular (supporting) cells and basal cells. Beneath the olfactory epithelium are mucous-producing glands (of Bowman) which bathe the epithelial surface.

The vestibular membranous labyrinth of the cochlear comprises three semicircular canals, which assume superior, posterior and horizontal positions, utricle and saccule. An area rich in vestibular receptors is found in a dilated region of the canal, the crista ampullaris, which contain hair cells and supporting cells. Hair cells of crista have a non-motile kinocilium and numerous apical stereocilia; hence E is the correct response. The hair cells of the crista respond to angular acceleration and deceleration.

5.32 A – Submandibular

Unlike the parotid gland, the submandibular gland has both serous and mucous acini, with serous being predominant. Serous cells have a prominent, purplish-stained cytoplasm with distinct eosinophilic zymogen granules. Mucous cells have a pale-stained clear cytoplasm where nuclei appear pushed against the basal cell membrane. The gland also contains mixed seromucous acini, where larger mucous cells surrounded by a lumen push against flattened, zymogen-rich serous cells forming a crescent-shaped demilune (as shown below). The secretory acini merge into intercalated ducts, which are lined by cuboidal or simple low cuboidal epithelium and surrounded by myoepithelial cells. These merge to form intralobular, or striated ducts characterised by tall columnar epithelium, which fuse to form larger interlobular ducts characterised by a non-striated, pseudostratified epithelium; hence A is the correct response. In contrast, sublingual and parotid glands have predominantly mucous and serous acini, respectively. The other glands do not have this histological appearance.

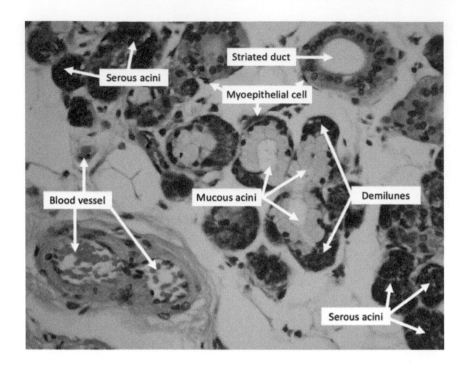

5.33 *C – Non-keratinised stratified squamous to simple columnar epithelium*

The transition in the epithelial lining between the stomach and the oesophagus is called the Z line. At this junction, simple columnar epithelium of the stomach changes to non-keratinised stratified squamous epithelium of the oesophagus, as shown below; hence C is the correct response. Clinically, this is an important transition zone as pathological abnormalities are common, such as oesophageal carcinoma.

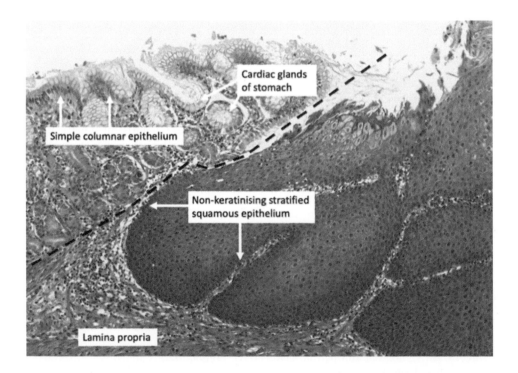

5.34 *E – Capsule*

The spleen is covered by an outer dense, thin fibrocollagenous capsule with distinct connective tissue trabeculae. This is not evident in this histological section; hence E is the correct response. Short septa extend into the parenchyma which support a network of reticular fibres. Unlike other lymphoid organs, spleen parenchyma consists of predominantly red pulp and white pulp, and not a cortex and medulla, as shown below. Red pulp contains sinusoid networks with interspersed vascular sinuses and splenic cords of Billroth. The term splenic cord is a misnomer since these are spaces between sinuses which contain erythrocytes, lymphocytes, macrophages, and reticular cells all trapped within a reticular fibre scaffold. White pulp contains aggregates of lymphoid tissue, often with a germinal centre and surrounding mantle, that surrounds a central arteriole forming a periarterial lymphatic sheath (PALS). Lymphoid nodules are regions of white pulp which may contain arterioles, but primary nodules (follicles) lack a germinal centre.

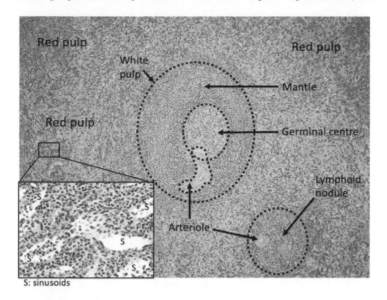

5.35 *D – Antibody production is rich in region 2*

Region 1 and region 2 correspond to the red pulp and white pulp, respectively. T and B cells are found in the white pulp, with T cells predominating in PALS and B cells in primary and secondary lymphoid nodules/follicles; hence D is the correct response. Macrophages and a smaller number of B cells are found in the outer aspect of the mantle, an area known as the marginal zone. Follicular dendritic cells predominate in white pulp, not red pulp. Small, immature lymphocytes are common in white pulp, not red pulp. Venous sinusoids or cords of Billroth are found in red pulp, not white pulp. Periarteriolar lymphoid sheaths (PALS) are found in white pulp, not equally abundant in white and red pulp.

5.36 *A – Penile urethra*

The urethra comprises three parts: prostatic, membranous and penile (spongy). Predominantly, the prostatic urethra is lined by transitional epithelium, the membranous urethra is lined by pseudostratified columnar epithelium, and the penile urethra is lined by stratified squamous epithelium. Upon urethral enlargement, the transition from columnar to non-keratinised stratified squamous epithelium occurs at the fossa navicularis. In the proximal penile urethra are Cowper's glands, whereas multiple, smaller glands of Littré span the entire penile urethra and drain into small epithelial folds called lacunae of Morgagni, as shown below. These are responsible for mucous secretion which lubricate the urethra for semen ejaculation; hence A is the correct response.

The penis consists of three cylindrical columns of erectile tissue: two dorsal corpora cavernosa (*sing.* corpus cavernosum) and one smaller ventral corpus spongiosum, through which the penile urethra runs. These are bound by a dense fibroelastic layer called the tunica albuginea. These erectile tissues are collections of labyrinthine trabeculae interconnected with fibroelastic connective tissue and vascular sinuses, which fill with blood during erection. The penis is highly vascularised via the dorsal and deep arteries, and convoluted helicine arteries which open into the sinuses.

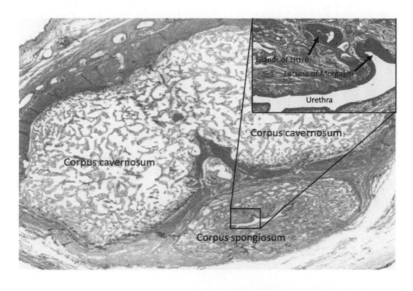

5.37 *D – Cervix*

The cervix is the inferior part of the uterus which consists of the cervical canal (endocervix) and the portio vaginalis (exocervix or ectocervix). The endocervix and exocervix are lined with simple columnar epithelium and non-keratinised stratified squamous epithelium, respectively; hence D is the correct response. This abrupt change at the external os is known as the transformation zone, or histologically, the squamocolumnar junction, as shown below. This zone is the site of many pathological changes, such as cervical carcinomas.

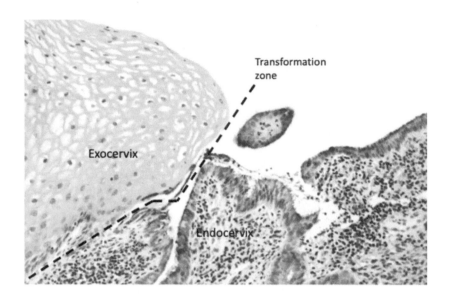

5.38 *C – Lens*

The lens is a soft transparent biconvex structure between the iris and vitreous body. It has an outer collagenous capsule composed of type IV collagen, laminin, entactin, perlecan and fibronectin, which acts as a barrier to diffusion. Anterior cuboidal epithelial cells lie beneath the capsule and contain numerous cytoskeleton proteins such as actin, myosin, vimentin and spectrin. Lens fibres make up the lens nucleus which are elongated columnar epithelial cells that form highly ordered concentric shells, as shown below. They lack a nucleus and become tightly packed by lens cytoplasmic proteins called crystallins. Posteriorly, the lens lacks an epithelium. The lens is suspended by suspensory fibres to the ciliary body by zonular fibres (zonule of Zinn), which are composed of fibrillin, proteoglycans and glycosaminoglycans, and play an important role in accommodation by affecting the curvature of the lens; hence C is the correct response.

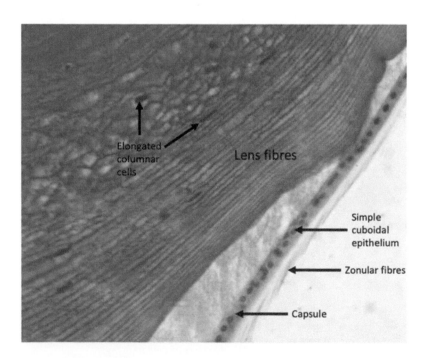

5.39 *E – Monocyte*

The most abundant cells of a blood film/smear are erythrocytes. These are anucleate biconcave discs which appear bright pink due to acidophilic haemoglobin. They are 6–10 µm in diameter and have a life span of 120 days. Interspersed between erythrocytes are basophilic platelets which appear as pale blue fragments with a central dark blue granulomere. These are the smallest cells with a diameter of 2–4 µm and lifespan of 10 days.

There are five main types of leucocytes. Granulocytes include neutrophils, eosinophils and basophils. Neutrophils are the most abundant and constitute 50–70% of the leucocyte count. They appear as a densely stained, segmented nucleus with multiple lobes, and a pale, finely granular cytoplasm, as shown in the three examples in the blood film below. They have a diameter of 8–12 µm. Eosinophils constitute 2–5% of the leucocyte count. They have a densely stained, bilobed nucleus with a large, coarse, homogenous granular cytoplasm which is characteristically red. They have a diameter of 12–15 µm. Basophils are the least common leucocyte which constitute less than 1% of the leucocyte count. They can have a bilobed or segmented nucleus with a char-acteristically large, intensely basophilic granular cytoplasm which appears blue. The nucleus can often be obscured and can often be confused with lymphocytes. They are 10–15 µm in diameter.

Agranulocytes are monocytes and lymphocytes. Monocytes constitute 2–10% of the leucocyte count. They are the largest of the blood cells with an indented, sometimes kidney-shaped pale nucleus and pale blue, agranular cytoplasm. They have a diameter of 10–20 µm; hence E is the correct response. Lymphocytes constitute 20–50% of the leucocyte count. They have a small round, slightly indented, dark-stained blue nucleus with an agranular slightly basophilic blue cytoplasm. The cytoplasm is small, and often only appears as a narrow rim. Small lymphocytes have a diameter of 6–10 µm, whereas larger lymphocytes can range from 11–18 µm.

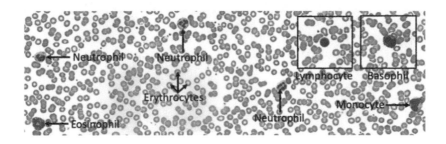

5.40 *D – Monocytes often have a reniform nucleus*

Monocytes are large, motile, agranular leucocytes that are phagocytic. They often have a vacuolated cytoplasm with a variably shaped nucleus which may appear oval, horseshoe-like, or kidney-shaped (reniform); hence D is the correct response. The most abundant protein in erythrocytes is haemoglobin (>98%), yet there are less abundant proteins also present such as carbonic anhy-drase, glycophorins, spectrin and a variety of membrane proteins. Neutrophils are granulocytes (not agranulocytes). Eosinophils contain eosinophilic (not basophilic) granules. Basophils, like mast cells have highly specific membrane receptors for IgE (not IgG).

Histopathology

5.41 *C – Coeliac disease*

The plicae of the small intestine are arranged into villi which protrude into the lumen, which increases the surface area for absorp-tion. This can be seen in a normal duodenal biopsy (A). Coeliac disease, or gluten enteropathy, results from damage to microvilli and villi, whereby gluten leads to immune-mediated inflammation and flattening of the intestinal surface causing loss of villi (B). Histological features include blunting of villi, and an abundance of intraepithelial lymphocytes and lymphocytes within the lamina propria (B). Figure C shows the return of villi, but an abundance of lymphocytes remain, as seen in partially treated coeliac disease where gluten has been excluded from the diet; hence C is the correct response.

5.42 *E – Barrett's oesophagus*

A history of chronic non-steroidal anti-inflammatory use with longstanding heartburn should always add Barrett's oesophagus to the differential diagnosis list. It is very likely that this started as gastro-oesophageal reflux disease (GORD) which has progressed. Histological features include metaplasia of the stratified squamous epithelium of the lower oesophagus into glandular epithelium with many goblet cells. There are often 'mucosal tongues' that extend proximally from the gastro-oesophageal junction. There are also many lymphocytes and plasma cells that infiltrate surrounding connective tissue; hence E is the correct response. Oesophageal adenocarcinoma can develop in patients with chronic Barrett's oesophagus. It should certainly be considered when the history includes progressive weight loss and dysphagia in a smoker, or in a patient who drinks alcohol to excess. Histologically, there may be focal regions of keratin (pearls) embedded within differentiated squamous cell carcinoma.

5.43a *B – Crohn's disease*

Crohn's disease is a chronic autoimmune inflammatory disease which can affect any location of the gastrointestinal tract, but is more common in the distal ileum and colon. It is characterised by asymmetric transmural inflammation and skip lesions (involved regions of abnormal bowel separated by uninvolved regions of normal bowel). Histological features include cryptitis (infiltration of neutrophils within crypts), circular non-caseating granulomas within the lamina propria, pseudopolyps, and extensive inflammation highlighted by an abundance of neutrophils; hence B is the correct response.

Ulcerative colitis is an inflammatory bowel disease which results in ulceration and destruction of the absorptive epithelium. Symptoms can include abdominal pain, bloody diarrhoea, weight loss, anaemia and passage of mucus. Histological features include inflammation confined to the mucosa and submucosa (compared to transmural inflammation seen in Crohn's disease), loss of goblet cells, crypt abscesses, pseudopolyps and glandular atrophy.

The micrograph shows a flat surface with many straight tubular glands extending down to the muscularis mucosae. There are a large population of cells at the bases of these glands, including stem cells, goblet cells, columnar cells and endocrine cells. This is typical of a colon biopsy. Coeliac disease affects the small intestine where there are long crypts with no villi. Giardiasis is a protozoan infection associated with chronic diarrhoea and malabsorption, often caused by *Giardia lamblia*. Histological features include villous blunting and increased inflammatory cells, with Giardial trophozoites appearing as teardrops along the surface of foveolar epithelial cells. This is not evident in this micrograph. Colon carcinoma is typically an adenocarcinoma arising from malignant mucosal glandular epithelium which often infiltrates the muscularis propria with progression. This is not evident in this micrograph.

5.43b *A – Tuberculosis*

The Ziehl-Neelsen (ZN) stain is a standard tuberculosis diagnostic tool used in acid-fast bacilli (AFB) staining of mycobacteria; hence A is the correct response. Acid-fast microorganisms have a high lipid content of mycolic acid in their cell walls which allows them to bind and retain carbol-fuchsin dye, even after decolourisation with acid-alcohol. Acid-fast bacteria stain bright red, while non-acid-fast bacteria stain blue/green with the counterstain methylene blue. Although AFB staining is highly specific, it is relatively insensitive. Owing to this, culture methods appear to be more sensitive than AFB smears, and modern immunofluorescence techniques have led to development of newer fluorochrome stains, such as rhodamine and auramine, which have improved sensitivity. These techniques, together with advances in endobronchial ultrasound-guided aspiration of lymph nodes may prove beneficial in cases of mycobacterial infection without necrosis and in children who do not expectorate sputum.

5.44 *D – Helicobacter pylori*

All options listed are known to cause gastritis. However, the spiral-shaped bacterium *H. pylori* can be seen in haematoxylin and eosin (H&E) staining in this histological section; hence D is the correct response. Several techniques have been developed for accurate detection of *H. pylori*, which include non-invasive methods (urea breath test, stool antigen test and serology), and invasive methods (rapid urease test, histology and culture). At higher magnifications, H&E stain has a high specificity and sensitivity. However, at lower magnification, it can often be difficult to visualise the organism, and special stains are preferred, such as Giemsa staining, Genta staining and immunohistochemistry. Using such stains can also significantly increase specificity.

5.45 *B – Seborrhoeic keratosis*

This histological section shows squamous cell carcinoma of the skin with neoplastic cells that have orangeophilic cytoplasm, and enlarged, hyperchromatic nuclei which are centrally positioned with angulated contours. Nuclei often have a tendency towards pyknosis. There are numerous anucleated squames, irregular cytoplasmic thinning in the form of spindle cells, elongated cells in the form of tadpole cells, and keratin pearls, which are concentric rings of squamous cells that gradually keratinise. SCC is the second most common form of skin cancer characterised by rough, reddish scaly patches with raised borders, which can appear ulcerated. These cancers are most often found in areas of prolonged sun exposure, such as the head, neck and arms. There are several risk factors for SCC, which include age and sex (more common in elderly men), previous SCC or another skin cancer (melanoma, basal cell carcinoma), actinic keratosis, smoking, inherited syndromes (xeroderma pigmentosum, epidermodysplasia verruciformis and albinism), and discoid lupus erythematosus. Bowen's disease is a form of skin cancer, also known as squamous cell carcinoma *in situ* and intraepidermal squamous cell carcinoma. Keratoacanthoma is a rapidly growing skin cancer which can often be indistinguishable from SCC which is more common in fair-skinned older men. Seborrhoeic keratosis is a benign, warty skin growth that appears with age. They are generally tan-coloured, have a 'stuck-on-appearance' and are not premalignant tumours; hence B is the correct response.

5.46 *C – Asthma*

This is a histological section of a bronchiole and lung interstitium. There are typical features of obstruction, which include:

1) mucus plugging filling the lumen due to hypersecretion from goblet cells and thick mucus layer on the epithelial surface
2) metastatic epithelial changes containing more goblet cells (bronchioles normally have far more club (Clara) cells than goblet cells)
3) thickening of the basement membrane
4) smooth muscle hypertrophy and hyperplasia
5) chronic lymphocytic inflammation and thickening of the adventitia

This picture is common in asthma, which is a chronic inflammatory airway disease caused by bronchoconstriction mediated by bronchial smooth muscle and excessive mucus production as a result of immune-mediate factors (allergens, infection, exercise). This causes narrowing of the airways and presents clinically with shortness of breath, wheezing, chest tightness and a cough often worse in the night and/or morning; hence C is the correct response.

COPD is also an obstructive airway disease, but notable histological differences include permanent destruction of the alveolar structures, with permanent enlargement of alveolar airspaces. There is associated loss of elasticity without fibrosis. There is an abundant of inflammatory cells, often with carbon pigment being evident. Bronchiectasis is a chronic lung disease characterised by persistent widening of bronchial airways and mucociliary transport dysfunction. As a result of repeated infections, there is significant bacterial invasion and mucus production throughout the airways. Histologically, there is predominant neutrophilic inflammation and infiltration with mucus gland hyperplasia, fibrosis and cartilage destruction. Idiopathic pulmonary fibrosis is a chronic interstitial lung disease often characterised by chronic shortness of breath, dry cough and finger clubbing. On chest auscultation, there are end inspiratory fine crackles in both lung bases. Histologically, within the interalveolar septa, there is an increase in the number of fibroblasts which secrete excess collagen and elastin and results in fibrocollagenous thickening. This can lead to destruction of alveolar architecture and often a honeycomb appearance where cystic spaces are lined by bronchial epithelium and a fibrotic wall. Eosinophilic pneumonia is a lung disease characterised by eosinophilia in the alveolar and interstitial spaces. There can be diffuse alveolar damage in acute phases, which tend to disappear in chronic disease. Mucus plugging, granulomatosis, and scattered histiocytes and plasma cells can also be seen. Clinical symptoms include fever, weight loss and shortness of breath. It is also known as Loeffler syndrome.

5.47 *D – Acute steatohepatitis*

This is a histological section of the liver which shows two main features: (1) the abnormal accumulation of triglycerides and fatty acids in hepatocytes in the form of large (macrovesicular) and small (microvesicular) lipid droplets (steatosis), and (2) predominantly neutrophilic inflammatory infiltration. In microvesicular steatosis, the cytoplasm is replaced by 'bubbles' of fat that do not displace the nucleus, whereas in macrovesicular steatosis, the cytoplasm is replaced by a large 'bubble' of fat that displaces the nucleus to the periphery of the cell. This histological pattern is often seen in acute alcoholic steatohepatitis, particularly binge drinking; hence D is the correct response. In addition, Mallory-Denk bodies (ropy eosinophilic material within the hepatocyte cytoplasm), central hyaline sclerosis, ballooning degeneration of hepatocytes, and apoptotic bodies (small cellular remnants with hyperchromatic condensed nuclei and eosinophilic rims) are also features of alcoholic steatohepatitis. Chronic alcoholic steatohepatitis is characterised by a predominance of lymphocytes rather than neutrophils, and lipogranulomas where chronic inflammatory cells surround extracellular lipids. Chronic excessive alcohol consumption can eventually lead to fibrosis, alcoholic hepatitis, cirrhosis and hepatocellular carcinoma. It can often be difficult distinguishing between alcoholic steatohepatitis and non-alcoholic steatohepatitis (NASH) on clinical history alone, and a liver biopsy can offer more clues. For example, there are far greater neutrophilic infiltrations, lipogranulomas and Mallory-Denk bodies seen in alcoholic steatohepatitis than NASH. In addition, cholestasis is more common in alcoholic steatohepatitis than NASH, and histologically, bile plugs and bile ductular proliferation within fibrotic portal tracts are evident. The presence of iron/haemosiderin is also far more frequent in alcoholic steatohepatitis than NASH. Fibrosis results from an abnormal continuation of fibrogenesis, especially excessive collagen deposition, which over time leads to cirrhosis. Histologically, cirrhosis is characterised by continual death of hepatocytes, collapse of normal histoarchitecture, and irregular scarring due to vascularised fibrotic septa that connect portal tracts with central hepatic veins and terminal venules. Portal hypertension usually results due to increased pressure in the portal venous system as blood cannot flow through the normal channels.

Autoimmune hepatitis is a chronic progressive liver disease where circulating autoantibodies are considered the hallmark, and liver biopsy is the gold standard for grading and staging. Histologically, it is characterised by interface hepatitis and/or lobular hepatitis, with lymphocyte and plasma cell infiltration in portal tracts (especially in clusters), hepatic rosette formation (hepatocytes encircling a lumen) and emperipolesis (lymphocytes/plasma cells within the cytoplasm of hepatocytes). Biliary changes and cholestasis are rarely seen in autoimmune hepatitis.

5.48 *B – Squamous cell carcinoma in situ*

Figure A shows an erythematous, irregular-bordered plaque with scale and surface erosion, typically seen in squamous cell carcinoma *in situ* (Bowen's disease). In some patients, surface erosions can be extensive and lead to ulceration. Lesions are slow growing over many years. It mainly affects middle-aged and elderly individuals and is associated with sun exposure. However, it can occur at any age, especially in immunocompromised patients, and it is the most common skin cancer caused by arsenic ingestion. Approximately 5% of cases have been shown to progress to invasive SCC. Histologically (Figure B), there is full-thickness disorganisation of the squamous epithelium with many large, atypical cells evident which leads to disordered surface maturation. There is dyskeratosis, parakeratosis and hyperkeratosis, and multiple mitotic figures within several layers of the epithelium. There is often involvement of associated pilosebaceous apparatus with an intact epidermal junction; hence B is the correct response.

Amelanotic melanoma is a subtype of cutaneous melanoma that has very little or no pigment and can often simulate various other skin lesions as they occur in sun-exposed areas of skin, particularly in the elderly. Histologically, there are often large numbers of dissociated cells showing nuclear pleomorphism with extensive mitotic activity. Absence of melanin pigment confirmed by Masson's Fontana stain leads to an extensive list of differential diagnoses, such as melanomas, carcinomas, sarcomas and lymphomas. Therefore, immunohistochemistry is needed to confirm the diagnosis.

BCC is the most common cancer type in fair-skinned people and in middle aged adults. It is common in sun-exposed areas, such as the head and trunk. Clinically, the nodular variant is more common which usually presents as a pink papule, or nodule with telangiectasia which can become ulcerated with rolled borders and giving rise to the term 'rodent ulcer'. BCC can also be superficial, keratotic, adenoid, infiltrative and pigmented.

Actinic keratosis is the most common precursor of invasive SCC of the skin. Clinically, it presents as single or multiple erythematous and hyperkeratotic macules or papules, which can be pigmented or ulcerated, and are more common in sun-exposed regions of the body such as the face, scalp and arms. Histologically, there are atypical basal keratinocytes which can progress into the mid and upper epidermal layers but is never full thickness. There can be mild acanthosis, focal parakeratosis, and dermal changes such as solar elastosis and mild inflammatory lymphocytic infiltration.

5.49 *E – Amyloidosis*

Amyloidosis is characterised by the deposition of abnormally folded proteins in various tissues of the body. These proteins are formed from soluble proteins that undergo misfolding, and lead to insoluble, fibrillar aggregates (anti-parallel β-sheet configuration) that ultimately cause organ damage. The most common form of systemic amyloidosis is that derived from immunoglobulin light chain, most commonly λ (AL). Approximately two-thirds of patients present with renal involvement, often with nephrotic syndrome, and cardiac involvement, often leading to heart failure. Amyloid often deposits in the mesangium and ultimately capillaries of the kidneys. Congo red is used to confirm and rule out amyloid deposits (as the mature fibrils have Congo red binding sites), and under polarised light, a characteristic apple-green birefringence can be seen; hence E is the correct response. In patients on long-term dialysis, amyloidosis derived from β_2-microglobulin (Aβ_2m) should also be considered.

In non-diabetic patients who present with multisystem symptoms, such as dyspnoea, diarrhoea, neuropathy, and unexplained weight loss with nephrotic syndrome (proteinuria and hypoalbuminaemia), amyloidosis should be suspected. AL amyloidosis and multiple myeloma (MM) share features such as clonal plasma cell proliferation and monoclonal immunoglobulin production. Approximately 10–20% of patients with Al amyloidosis also present with MM. However, in MM nephrotic syndrome is rare and predominantly Bence-Jones protein is found in the urine. Histologically, in myeloma-induced nephropathy there are hyaline fractured casts deposited in the distal convoluted tubules and collecting ducts, whereas in AL these are deposited in the mesangium and capillaries.

Glomerulonephritis (GN) is inflammation within the glomerulus caused by various immune-mediated mechanisms. It can include minimal change, diffuse, focal and segmental. Post-infectious GN is a diffuse proliferative type that affects mesangial and endothelial cells provoked commonly by immune complexes deposited by Streptococcal bacteria, viruses or parasitic agents. Histologically, this is an endocapillary GN where glomeruli appear large and hypercellular with nuclei of varying size and form. There are often subepithelial deposits termed 'humps'. In membranoproliferative GN (focal or diffuse), as seen in IgA nephropathy, there is proliferation (endocapillary and/or mesangial) and thickening of the capillary walls by subendothelial immune/complement deposits. Idiopathic crescentic GN, microscopic polyangiitis and granulomatosis with polyangiitis are examples of a focal or diffuse proliferative GN with extensive crescent formation in glomeruli. Antiglomerular basement membrane disease (anti-GBM) is a focal segmental GN with necrosis which can progress to extensive crescent formation caused by immunoglobulins to type IV collagen.

Sarcoidosis is a multisystem disease that predominantly involves the lungs, lymph nodes, liver, bone, skin and eyes. Renal involvement is rare in sarcoidosis. Histologically, non-caseating epithelioid granulomas with tightly packed epithelioid cells and Langhans giant cells are present in the interstitium surrounding bronchioles and blood vessels. Although not specific to sarcoidosis, laminated concretions of calcium and protein, known as Schaumann bodies, and asteroid bodies, spindly radiating star-like structures within the epithelioid cells may also be present.

5.50 *C – Gout*

Crystal arthropathies are joint disorders characterised by accumulation of crystals in one or more joints. Monosodium urate crystal deposition is the central pathophysiological cause of gout. Needle-shaped or rod-shaped crystals are seen under the light microscope, and under polarising light they show negative birefringence; hence C is the correct response. Calcium pyrophosphate dihydrate (CPPD) crystal deposition causes pseudogout and is characterised by rhomboid-shaped crystals seen under the light microscope, and weak, positive birefringence under polarising light. Radiographically in elderly patients, there is often evidence of CPPD deposition known as chondrocalcinosis. CPPD crystal deposition is present in approximately 20% of patients with osteoarthritis. In contrast, concurrent CPPD crystal deposition and rheumatoid arthritis is very rare. Similarly, acute gout or pseudogout are rarely seen with clinical and laboratory findings suggestive of septic arthritis. Although patients with chronic diseases and immunosuppression are more likely to have septic arthritis. Gram staining and microbial culture can be used to distinguish between septic arthritis and crystal arthropathies. Oxalate arthropathy is a rare cause of arthritis characterised by calcium oxalate crystal deposition within synovial fluid. Calcium oxalate monohydrate crystals appear as irregular squares or rods, whereas calcium oxalate dihydrate crystals have an envelope-like shape. Both types of crystals exhibit positive birefringence under polarised light (similar to CPPD).

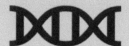

CHAPTER 6
Anatomy

I profess to learn and to teach anatomy not from books but from dissections, not from the tenets of Philosophers but from the fabric of Nature.

William Harvey

6.1   Neuroanatomy, head and neck

6.1.1 Which of the following muscles is innervated by the facial nerve?
A   Mylohyoid
B   Anterior belly of digastric
C   Omohyoid
D   Sternohyoid
E   Stylohyoid

6.1.2 Which of the following are boundaries of the posterior triangle in the neck?
A   Anterior border of sternocleidomastoid and trapezius, and inferior border of mandible
B   Anterior border of trapezius, middle third of clavicle and posterior midline of the neck
C   Posterior border of sternocleidomastoid, anterior border of trapezius and middle third of clavicle
D   Inferior belly of omohyoid muscle, proximal third of clavicle and occipital bone
E   Posterior border of sternocleidomastoid, posterior belly of digastric muscle and middle third of clavicle

6.1.3 Which of the following is **not** correct regarding the jugular foramen?
A   The vagus nerve lies most medial
B   Inferior petrosal sinus exits from the anterior compartment
C   Accessory nerve exits from the middle compartment
D   Hypoglossal nerve passes medial to internal and external carotid arteries
E   Sigmoid and inferior petrosal sinuses join to become the internal jugular vein

6.1.4 Which of the following regarding the trigeminal nerve and its branches is correct?
A   At the medulla, the sensory root expands into the trigeminal ganglion
B   Lingual nerve supplies sensory innervation to the posterior one-third of the tongue
C   Zygomatic nerve enters the orbit via the superior orbital fissure
D   Pterygopalatine ganglion is a branch of the ophthalmic nerve
E   The maxillary division exits the skull through the foramen rotundum

6.1.5 Which of the following nerves does **not** exit the skull via the superior orbital fissure?
A   Glossopharyngeal
B   Oculomotor
C   Trochlear
D   Ophthalmic
E   Abducens

6.1.6 Which of the following statements regarding the brain is correct?
A   The precentral gyrus is found in the parietal lobe
B   The cingulate sulcus is found on the lateral aspect of the cerebrum
C   The caudate nucleus lies in the wall of the lateral ventricle
D   The occipital lobe contains the primary auditory cortex
E   The cerebellum forms part of the forebrain

6.1.7 Which of the following is the boundary between the frontal and parietal lobes?
A   Central sulcus
B   Calcarine sulcus
C   Lateral sulcus
D   Cingulate sulcus
E   Lunate sulcus

6.1.8 Which of the following synthesises cerebrospinal fluid?
A   Superior sagittal sinus
B   Cisterna magna
C   Pineal gland
D   Choroid plexus
E   Pontine cistern

6.1.9 Which of the following does the anterior cerebral artery arch around posteromedially?
A   Pons
B   Medulla
C   Hypothalamus
D   Cerebellum
E   Corpus callosum

6.1.10 Which of the following sinuses <u>directly</u> drain into the internal jugular vein?
A   Inferior sagittal
B   Straight
C   Transverse
D   Sigmoid
E   Superior sagittal

6.1.11 Which of the following partially separates the caudate nucleus and putamen?
A   Internal capsule
B   Insula
C   Septum pellucidum
D   Lentiform nucleus
E   Globus pallidus

6.1.12 In a coronal plane, which of the following is the correct sequence of structures found within the brain rostrocaudally?
A   Corona radiata – claustrum – caudate head – lateral ventricle
B   Lateral ventricle – caudate head – claustrum – corona radiata
C   Claustrum – lateral ventricle – caudate head – corona radiata
D   Caudate head – claustrum – lateral ventricle – corona radiata
E   Lateral ventricle – claustrum – corona radiata – caudate head

6.1.13 How many colliculi are present in the midbrain?
A   2
B   3
C   4
D   5
E   6

6.1.14 Which of the following structures does the corticospinal tract pass anteriorly?
A   Dentate nucleus
B   Subthalamic nucleus
C   Vestibular nucleus
D   Red nucleus
E   Emboliform nucleus

6.1.15 Which of the following is **not** a motor pathway associated with the extrapyramidal system?
A   Tectospinal tract
B   Spinothalamic tract
C   Reticulospinal tract
D   Vestibulospinal tract
E   Rubrospinal tract

6.1.16 Which of the following is associated with the dorsal (posterior) columns of the spinal cord?
A   Pyramids
B   Medial lemniscus
C   Central canal
D   Pontine nuclei
E   Superior cerebellar peduncle

6.1.17 Which of the following (A–E) matches tracts (1–4)?

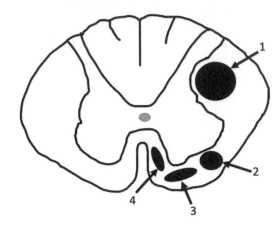

	(1)	(2)	(3)	(4)
A	Spinocerebellar	Later spinothalamic	Anterior corticospinal	Anterior spinothalamic
B	Lateral corticospinal	Lateral spinothalamic	Anterior spinothalamic	Anterior corticospinal
C	Corticobulbar	Anterior corticospinal	Lateral spinothalamic	Rubrospinal
D	Spinocerebellar	Rubrospinal	Lateral spinothalamic	Anterior corticospinal
E	Lateral corticospinal	Lateral spinothalamic	Rubrospinal	Anterior corticospinal

6.1.18 Which of the following statements regarding the cerebellar peduncles is **not** correct?
A The inferior cerebellar peduncle connects the cerebellum and pons
B The middle cerebellar peduncle is the largest
C The superior cerebellar peduncle contains efferent fibres
D The juxtarestiform body co-ordinates communication between the cerebellum and vestibular system
E The restiform body contains afferent fibres

6.1.19 Which of the following regarding boundaries of the diencephalon is correct?
A The third ventricle lies superiorly
B The optic chiasm lies posteriorly
C The pineal gland lies inferiorly
D The lamina terminalis lies anteriorly
E The fornix lies medially

6.1.20 Which of the following structures of the brain is matched correctly with the region that it is found?
A Fourth ventricle – midbrain
B Olive – spinal cord
C Basilar artery – pons
D Central canal – medulla
E Anterior median fissure – pons

6.1.21 Which of the following correctly matches the missing words (1–3) of the following sentence?
When secondary axons decussate in the anterior commissure of the cord, they ascend to the ......(1)...... in the ....(2)......... tract on the ......(3)...... side.

	(1)	(2)	(3)
A	pons	anterior spinothalamic	ipsilateral
B	medulla	lateral spinothalamic	ipsilateral
C	pons	anterior spinothalamic	ipsilateral
D	thalamus	lateral spinothalamic	contralateral
E	thalamus	anterior spinothalamic	contralateral

6.1.22 Which of the following motor components of each cranial nerve is correct?

	III			VII			XI		
	S	B	V	S	B	V	S	B	V
A	✓		✓	✓				✓	✓
B	✓	✓			✓	✓		✓	
C		✓	✓	✓		✓	✓	✓	
D			✓	✓	✓		✓		✓
E	✓		✓		✓	✓		✓	

Key: S: somatic; B: branchial; V: visceral

6.1.23 Which of the following cranial nerves is the only one to exit from the posterior aspect of the brainstem?
  A Trochlear
  B Abducens
  C Trigeminal
  D Hypoglossal
  E Optic

6.1.24 Which of the following would result from a lesion close to the origin of the vagus nerve?
  A Bronchoconstriction
  B Pupillary constriction
  C Increased gastric motility
  D Decreased gastric motility
  E Decreased heart rate

6.1.25 Which cranial nerve is associated with decreased lacrimation <u>and</u> loss of the efferent limb of the corneal reflex?
  A V
  B IX
  C VII
  D III
  E VI

6.1.26 Which of the following regarding the shaded area X is **not** correct?

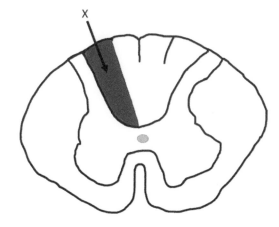

  A It contains afferent fibres from the upper trunk and extremities
  B It is formed from afferent fibres that enter the spinal cord above T6
  C It is responsible for transmitting vibration, fine touch and proprioception
  D It receives its blood supply from the posterior spinal artery
  E It is present throughout the length of the spinal cord

6.1.27 Which of the following diagrams represent one possible lesion site (X) based on the following scenario?

> *A patient repeatedly burns his fingers on both hands when cooking because they did not recognise when the handle of the pan was too hot. Although the fingers were seriously injured, the patient did not feel pain in them.*

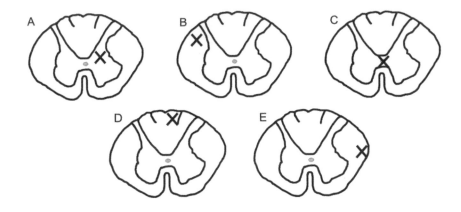

Questions 6.1.28 to 6.1.31 relate to the following MRI figure of the head and neck.

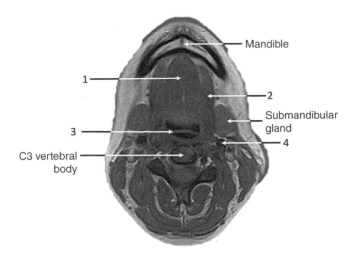

6.1.28 Which of the following muscles corresponds to label 1?
  A Mylohyoid
  B Hyoglossus
  C Stylohyoid
  D Genioglossus
  E Posterior belly of digastric

6.1.29 Which of the following muscles corresponds to label 2?
  A Mylohyoid
  B Hyoglossus
  C Styloglossus
  D Geniohyoid
  E Superior belly of omohyoid

6.1.30 Which of the following is the function of label 3?
  A Traps saliva and prevents the swallowing reflex
  B Protects the airway and prevents aspiration
  C Acts as attachment site for anterior neck muscles
  D Contract so that a food bolus can pass into the oesophagus
  E Supports the vocal cords

6.1.31 Which of the following blood vessels corresponds to label 4?
    A Facial artery
    B Internal jugular vein
    C External jugular vein
    D Vertebral artery
    E Common carotid artery

Questions 6.1.32 to 6.1.37 relate to the following figures of the skull and lateral wall of the nasal cavity.

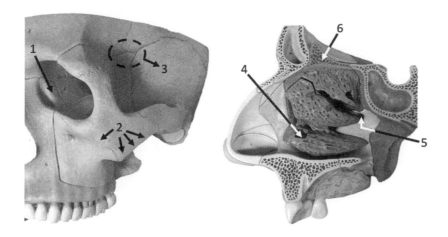

6.1.32 Which of the following bones corresponds to label 1?
    A Ethmoid
    B Sphenoid
    C Lacrimal
    D Zygomatic
    E Nasal

6.1.33 Which of the following muscles originates at region labelled 2?
    A Masseter
    B Medial pterygoid
    C Lateral pterygoid
    D Temporalis
    E Middle pharyngeal constrictor

6.1.34 Which of the following bones is **not** in close proximity at region labelled 3?
    A Frontal
    B Parietal
    C Sphenoid
    D Temporal
    E Ethmoid

6.1.35 Which of the following opens under the anterior lip of structure labelled 4?
    A Maxillary sinus
    B Nasolacrimal duct
    C Sphenoidal sinus
    D Middle ethmoidal cells
    E Frontonasal duct

6.1.36 Which of the following structures does **not** pass through label 5?
    A Sphenopalatine artery
    B Sphenopalatine vein
    C Descending palatine artery
    D Posterior superior lateral nasal nerve
    E Nasopalatine nerve

6.1.37 Which of the following nerves enters the nasal and cranial cavity through structure labelled 6?
  A Greater petrosal
  B Zygomaticofacial
  C Infra-orbital
  D Olfactory
  E Optic

Questions 6.1.38 to 6.1.44 relate to the following figures of the skull, brain and facial muscles.

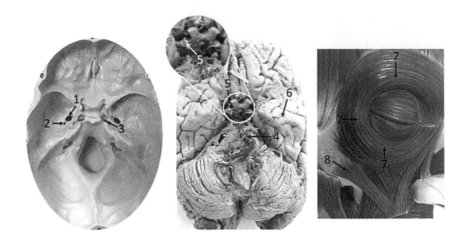

6.1.38 Which of the following structures passes through region labelled 1?
  A Mandibular division of trigeminal nerve
  B Maxillary division of trigeminal nerve
  C Middle meningeal artery
  D Optic nerve
  E Internal jugular vein

6.1.39 Which of the following correctly identifies foramina/fissures of the cranial cavity?

	Label 2	Label 3
A	Foramen rotundum	Carotid canal
B	Hypoglossal canal	Foramen ovale
C	Foramen spinosum	Carotid canal
D	Optic canal	Foramen spinosum
E	Superior orbital fissure	Internal acoustic meatus

6.1.40 Which of the following arise from a rostral bifurcation of structure labelled 4?
  A Vertebral arteries
  B Anterior inferior cerebellar arteries
  C Posterior cerebral arteries
  D Anterior cerebral arteries
  E Superior cerebellar arteries

6.1.41 Which of the following is **not** supplied by structure labelled 5?
  A Superior portion of parietal lobe
  B Basal ganglia
  C Broca's area
  D Lateral inferior portion of frontal lobe
  E Wernicke's area

6.1.42 Which of the following is **not** controlled by lobe labelled 6?
  A Emotions
  B Memory
  C Feelings
  D Learning
  E Anticipation

6.1.43 Which of the following muscles is the major antagonist of muscle labelled 7?
  A Superior oblique
  B Superior rectus
  C Levator palpebrae superioris
  D Corrugator supercilii
  E Levator labii superioris

6.1.44 Which of the following is the function of muscle labelled 8?
  A Protrudes the lower lip
  B Draws the corner of the mouth down and laterally
  C Retracts the corner of the mouth
  D Draws the upper lip upward
  E Draws the corner of the mouth upward and laterally

Questions 6.1.45 to 6.1.47 relate to the following figure of the neck.

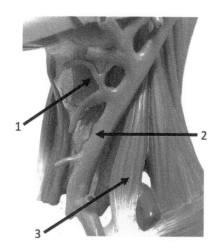

6.1.45 Which of the following muscles corresponds to label 1?
  A Sternohyoid
  B Sternothyroid
  C Superior belly of omohyoid
  D Inferior belly of omohyoid
  E Thyrohyoid

6.1.46 Which of the following is correct regarding vessel labelled 2?

	Origin	Unites with	Terminal tributary in neck	Runs parallel with
A	Transverse and inferior petrosal sinus	Subclavian vein	Superior thyroid vein	Phrenic nerve
B	Transverse and sigmoid sinus	Brachiocephalic vein	Middle thyroid vein	Vagus nerve
C	Sigmoid and cavernous sinus	Brachiocephalic vein	Inferior thyroid vein	Phrenic nerve
D	Sigmoid and inferior petrosal sinus	Subclavian vein	Middle thyroid vein	Vagus nerve
E	Sigmoid and inferior petrosal sinus	Subclavian vein	Inferior thyroid vein	Vagus nerve

6.1.47 Which of the following is the correct function and innervation of muscle labelled3?
  A Elevation of rib I; anterior rami of C3–C7
  B Elevation of rib I; anterior rami of C4–C7
  C Elevation of rib II; anterior rami of C5–C7
  D Depression of hyoid bone; anterior rami of C1–C3
  E Flexion of head; anterior rami of C1–C3

6.1.48 Which of the following muscles tenses the vocal ligaments and aids in phonation?
  A Aryepiglottic
  B Cricothyroid
  C Lateral cricoarytenoid
  D Salpingopharyngeus
  E Posterior cricoarytenoid

6.1.49 Which of the following regarding lymphatic drainage of the head and neck is **not** correct?

	Site	Lymph nodes into which it drains
A	Lateral border of eye lids	Parotid
B	Floor of mouth	Submental
C	Anterior tongue	Submandibular
D	Nasopharynx	Superficial cervical
E	Helix of ear	Posterior auricular

6.1.50 Which of the following arteries is **not** a branch of the external carotid artery?
  A Facial
  B Lingual
  C Occipital
  D Ophthalmic
  E Maxillary

6.2   Special senses

6.2.1 Which of the following regarding special senses is correct?
  A The organ of Corti is a specialised receptor organ for hearing supported by Deiter's and Claudius cells
  B Müller cells of the retina relay information from cones to rods
  C Cones contain photopsin and are more sensitive to light than rods
  D Only type II hair cells found in the maculae of the ear contain kinocilium
  E Most of the external layers of the retina including the pigment epithelium have vasculature supplied by the central retinal artery

6.2.2 Which of the following regarding special senses is correct?
  A The superior ophthalmic vein joins with the pterygoid plexus
  B The ciliary ganglion is a sympathetic ganglion of the oculomotor nerve
  C The tympanic nerve is a branch of the vagus nerve
  D The abducens nerve enters the orbit through the superior orbital fissure
  E The sphenoethmoidal recess is found between the inferior concha and nasal roof

6.2.3 Which of the following regarding special senses is correct?
  A Chorda tympani joins the maxillary nerve in the infratemporal fossa
  B Palatoglossus is innervated by the glossopharyngeal nerve
  C Alae of vomer form the lateral wall of the nasal cavity
  D Filiform papillae contain no taste buds
  E Lamina of modiolus is found in the semicircular canals

6.2.4 Which of the following regarding the orbit is **not** correct?
  A Lateral rectus muscle medially rotates the eyeball
  B Orbicularis oculi is innervated by the facial nerve
  C Photoreceptors are absent from the optic disc
  D Loss of oculomotor nerve function results in ptosis
  E Ciliary muscles are innervated by sympathetics from the oculomotor nerve

6.2.5 Which of the following regarding the eyelids is correct?
  A The supra-orbital artery is a branch of the superficial temporal artery
  B The infratrochlear nerve is a branch of the maxillary nerve
  C Lymphatic drainage is primarily to the parotid and pre-auricular nodes
  D Loss of innervation of the superior tarsal muscle causes an inability to close the eyelids
  E The trochlear nerve innervates levator palpebrae superioris

6.2.6 Which of the following anatomical muscle actions is correctly matched to the eye movement when specific muscles are being clinically tested?
  A Medial rectus – look laterally
  B Superior oblique – look laterally and downward
  C Inferior oblique – look medially and upward
  D Superior rectus – look medially and downward
  E Inferior rectus – look laterally and upward

6.2.7 Which of the following muscles originates lateral to the nasolacrimal groove and inserts into the posterior inferolateral surface of the eyeball?
  A Superior rectus
  B Inferior rectus
  C Lateral rectus
  D Superior oblique
  E Inferior oblique

6.2.8 Which of the following is **not** correct regarding the formation of the orbital rim (base)?
  A Superiorly is the frontal bone
  B Inferiorly is the zygomatic process of the maxilla
  C Medially is the frontal process of the maxilla
  D Posteriorly, the orbital process of the palatine bone contributes to the roof
  E Laterally is the zygomatic bone

6.2.9 Which of the following is the correct order of light passage through the eye?
  A Cornea → Vitreous humour → Lens → Pupil → Aqueous humour → Retina
  B Vitreous humour → Cornea → Lens → Pupil → Aqueous humour → Retina
  C Aqueous humour → Cornea → Pupil → Lens → Vitreous humour → Retina
  D Cornea → Aqueous humour → Pupil → Lens → Vitreous humour → Retina
  E Cornea → Pupil → Aqueous humour → Lens → Vitreous humour → Retina

6.2.10 Which of the following can become more opaque with increasing age and lead to cataracts?
  A Lens
  B Retina
  C Conjunctiva
  D Iris
  E Pupil

6.2.11 Which of the following are holocrine glands found along the eyelid rim embedded in the tarsal plate?
  A Krause
  B Meibomian
  C Wolfring
  D Moll
  E Zeis

6.2.12 Which of the following nerves enter the orbit through the annulus of Zinn?

A Lacrimal and optic

B Frontal and lacrimal

C Trochlear and frontal

D Nasociliary and trochlear

E Nasociliary and abducens

6.2.13 Which of the following regarding the blood supply of the eye is correct?

A The ophthalmic artery enters the orbit above the optic nerve

B The ophthalmic artery arises from the external carotid artery

C The central retinal artery is the largest branch of the ophthalmic artery

D The largest proportion of blood flow in the eye passes through the choroid

E The lacrimal artery runs along the upper border of the medial rectus muscle

6.2.14 Which of the following regarding the pupillary light reflex is correct?

A Its afferent limb is carried in the oculomotor nerve

B Its efferent limb is carried in the optic nerve

C It is mediated by the inferior colliculi in the midbrain

D In bright light, pupils constrict as radial muscles contract

E In dim light, pupils dilate as circular muscles relax

6.2.15 Which of the following would result from direct paralysis of the superior tarsal muscle?

A Ptosis

B Miosis

C Mydriasis

D Diplopia

E Proptosis

6.2.16 Which of the following regarding innervation of the lacrimal gland is correct?

A Parasympathetic fibres continue as the deep petrosal nerve

B Pterygopalatine ganglion contain no sympathetic fibres

C Parasympathetic preganglionic fibres enter the greater petrosal nerve

D The zygomaticofacial nerve joins the lacrimal nerve

E The pterygoid canal transmits the maxillary nerve

6.2.17 Which of the following regarding the macula lutea is correct?

A It is approximately 50 μm in diameter

B It is located on the anterior pole of the retina

C It appears yellow due to high concentrations of lutein and zeaxanthin

D It is rich in rods

E It is commonly referred to as the blind spot

6.2.18 Which of the following regarding the external ear is correct?

A The tragus is the non-cartilaginous part of the auricle

B The superficial part of the auricle is supplied by the auricular branch of vagus nerve

C The external carotid artery supplies the anterior auricular artery

D Sensory innervation of the tympanic membrane inner surface is carried entirely by the glossopharyngeal nerve

E Sensory innervation of the external acoustic meatus is carried entirely by the mandibular nerve

6.2.19 Which of the following regarding the middle ear is correct?

A The tegmental wall is the floor of the middle ear

B The oval window is attached to the base of the incus

C Tensor tympani is innervated by a branch of the facial nerve

D The stapes is the largest of the auditory ossicles

E The tympanic nerve forms the tympanic plexus, of which, the lesser petrosal nerve is a major branch

6.2.20 Which of the following regarding the inner ear is correct?
    A There are three semicircular canals
    B The helicotrema of the cochlea connects perilymph with the subarachnoid space
    C There are two ducts within the membranous labyrinth
    D The vestibulocochlear nerve exits the skull through the stylomastoid foramen
    E The greater petrosal nerve carries parasympathetic fibres to the geniculate ganglion

Questions 6.2.21 to 6.2.25 relate to the following figures of the ear.

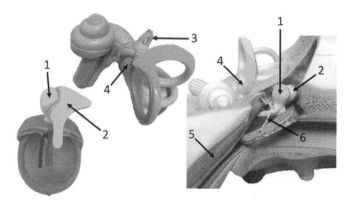

6.2.21 Which of the following (A–E) corresponds to labels (1–4)?

	Label 1	Label 2	Label 3	Label 4
A	Incus	Utricle	Malleus	Stapes
B	Incus	Stapes	Malleus	Saccule
C	Malleus	Incus	Stapes	Saccule
D	Malleus	Incus	Stapes	Utricle
E	Incus	Malleus	Stapes	Utricle

6.2.22 Which of the following is **not** correct regarding the muscle which attaches to structure labelled 3?
    A It originates from inside the pyramidal eminence within the petrous temporal bone
    B It is supplied by a branch from the facial nerve
    C Paralysis leads to hyperacusis
    D It contracts reflexively in response to loudness of sound
    E It inserts into the base of structure labelled 3

6.2.23 Which of the following empties into structure labelled 4?
    A Cochlear duct
    B Endolymphatic duct
    C Utriculosaccular duct
    D Vestibular aqueduct
    E Semicircular ducts

6.2.24 Which of the following innervates muscle labelled 5?
    A Branch of maxillary nerve
    B Branch of mandibular nerve
    C Branch of facial nerve
    D Branch of vestibulocochlear nerve
    E Branch of cochlear nerve

6.2.25 Which of the following regarding label 6 is correct?

	Arises from	Merges with	Exits through
A	Glossopharyngeal nerve	Maxillary nerve	Pterygomaxillary fissure
B	Glossopharyngeal nerve	Lingual nerve	Fissures of Santorini
C	Facial nerve	Maxillary nerve	Petrotympanic fissure
D	Hypoglossal nerve	Lesser petrosal nerve	Pterygomaxillary fissure
E	Facial nerve	Lingual nerve	Petrotympanic fissure

6.2.26 Which of the following is **not** concerned with balance?
   A Posterior semicircular duct
   B Saccule
   C Utricle
   D Cochlear duct
   E Lateral semicircular duct

6.2.27 Which of the following arteries give rise to the labyrinthine artery?
   A Superior cerebellar and basilar
   B Anterior inferior cerebellar and vertebral
   C Anterior inferior cerebellar and basilar
   D Posterior inferior cerebellar and basilar
   E Superior cerebellar and anterior spinal

6.2.28 Which of the following does the labyrinthine vein drain into?
   A Straight or occipital sinus
   B Superior petrosal or inferior petrosal sinus
   C Inferior petrosal or transverse sinus
   D Sigmoid or transverse sinus
   E Sigmoid or inferior petrosal sinus

6.2.29 Which of the following muscles of the soft palate is innervated by the mandibular nerve?
   A Tensor veli palatini
   B Levator veli palatini
   C Musculus uvulae
   D Palatopharyngeus
   E Palatoglossus

6.2.30 Which of the following nerves innervates the upper oral cavity and upper teeth?
   A Facial
   B Maxillary branch of trigeminal
   C Mandibular branch of trigeminal
   D Hypoglossal
   E Glossopharyngeal

6.2.31 Which of the following regarding the tongue is **not** correct?
   A Vallate papillae are the largest
   B The lingual vein is located on each side of the frenulum
   C There are four extrinsic muscles
   D The deep and dorsal lingual veins drain into the external jugular vein
   E Taste from the oral part is carried by the facial nerve

6.2.32 Which of the following nodes do the lymphatic vessels of the palate drain into?
   A Anterior cervical
   B Posterior cervical
   C Deep cervical
   D Superficial cervical
   E Submandibular

6.2.33 Which of the following muscles shorten the tongue and elevates the tip?
   A Vertical
   B Transverse
   C Inferior longitudinal
   D Superior longitudinal
   E Palatoglossus

6.2.34 Which of the following types of taste sensation is detected by gustatory receptors predominantly found at the base of the tongue?
   A Sweetness
   B Sourness
   C Bitterness
   D Saltiness
   E Umami

6.2.35 Which of the following is the site of development of the thyroid?
   A Foramen caecum
   B Sulcus terminalis
   C Median raphe
   D Epiglottis
   E Tuberculum impar

Questions 6.2.36 to 6.2.38 relate to the following figure.

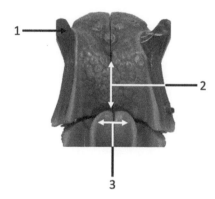

6.2.36 Which of the following regarding structure labelled 1 is **not** correct?
   A It is an extrinsic muscle of the tongue
   B It is innervated by the hypoglossal nerve
   C It arises from the greater cornu of the hyoid
   D It helps elevate and retract the tongue
   E It passes between internal and external carotid arteries

6.2.37 Which of the following regarding region labelled 2 is correct?
   A Is usually associated with fungiform papillae
   B Does not form part of Waldeyer's ring
   C Histologically, no crypts are found
   D It is supplied by the dorsal lingual artery
   E It is covered by ciliated pseudostratified columnar epithelium

6.2.38 Which of the following solely connects structure labelled 3 to the tongue?
   A Lateral glossoepiglottic fold
   B Median glossoepiglottic fold
   C Aryepiglottic folds
   D Valleculae
   E Aryepiglotticus

6.2.39 Which of the following nerves does **not** innervate the nasal cavities?
A Mandibular division of trigeminal
B Maxillary division of trigeminal
C Ophthalmic division of trigeminal
D Olfactory
E Facial

6.2.40 Which of the following articulates with the inferior concha in the ethmoid bone?
A Cribriform plate
B Crista galli
C Superior concha
D Uncinate process
E Orbital plate of ethmoidal labyrinth

6.2.41 Which of the following does **not** drain onto the lateral wall of the nasal cavity?
A Nasolacrimal duct
B Middle ethmoidal cells
C Posterior ethmoidal cells
D Frontal sinus
E Sphenoidal sinus

6.2.42 Which of the following are **not** margins of the choanae?
A Posteriorly by the sphenoid bone
B Anteriorly by the ala of the vomer
C Inferiorly by the palatine bone
D Medially by the posterior aspect of the vomer
E Laterally by the vaginal process of the pterygoid process

6.2.43 Which of the following pass through the sphenopalatine foramen?
A Greater palatine branch of maxillary nerve
B Infra-orbital nerve
C Superior nasal branches of the maxillary nerve
D Anterior ethmoidal nerve
E Fibres of the olfactory nerve

6.2.44 Which of the following is **not** a component of the infratemporal fossa?
A Lateral pterygoid
B Tendon of masseter
C Chorda tympani
D Maxillary artery
E Pterygoid venous plexus

Question 6.2.45 to 6.2.48 relate to the following CT figure of the head.

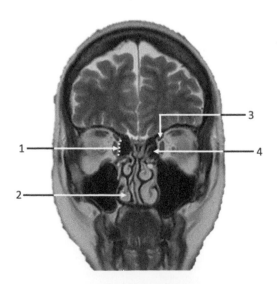

6.2.45 Which of the following is **not** a correct articulation of structure labelled 1?
  A Anteriorly with the lacrimal bone
  B Posteriorly with the sphenoid bone
  C Superiorly with the orbital plate of the frontal bone
  D Inferiorly with the orbital process of the palatine bone
  E Medially with the maxilla

6.2.46 Which of the following corresponds to structure labelled 2?
  A Inferior concha
  B Vomer
  C Middle concha
  D Inferior meatus
  E Hiatus semilunaris

6.2.47 Which of the following regarding structure labelled 3 is correct?
  A It is innervated by the abducens nerve
  B It is responsible for outward gaze
  C It primarily elevates the upper eyelid and adducts the eyeball
  D It receives its blood supply from the ophthalmic artery
  E It originates from the maxillary bone

6.2.48 Which of the following corresponds to structure labelled 4?
  A Maxillary sinus
  B Ethmoid bulla
  C Uncinate process
  D Superior concha
  E Vomer

6.2.49 Which of the following regarding paranasal sinuses is **not** correct?
  A Frontal sinuses are supplied by branches of the anterior ethmoidal arteries
  B There are three divisions of ethmoidal cells
  C Maxillary sinuses are the largest
  D The pituitary gland can be surgically approached via the frontal sinuses
  E Sphenoidal sinuses are related laterally to the cavernous sinuses

6.2.50 Which of the following muscles does **not** help widen the nares?
  A Dilator naris
  B Compressor naris
  C Depressor septi nasi
  D Depressor supercilii
  E Levator labii superioris alaeque nasi

6.3   Upper limb

6.3.1 Which of the following nerves is a terminal branch of the lateral cord of the brachial plexus and receives fibres from C5?
  A Lateral pectoral
  B Suprascapular
  C Axillary
  D Radial
  E Musculocutaneous

6.3.2 Which of the following regarding the brachial plexus is correct?
  A C5 and C6 roots unite to form the middle trunk
  B Roots of the brachial plexus usually pass through the gap between the middle and posterior scalene muscles
  C Only the posterior division of the superior and middle trunks form the posterior cord
  D The medial cord is a continuation of the anterior division of the inferior trunk
  E The long thoracic nerve originates from the ventral rami of C8 and T1

6.3.3   Which of the following regarding boundaries of the axilla is correct?

     A   The lateral wall is formed by the intertubercular sulcus of the humerus

     B   The medial margin of the axillary inlet is the lateral border of the 2nd rib

     C   The anterior wall is formed by the pectoralis major and minor muscles and supraspinatus

     D   The posterior wall is formed by latissimus dorsi, subscapularis and the short head of triceps brachii muscle

     E   The floor is formed by the concave skin only

6.3.4   Which of the following arteries passes through the triangular space and enters the infraspinous fossa?

     A   Internal thoracic

     B   Suprascapular

     C   Circumflex scapular

     D   Subscapular

     E   Thoracodorsal

6.3.5   Which of the following cutaneous nerves of the upper limb is a branch from T2 and supplies the skin on the medial surface of the arm?

     A   Supraclavicular

     B   Superior lateral cutaneous nerve of arm

     C   Intercostobrachial

     D   Lateral cutaneous nerve of forearm

     E   Inferior lateral cutaneous nerve of arm

Questions 6.3.6 to 6.3.8 relate to the following figure.

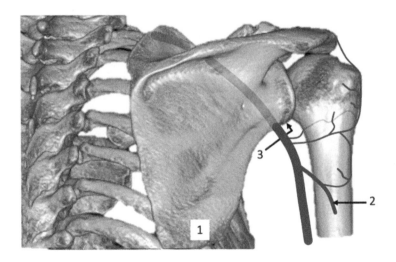

6.3.6   Which of the following nerves innervates the muscle which originates in region labelled 1?

     A   Thoracodorsal

     B   Axillary

     C   Inferior subscapular

     D   Superior subscapular

     E   Dorsal scapular

6.3.7   Which of the following arteries corresponds to structure labelled 2?

     A   Superior ulnar collateral

     B   Profunda brachii

     C   Anterior circumflex humeral

     D   Posterior circumflex humeral

     E   Brachial

6.3.8   Which of the following is **not** correct regarding the muscle that originates at region label 3?
   A   It is innervated by the radial nerve
   B   It inserts into the olecranon process of the ulna
   C   It is a primary extensor of the forearm at the elbow joint
   D   Venous drainage is via the brachial veins
   E   It is an accessory abductor at the glenohumeral joint

6.3.9   Which of the following regarding dermatomes of the upper limb is **not** correct?
   A   Upper lateral arm tests for C5
   B   Palmar aspect of thumb tests for C6
   C   Index finger tests for C7
   D   Little finger tests for C8
   E   Skin on lateral aspect of the elbow tests for T1

6.3.10   Which of the following ligaments of the shoulder attach to the conoid tubercle and trapezoid line?
   A   Coracoclavicular
   B   Acromioclavicular
   C   Coracoacromial
   D   Coracohumeral
   E   Glenohumeral

Questions 6.3.11 to 6.3.16 relate to the following MRI figure of the shoulder.

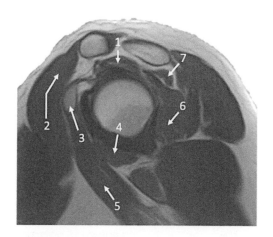

6.3.11   Which of the following muscle labels is **not** a component of the rotator cuff?
   A   1
   B   2
   C   4
   D   6
   E   7

6.3.12   Which of the following corresponds to structure labelled 3?
   A   Supraglenoid tubercle
   B   Spine of scapula
   C   Clavicle
   D   Acromion
   E   Coracoid process

6.3.13   Which of the following muscle labels is innervated by the suprascapular nerve?
   A   2
   B   4
   C   5
   D   6
   E   7

6.3.14 Which of the following muscle labels initiates abduction of the arm at the glenohumeral joint?
- A 1
- B 2
- C 5
- D 6
- E 7

6.3.15 Which of the following muscles originate from the apex of structure labelled 3?
- A Brachialis and long head of triceps brachii
- B Brachialis and short head of biceps brachii
- C Coracobrachialis and short head of biceps brachii
- D Coracobrachialis and long head of biceps brachii
- E Coracobrachialis and long head of triceps brachii

6.3.16 Which of the following arteries supplies muscle labelled 2?
- A Suprascapular
- B Dorsal scapular
- C Circumflex scapular
- D Posterior humeral circumflex
- E Thoracodorsal

6.3.17 Which of the following regarding spaces within the shoulder is correct?
- A The circumflex scapular vein passes through the quadrangular space
- B The teres minor muscle is an inferior boundary of the quadrangular space
- C The teres major muscle is a superior boundary of the triangular space
- D The profunda brachii artery passes through the triangular interval
- E The triangular space is lateral to the quadrangular space

6.3.18 Which of the following nerves passes through the triangular interval?
- A Radial
- B Axillary
- C Superior subscapular
- D Thoracodorsal
- E Posterior brachial cutaneous

Questions 6.3.19 to 6.3.22 relate to the following 3D reconstruction and radiograph of the shoulder.

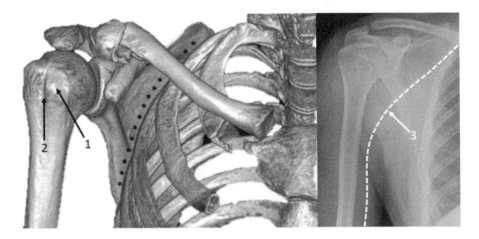

6.3.19 Which of the following muscles inserts into region labelled 1?
- A Teres minor
- B Teres major
- C Latissimus dorsi
- D Subscapularis
- E Subclavius

6.3.20 Which of the following nerves innervates the muscle that inserts into the region denoted by asterisks (*)?
   A Medial pectoral nerve
   B Long thoracic
   C Inferior subscapular
   D Lower subscapular
   E Intercostal

6.3.21 Which of the following is correct regarding the tendon which crosses at label 2?

	Insertion	Innervation	Action
A	Radial tuberosity	Musculocutaneous nerve	Pronation of forearm
B	Lateral epicondyle of humerus	Radial nerve	Pronation of forearm
C	Radial tuberosity	Radial nerve	Flexion of forearm at elbow
D	Medial epicondyle of humerus	Musculocutaneous nerve	Flexion of forearm at elbow
E	Radial tuberosity	Musculocutaneous nerve	Flexion of forearm at elbow

6.3.22 Which of the following nerves would line labelled 3 **not** likely represent?
   A Ulnar
   B Median
   C Medial cutaneous nerve of forearm
   D Lateral cutaneous nerve of forearm
   E Medial cutaneous nerve of arm

Questions 6.3.23 to 6.3.25 relate to the following CT figure of the shoulder.

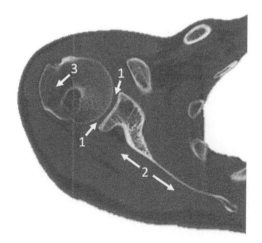

6.3.23 Which of the following corresponds with region labelled 1?
   A Subacromial bursa
   B Subcoracoid bursa
   C Glenoid fossa
   D Glenoid labrum
   E Articular capsule

6.3.24 Which of the following muscles corresponds with region labelled 2?
   A Deltoid
   B Supraspinatus
   C Infraspinatus
   D Subscapularis
   E Teres minor

6.3.25 Which of the following corresponds with region labelled 3?
  A Inferior facet of greater tubercle
  B Superior facet of greater tubercle
  C Intertubercular groove
  D Lesser tubercle
  E Greater tubercle

Questions 6.3.26 to 6.3.31 relate to the following MRI figures of the elbow.

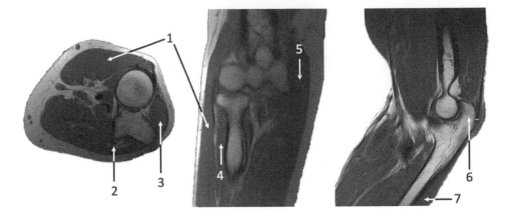

6.3.26 Which of the following corresponds to muscle labelled 1?
  A Extensor digitorum
  B Extensor carpi radialis longus
  C Extensor carpi radialis brevis
  D Brachioradialis
  E Extensor carpi ulnaris

6.3.27 Which of the following is found within region labelled 2?
  A Ulnar nerve
  B Annular ligament
  C Radial nerve
  D Collateral ligament
  E Basilic vein

6.3.28 Which of the following arteries and nerves supply and innervate muscle labelled 3 respectively?
  A Posterior interosseous recurrent artery and radial nerve
  B Medial collateral artery and ulnar nerve
  C Deep brachial artery and musculocutaneous nerve
  D Ulnar artery and radial nerve
  E Brachial artery and median nerve

6.3.29 Which of the following regarding muscles labelled 4 and 5 is correct?
  A 4 belongs to the posterior and 5 belongs to the lateral compartments of the forearm, respectively
  B 4 and 5 receive a blood supply from both the ulnar and radial arteries
  C 4 proximally attaches to the medial epicondyle of the humerus and 5 proximally attaches to the anterior surface of the radius
  D 4 flexes the elbow and 5 pronates the forearm
  E 4 is innervated by the deep branch of the radial nerve and 5 receives a blood supply from the ulnar artery

6.3.30 Which of the following corresponds to region labelled 6?
  A Capitellum
  B Trochlea
  C Coronoid process
  D Olecranon
  E Radial notch

6.3.31 Which of the following is the action of muscle labelled 7?
    A Flexes and adducts the hand at the wrist
    B Flexes and abducts the hand at the wrist
    C Flexes distal phalanges at distal interphalangeal joints of medial four digits
    D Flexes proximal phalanges at proximal interphalangeal and metacarpophalangeal joints of medial four digits
    E Flexes interphalangeal joint of 1st digit

6.3.32 Which of the following is **not** contained within the antecubital fossa?
    A Median nerve
    B Bifurcation of brachial artery
    C Biceps brachii tendon
    D Radial nerve
    E Median cubital vein

6.3.33 Which of the following ligaments attaches the medial epicondyle of the humerus to the coronoid process?
    A Quadrate
    B Accessory collateral
    C Annular
    D Radial collateral
    E Ulnar collateral

6.3.34 Which of the following is **not** innervated by the posterior interosseous nerve?
    A Extensor digitorum
    B Extensor carpi ulnaris
    C Abductor pollicis longus
    D Supinator
    E Extensor carpi radialis longus

6.3.35 Which of the following is a superficial forearm muscle that attaches to the medial epicondyle of the humerus proximally?
    A Flexor pollicis longus
    B Flexor digitorum profundus
    C Palmaris longus
    D Supinator
    E Brachioradialis

6.3.36 Which of the following muscles is likely to be affected by compression of the median nerve in the carpal tunnel?
    A Flexor pollicis longus
    B Flexor pollicis brevis
    C Opponens digiti minimi
    D Flexor carpi radialis
    E Dorsal interossei

Questions 6.3.37 to 6.3.41 relate to the following MRI figures of the forearm, wrist and hand.

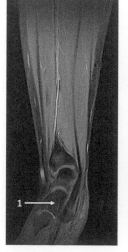 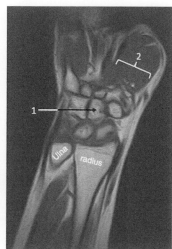 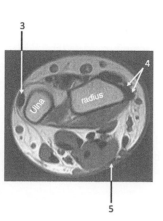

6.3.37 Which of the following corresponds to structure labelled 1?
    A Hamate
    B Capitate
    C Triquetrum
    D Trapezoid
    E Scaphoid

6.3.38 Which of the following structures is part of region labelled 2?
    A Pisometacarpal ligament
    B Guyon's canal
    C Hook of hamate
    D Opponens digiti minimi
    E Opponens pollicis

6.3.39 Which of the following is main action of muscle labelled 3?
    A Flexes and adducts the wrist
    B Flexes and abducts the wrist
    C Extends and adducts the wrist
    D Extends and abducts the wrist
    E Extends the little finger

6.3.40 Which of the following arteries supplies muscle labelled 4?
    A Posterior interosseous
    B Anterior interosseous
    C Recurrent interosseous
    D Posterior ulnar recurrent
    E Anterior ulnar recurrent

6.3.41 Which of the following correspond to muscle tendon labelled 5?
    A Flexor carpi radialis
    B Palmaris longus
    C Abductor pollicis longus
    D Flexor pollicis longus
    E Flexor carpi ulnaris

6.3.42 Which of the following is **not** found in the carpal tunnel?
    A Median nerve
    B Flexor pollicis longus tendon
    C Flexor digitorum superficialis tendons
    D Flexor digitorum profundus tendons
    E Flexor carpi radialis tendon

6.3.43 Which of the following boundaries of Guyon's canal is **not** correct?
    A Pisiform forms the medial wall
    B Volar carpal ligament forms the roof
    C Adductor digiti minimi forms the lateral (radial) wall and floor
    D Flexor retinaculum forms the floor
    E Hook of hamate forms the lateral wall

6.3.44 Which of the following intrinsic muscles of the hand adducts the thumb, index, ring and little fingers at the metacarpophalangeal joints?
    A Palmaris brevis
    B Adductor pollicis
    C Lumbricals
    D Palmar interossei
    E Dorsal interossei

6.3.45 Which of the following regarding the hand and wrist is **not** correct?
    A The wrist is composed of eight carpal bones
    B The radial collateral ligament stabilizes proximal carpal bones
    C The palmar ligament (plate) at the interphalangeal joints prevents hyperextension
    D There are seven extensor compartments of the wrist
    E Palmar interossei are unipennate

6.3.46 Which of the following intrinsic hand muscles attaches proximally to the hook of hamate?
    A Abductor digiti minimi
    B Flexor digiti minimi
    C Adductor pollicis
    D Opponens pollicis
    E Lumbricals 1 and 2

6.3.47 Which of the following muscles is **not** involved in extension?
    A Biceps brachii
    B Latissimus dorsi
    C Triceps brachii
    D Teres major
    E Interossei

6.3.48 Which of the following regarding blood supply to the upper limb is correct?
    A The right subclavian artery arises from the aortic arch
    B The brachial artery usually bifurcates superior to the trochlea of humerus
    C Anastomoses occur in the shoulder, elbow, and hand
    D Cephalic and basilic veins are deep veins
    E The ulnar artery predominantly gives rise to the deep palmar arch

Questions 6.3.49 to 6.3.50 relate to the following figure of the hand.

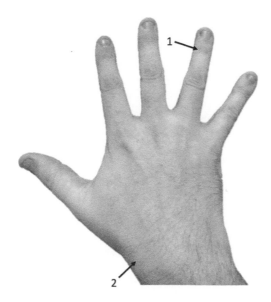

6.3.49 Which of the following nerves and arteries innervate and supply region labelled 1 respectively?
    A Ulnar nerve and radial artery
    B Median nerve and radial artery
    C Ulnar nerve and ulnar artery
    D Radial nerve and ulnar artery
    E Median nerve and ulnar artery

6.3.50 Which of the following is **not** located in region labelled 2?
A   Palmar branch of median nerve
B   Extensor pollicis brevis tendon
C   Cephalic vein
D   Abductor pollicis longus tendon
E   Radial artery

6.4   Thorax, mediastinum and back

6.4.1 At which vertebral level does the azygos vein curve anteriorly over the hilum of the right lung and drains into the superior vena cava?
A   T2
B   T3
C   T4
D   T5
E   T6

6.4.2 Which of the following muscles attaches to the coracoid process of the scapula?
A   Subclavius
B   Pectoralis major
C   Pectoralis minor
D   Subscapularis
E   Trapezius

6.4.3 Which of the following regarding passage of structures through the diaphragm is **not** correct?
A   The inferior vena cava enters the abdomen through the central tendon of the diaphragm at approximately T8
B   The thoracic duct passes behind the diaphragm with the aorta
C   The hemiazygos vein may enter through the aortic hiatus or left crus
D   The oesophagus passes through the oesophageal hiatus at T12
E   The vagus nerve passes through the diaphragm at T10

6.4.4 Which of the following is **not** contained within the coronary sulcus?
A   Great cardiac vein
B   Small cardiac vein
C   Coronary sinus
D   Circumflex branch of left coronary artery
E   Right coronary artery

6.4.5 Which of the following regarding the internal structure of the heart is correct?
A   Crista terminalis is smooth myocardium within the left atrium
B   Pectinate muscles are found on the inner walls of the ventricles
C   The septomarginal trabecula is found in the right ventricle
D   The septal papillary muscle is the largest
E   Conus arteriosus derives from the embryonic primitive ventricle

6.4.6 Which of the following is a branch of the right coronary artery?
A   Circumflex
B   Marginal
C   Anterior interventricular
D   Diagonal
E   Posterior interventricular branch of circumflex branch

6.4.7 Which of the following structures is **not** found in the superior mediastinum?
A   Thymus
B   Left brachiocephalic vein
C   Superior vena cava
D   Left recurrent laryngeal nerve
E   Oesophageal plexus

6.4.8 Which of the following are **not** correctly matched relationships of the sternum to the vertebral column?
  A Manubrium T3–T4
  B Sternal angle T4–T5
  C Body of sternum T5–T9
  D Xiphisternal joint T9
  E Xiphoid process T12

6.4.9 Which of the following joints of the thoracic wall is a symphysis?
  A Manubriosternal
  B Xiphisternal
  C Interchondral
  D Costochondral
  E Sternocostal

6.4.10 Which of the following arteries does **not** supply an arterial branch to the breast?
  A Subclavian
  B Internal thoracic
  C Lateral thoracic
  D Brachial
  E Axillary

6.4.11 Which of the following lymph nodes are **not** axillary?
  A Apical
  B Supraclavicular
  C Pectoral
  D Humeral
  E Subscapular

6.4.12 Which of the following muscles of the thorax attaches to the nuchal ligament superiorly and to the superior borders of 2nd – 5th ribs inferiorly?
  A Transversus thoracis
  B Subcostalis
  C Levatores costarum
  D Serratus posterior superior
  E Serratus posterior inferior

6.4.13 Which of the following regarding the lungs is **not** correct?
  A Bifurcation of the trachea occurs at the level of the sternal angle
  B Right main bronchus passes directly to the hilum of the right lung
  C Left main bronchus passes superior to the aortic arch and posterior to the oesophagus
  D Left bronchial arteries arise from the thoracic aorta
  E Nerves of the lungs contain parasympathetic fibres from the vagus nerve

6.4.14 Which of the following regarding the pericardium is correct?
  A Serous pericardium is continuous with the central tendon of the diaphragm
  B Sternopericardial ligaments attach fibrous pericardium to the posterior surface of the sternum
  C Pericardiacophrenic arteries are branches of the aortic arch
  D Myocardium is composed of visceral serous pericardium
  E Nerve supply of the pericardium is predominantly from the vagus nerve

6.4.15 Which of the following regarding ligaments of the back is **not** correct?
  A The anterior longitudinal ligament is attached superiorly to the base of the skull and anteriorly to the sacrum
  B The posterior longitudinal ligament lines the anterior surface of the vertebral canal
  C The ligamentum flava forms part of the posterior surface of the vertebral canal
  D The ligamentum nuchae extends from the external occipital protuberance to the foramen magnum, and then extends inferiorly, where the apex is attached to the spinous process of C4
  E Interspinous ligaments blend with supraspinous ligaments posteriorly and the ligamentum flava anteriorly

6.4.16 Which of the following muscles is innervated by the thoracodorsal nerve?
A Latissimus dorsi
B Trapezius
C Rhomboid major
D Rhomboid minor
E Levator scapulae

6.4.17 Which of the following muscles is **not** involved in adduction?
A Latissimus dorsi
B Trapezius
C Rhomboid major
D Rhomboid minor
E Levator scapulae

6.4.18 Which of the following vertebrae contain an uncinate process?
A C6
B T3
C T9
D L4
E S2

6.4.19 Which of the following arteries does **not** supply the spinal cord?
A Posterior intercostal
B Segmental spinal
C Superior radicular
D Segmental medullary
E Posterior spinal

Questions 6.4.20 to 6.4.23 relate to the following figure.

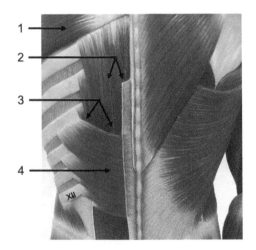

6.4.20 Which of the following nerves supplies muscle labelled 1?
A Thoracodorsal
B Accessory
C Suprascapular
D Dorsal scapular
E Axillary

6.4.21 Which of the following muscles corresponds to label 2?
A Splenius cervicis
B Spinalis
C Longissimus
D Iliocostalis
E Multifidus

6.4.22 Which of the following arteries supplies muscle labelled 3?
A Musculophrenic
B Lateral thoracic
C Superior intercostal
D Anterior intercostal
E Lumbar

6.4.23 Which of the following functions of muscle labelled 4 is correct?
A Depresses ribs
B Elevates ribs
C Moves ribs superiorly
D Move ribs inferiorly
E Depresses costal cartilages

Questions 6.4.24 to 6.4.29 relate to the following structures.

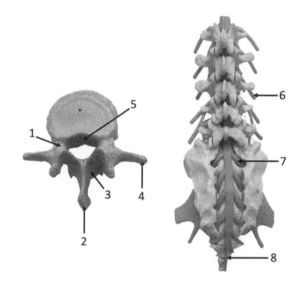

6.4.24 Which of the following vertebral structures match labels 1–4?

	1	2	3	4
A	Lamina	Spinous process	Pedicle	Transverse process
B	Pedicle	Spinous process	Lamina	Transverse process
C	Pedicle	Transverse process	Lamina	Spinous process
D	Lamina	Pedicle	Spinous process	Transverse process
E	Pedicle	Lamina	Transverse process	Spinous process

6.4.25 Which of the following ligaments, which runs almost the entire length of the spine, is found in region labelled 5?
A Ligamentum flavum
B Anterior longitudinal ligament
C Posterior longitudinal ligament
D Supraspinous ligament
E Interspinous ligament

6.4.26 Which of the following nerve roots is **not** a division of nerve labelled 6?
A Genitofemoral
B Femoral
C Obturator
D Accessory obturator
E Lateral femoral cutaneous

6.4.27 Which of the following would result from compression of nerve root labelled 7?
  A Diminished knee extension
  B Diminished toe adduction
  C Diminished great toe extension
  D Diminished ankle plantarflexion
  E Diminished toe dorsiflexion

6.4.28 Which of the following is structure labelled 8 a continuation of?
  A Arachnoid mater
  B Dura mater
  C Pia mater
  D Glia limitans
  E Subdural space

6.4.29 Which of the following is the vertebrae shown (left) most likely to represent?
  A C2
  B C6
  C T4
  D T11
  E L3

Questions 6.4.30 to 6.4.36 relate to the following CT figures.

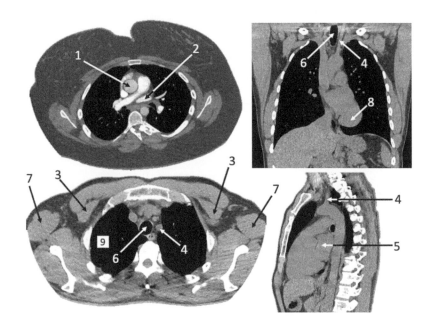

6.4.30 Which of the following corresponds to structure labelled 1?
  A Superior vena cava
  B Inferior vena cava
  C Ascending aorta
  D Descending aorta
  E Trachea

6.4.31 Which of the following corresponds to structure labelled 2?
  A Pulmonary vein
  B Pulmonary artery
  C Descending aorta
  D Ascending aorta
  E Superior vena cava

6.4.32 Which of the following muscles corresponds to label 3?
A Pectoralis minor
B Pectoralis major
C Serratus anterior
D Platysma
E Sternocleidomastoid

6.4.33 Which of the following corresponds to structures labelled 4–6?

	4	5	6	7
A	Left common carotid artery	Left atrium	Oesophagus	Teres major
B	Left subclavian artery	Left ventricle	Trachea	Deltoid
C	Left common carotid artery	Left ventricle	Trachea	Subscapularis
D	Left subclavian artery	Left atrium	Trachea	Deltoid
E	Left subclavian artery	Left atrium	Oesophagus	Teres major

6.4.34 Which of the following vertebral levels is shown in the top left figure?
A T3
B T6
C T8
D T10
E T12

6.4.35 Which of the following is correct regarding structure labelled 8?
A Coarse but fewer trabeculations are evident in the myocardium
B There are three papillary muscles which attach to valves via chordae tendineae
C It is the most anterior of the four chambers
D Bachmann's bundle is present
E Perimysial tendons increase in diameter in the hypertrophied heart

6.4.36 Which of the following lung segments corresponds to label 9 at this vertebral level?
A Lateral middle lobe
B Superior lower lobe
C Lateral lower lobe
D Apical upper lobe
E Posterior upper lobe

6.4.37 Which of the following regarding the phrenic nerve is correct?
A It originates in the spinal cervical roots C4–C6
B It contains only motor fibres
C The right is longer than the left
D The oesophageal hiatus transmits the right phrenic nerve
E The left phrenic nerve descends between the left common carotid and left subclavian arteries

Questions 6.4.38 to 6.4.40 relate to the following figure.

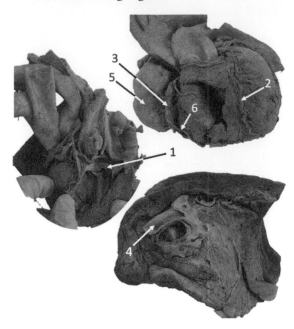

6.4.38 Which of the following structures correspond to labels 1–4?

	1	2	3	4
A	Mitral valve	Left marginal artery	Right coronary artery	Left bronchus
B	Mitral valve	Anterior interventricular artery	Conal artery	Right pulmonary artery
C	Tricuspid valve	Anterior interventricular artery	Right coronary artery	Right bronchus
D	Aortic valve	Circumflex artery	Posterior interventricular artery	Left pulmonary artery
E	Tricuspid valve	Anterior interventricular artery	Right marginal artery	Right bronchus

6.4.39 Which of the following is found within structure labelled 5?
  A Crista terminalis
  B Chordae tendineae
  C Trabeculae carneae
  D Conus arteriosus
  E Moderator band

6.4.40 Which of the following ECG leads is most likely to show acute changes (ST-segment elevation) in electrical activity resulting from occlusion of structure labelled 6?
  A Lead I
  B Lead III
  C Lead aVL
  D Lead V2
  E Lead V4

6.4.41 Which of the following regarding ribs is **not** correct?
  A Subclavius attaches to the first rib
  B Ribs eleven and twelve have no tubercles
  C Internal intercostal muscle fibres extend anteroinferiorly
  D Transversus thoracis attaches to the inferior aspect of the xiphoid process
  E Serratus anterior attaches to the tuberosity of the second rib

6.4.42 Which of the following is **not** correct regarding the thymus?
A Venous drainage is usually via the right brachiocephalic vein
B It lies posterior to the manubrium
C Arterial supply is primarily from branches of the internal thoracic arteries
D With age, it diminishes in size and is largely replaced by adipose tissue
E Lymphatic drainage is via parasternal lymph nodes

6.4.43 Which of the following is correct regarding the ligamentum arteriosum?
A It is an embryological remnant of the truncus arteriosus
B It is the level at which the left recurrent laryngeal nerve curves behind and below the aortic arch
C It is often obliterated in adults
D It is located at the level of the transpyloric plane
E It connects the pulmonary trunk and ascending aorta

Questions 6.4.44 to 6.4.46 relate to the following figure.

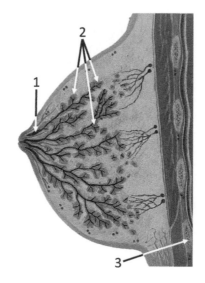

6.4.44 Which of the following corresponds to structure label 1?
A Alveoli
B Suspensory ligament
C Lactiferous sinus
D Lactiferous duct
E Lobule

6.4.45 Which of the following is secreted from structures labelled 2?
A Sweat
B Oxytocin
C Milk
D Prolactin
E Oestrogen

6.4.46 Which of the following ribs corresponds to label 3?
A Fourth rib
B Fifth rib
C Sixth rib
D Seventh rib
E Eighth rib

6.4.47 Which of the following regarding the lungs is correct?
   A The vagus and phrenic nerves pass anterior and posterior to the lung roots, respectively
   B The lingula is found in the right lung
   C The right lung is smaller than the left lung
   D There are ten bronchopulmonary segments in the right lung
   E Each lung has four surfaces

6.4.48 Which of the following rib levels do pleural reflections extend in the midaxillary line?
   A 6th rib
   B 7th rib
   C 8th rib
   D 10th rib
   E 12th rib

6.4.49 Which of the following regarding the oesophagus is correct?
   A Anteriorly are the right pulmonary artery and left main bronchus
   B It begins at C8
   C It passes through the central tendon at T10
   D It is partly innervated by the phrenic nerve
   E It lies posterior to the left atrium

6.4.50 Which of the following regarding cardiac veins is correct?
   A The middle cardiac vein begins between the right atrium and ventricle
   B The anterior cardiac vein enters the right atrium
   C The small cardiac vein ascends in the posterior interventricular sulcus
   D The posterior cardiac vein lies on the posterior surface of the left atrium
   E Venae cordis minimae are mostly associated with the left ventricle

6.5   Abdomen, pelvis and reproductive organs

6.5.1 Which of the following abdominal incisions (1–5) correctly matches the name?

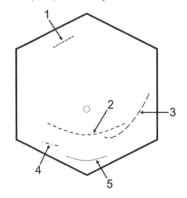

	1	2	3	4	5
A	Lanz	Maylard	Rutherford-Morison	Kocher	Pfannenstiel
B	Rutherford-Morison	Pfannenstiel	Maylard	Kocher	Lanz
C	Kocher	Maylard	Rutherford-Morison	Lanz	Pfannenstiel
D	Kocher	Rutherford-Morison	Lanz	Maylard	Pfannenstiel
E	Kocher	Pfannenstiel	Rutherford-Morison	Lanz	Maylard

6.5.2 Which of the following does **not** drain into inferior mesenteric lymph nodes?
   A Distal third of transverse colon
   B Sigmoid colon
   C Rectum
   D Ascending colon
   E Descending colon

6.5.3 Which of the following arteries is a direct branch of the coeliac trunk?
  A Gastroduodenal
  B Left gastric
  C Right gastric
  D Short gastric
  E Dorsal pancreatic

6.5.4 Which of the following is **not** contained within the spermatic cord?
  A Ductus deferens
  B Testicular artery
  C Cremasteric vein
  D Ilioinguinal nerve
  E Pampiniform plexus

6.5.5 Which of the following arteries arises superior to the inguinal ligament and enters the rectus sheath below the arcuate line?
  A Superior epigastric
  B Inferior epigastric
  C Superficial epigastric
  D Superficial circumflex iliac
  E Deep circumflex iliac

6.5.6 Which of the following structures forms the posterior (medial) wall of the superficial inguinal ring?
  A Lacunar ligament
  B Aponeurosis of external oblique
  C Conjoint tendon
  D Transversalis fascia
  E Inguinal ligament

6.5.7 Which of the following nerves innervates the cremaster muscle?
  A Ilioinguinal nerve
  B Posterior femoral cutaneous nerve
  C Anterior scrotal nerve
  D Posterior perineal nerve
  E Genitofemoral nerve

6.5.8 Which of the following muscles is innervated by the anterior rami of S1 and S2 and attaches to the greater trochanter of the femur?
  A Piriformis
  B Obturator internus
  C Coccygeus
  D Pubococcygeus
  E Iliococcygeus

6.5.9 Which of the following muscles' origin is the lateral one third of the inguinal ligament?
  A External oblique
  B Internal oblique
  C Transversus abdominis
  D Rectus abdominis
  E Pyramidalis

6.5.10 Which of the following arteries does **not** supply deeper structures of the anterolateral abdominal wall?
  A Superior epigastric
  B Musculophrenic
  C Subcostal
  D Inferior epigastric
  E Deep circumflex iliac

6.5.11 Which of the following arteries gives rise to the inferior epigastric artery?
   A Common iliac
   B Inferior mesenteric
   C External iliac
   D Femoral
   E Median sacral

6.5.12 Which of the following arteries is **not** a branch of the abdominal aorta?
   A Superior mesenteric
   B Middle suprarenal
   C Testicular
   D Superior phrenic
   E Inferior phrenic

6.5.13 Which of the following regarding structures labelled (1–5) is correct?

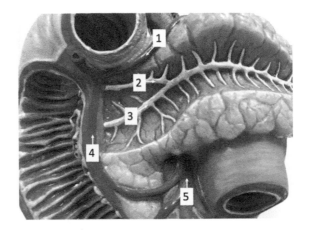

   A The origin of (1) arises anterior to the lower part of L1
   B (2) drains into the major duodenal papilla
   C (3) unites with the common bile duct via the ampulla of Vater
   D Terminal branches of (4) anastomose with the splenic artery
   E The first branch of (5) is the middle colic artery

6.5.14 Which of the following branches of the lumbar plexus is **not** correctly matched to the associated spinal segments?
   A Femoral nerve – L4
   B Iliohypogastric nerve – L1
   C Obturator nerve – L3
   D Genitofemoral nerve – L3
   E Ilioinguinal nerve – L1

6.5.15 Which of the following branches of the lumbar plexus emerges medial to psoas major?
   A Femoral nerve
   B Iliohypogastric nerve
   C Obturator nerve
   D Genitofemoral nerve
   E Ilioinguinal nerve

6.5.16 Which of the following vertebral levels is the transpyloric plane located?
   A T10
   B T11
   C T12
   D L1
   E L2

6.5.17 Which of the following regarding blood supply to the stomach is correct?
  A The left gastric artery supplies the greater curvature
  B The right gastric artery is a branch of the hepatic artery proper
  C The right gastroepiploic artery is a branch of the splenic artery
  D Short gastric arteries supply the pylorus
  E The posterior gastric artery is a branch of the right gastric artery

6.5.18 Which of the following is a direct continuation of the omental bursa?
  A Left paracolic gutter
  B Pouch of Morison
  C Left subphrenic space
  D Right subphrenic recess
  E Infracolic compartment

6.5.19 Which of the following regarding blood supply to the abdominal viscera is correct?
  A Ileocolic artery from the inferior mesenteric artery supplies the ileum
  B Anterior and posterior caecal arteries supply the caecum and ascending colon
  C Left colic artery from the superior mesenteric artery supplies the transverse colon
  D Middle rectal arteries from the internal pudendal artery supply the rectum and anal canal
  E Superior rectal artery is a direct branch of the internal iliac artery

6.5.20 Which of the following structures is retroperitoneal?
  A Oesophagus
  B Transverse colon
  C Stomach
  D Tail of pancreas
  E First part of duodenum

6.5.21 Which of the following ligaments of the liver results from the union of the coronary ligaments on the posteroinferior surface?
  A Falciform
  B Hepatogastric
  C Hepatoduodenal
  D Triangular
  E Ligamentum teres

6.5.22 Which of the following arteries divide into the hepatic arteries close to the porta hepatis?
  A Common hepatic
  B Hepatic artery proper
  C Gastroduodenal
  D Cystic
  E Supraduodenal

6.5.23 Which of the following structures does **not** drain into the inferior mesenteric vein?
  A Splenic flexure
  B Sigmoid colon
  C Rectum
  D Descending colon
  E Transverse colon

6.5.24 Which of the following is the correct sequence of artery branches from the abdominal aorta?
  A Coeliac trunk → common hepatic → cystic
  B Coeliac trunk → right gastric → gastroduodenal
  C Inferior mesenteric → right colic → superior rectal
  D Superior mesenteric → ileocolic → appendicular
  E Superior mesenteric → anterior superior pancreaticoduodenal → inferior pancreaticoduodenal

6.5.25 Which of the following vessels does the left suprarenal vein drain into?

A Azygos vein

B Hemiazygos vein

C Superior mesenteric vein

D Inferior vena cava

E Left renal vein

6.5.26 Which of the following vessels (1–3) and muscle to which (4) supplies is correct?

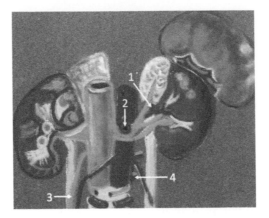

	1	2	3	4
	Artery	Artery	Vein	Supplies
A	Renal	Coeliac	Gonadal	Psoas minor
B	Inferior suprarenal	Superior mesenteric	Gonadal	Quadratus lumborum
C	Middle suprarenal	Coeliac	2nd lumbar	Psoas minor
D	Middle suprarenal	Inferior mesenteric	Gonadal	Quadratus lumborum
E	Inferior suprarenal	Superior mesenteric	3rd lumbar	Psoas major

6.5.27 Which of the following splanchnic nerves travels to the renal plexus?

A Greater

B Lesser

C Least

D Lumbar

E Sacral

6.5.28 Which of the following structures match the sites to which they attach (1–4)?

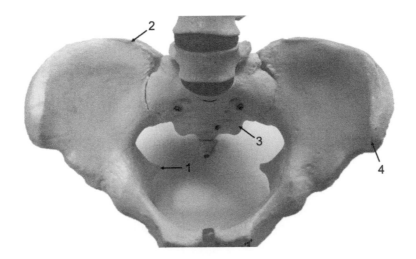

	1	2	3	4
A	Coccygeus	External oblique	Obturator internus	Sartorius
B	Inferior gamellus	Transversus abdominis	Sacrotuberous ligament	Internal oblique
C	Superior gamellus	External oblique	Sacrospinous ligament	Tensor fascia lata
D	Sacrospinous ligament	Quadratus lumborum	Piriformis	Sartorius
E	Sacrospinous ligament	Erector spinae	Piriformis	Transversus abdominus

6.5.29 Which of the following regarding the pelvis is correct?
A The pectineal line forms the posterior border of the superior pubic ramus
B The pelvic outlet (inferior aperture) is bound by the sacrotuberous ligament anteriorly
C The false pelvis lies between the pelvic inlet and outlet
D In males, the pubic arch is wider, and the obturator foramen is oval- shaped
E In females, the acetabulum is smaller, and the greater sciatic notch is wider

6.5.30 Which of the following muscles forms the boundary of the anterolateral wall of the pelvis?
A Piriformis
B Obturator internus
C Obturator externus
D Coccygeus
E Levator ani

6.5.31 Which of the following nerves is **not** a branch of the sacral plexus?
A Sciatic
B Pudendal
C Lateral femoral cutaneous
D Superior gluteal
E Inferior gluteal

6.5.32 Which of the following regarding arteries of the pelvis is **not** correct?
A The obturator artery exits the obturator canal and supplies muscles of the medial thigh
B The inferior vesical artery in males is homologous to the vaginal artery in females
C The uterine artery enters the root of the broad ligament
D The internal pudendal artery enters the ischioanal fossa through the greater sciatic foramen
E The superior gluteal artery supplies gluteus minimus

6.5.33 Which of the following structures are **not** correctly matched to the lymph nodes into which they drain?
A Epididymis – external iliac lymph nodes
B Ovaries – lumbar lymph nodes
C Prostate – internal iliac lymph nodes
D Glans of clitoris – deep inguinal lymph nodes
E Sigmoid colon – inferior mesenteric lymph nodes

6.5.34 Which of the following is **not** a boundary of the lesser sciatic foramen?
A Anteriorly, ischial tuberosity
B Posteriorly, sacrotuberous ligament
C Superiorly, sacrospinous ligament
D Inferiorly, nerve to obturator internus
E Superiorly, ischial spine

6.5.35 Which of the following arteries supplies the seminal vesicles?
A Superior vesical
B Inferior vesical
C Obturator
D Superior rectal
E Inferior gluteal

6.5.36 Which of the following veins directly drain the anterior aspect of the labia majora in women and scrotum in men?

A   Inferior rectal

B   Internal pudendal

C   External pudendal

D   Femoral

E   Great saphenous

6.5.37 Which of the following regarding the perineum is correct?

A   In males, the superficial perineal pouch contains no erectile tissue

B   It is bound laterally by the ischial spines

C   The dorsal nerve of the clitoris is a branch of the perineal nerve

D   Lymphatics from skin of the penis drain into superficial inguinal nodes

E   In females, cremasteric arteries are absent

6.5.38 Which of the following describes the correct relation of the fundus of the bladder to the vagina?

A   Anterior

B   Posterior

C   Superior

D   Inferior

E   Lateral

6.5.39 Which of the following regarding the uterus is correct?

A   The vesicouterine pouch separates the body of the uterus and bladder

B   The pouch of Douglas lies in close proximity to the anterior fornix of the vagina

C   The broad ligament is a remnant of the ovarian gubernaculum

D   The largest part of the broad ligament is the mesovarium

E   A normal uterus rests in a retroverted, retroflexed position

6.5.40 Which of the following lines demarcate the visceral–parietal transition point in the anal canal?

A   Shenton's

B   Arcuate

C   Hilton's

D   Pectineal

E   Dentate

6.5.41 Which of the following regarding the urogenital triangle is correct?

A   It is bound posteriorly by the ischiopubic rami

B   Bartholin's glands are present in males

C   Skene's glands open into the vulvar vestibule

D   Muscle development is greater in females

E   Corpus spongiosum is found on either side

Questions 6.5.42 to 6.5.43 relate to the following figure.

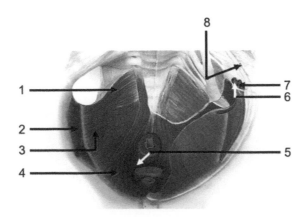

6.5.42 Which of the following muscles match labels (1–5)?

	1	2	3	4	5
A	Coccygeus	Obturator internus	Iliococcygeus	Pubococcygeus	Puborectalis
B	Coccygeus	Piriformis	Pubococcygeus	Iliococcygeus	Puborectalis
C	Piriformis	Obturator internus	Iliococcygeus	Pubococcygeus	Puborectalis
D	Obturator internus	Piriformis	Iliococcygeus	Pubococcygeus	Puborectalis
E	Coccygeus	Obturator internus	Pubococcygeus	Puborectalis	Iliococcygeus

6.5.43 Which of the following regarding labels (6–8) is correct?
A The terminal branch of (8) innervates the skin of the penis/clitoris
B (6) re-enters the pelvis via the greater sciatic foramen and then drains into the internal iliac vein
C (8) arises from the anterior rami of L2–L4 and accompanies (6–7) to supply the medial compartment of the thigh
D A branch of (7) supplies the scrotum in males and labia in females
E (6–7) leave the pelvis through the greater sciatic foramen inferior to piriformis

6.5.44 Which of the following is **not** a correct boundary of the anal triangle?
A Anteriorly, horizontal line between ischial tuberosities
B Posteriorly, tip of coccyx
C Roof, levator ani
D Laterally, sacrotuberous ligament
E Base, inferior pubic rami

6.5.45 Which of the following regarding the genitourinary system is correct?
A The seminal colliculus is located within the membranous urethra
B In the female pelvis, the uterine artery crosses the ureter
C Medial to the infundibulum of the uterine tubes is the expanded isthmus
D The prostate lies posterior to the bladder
E In males, the pubovesical ligaments support the bladder

6.5.46 Which of the following is most ventral in the penis?
A Corpus cavernosum
B Corpus spongiosum
C Urethra
D Deep artery of penis
E Superficial dorsal vein

6.5.47 Which of the following is **not** innervated by the perineal branch of the pudendal nerve?
A Bulbospongiosus
B Ischiocavernosus
C Superficial transverse perineal muscles
D External anal sphincter
E External urethral sphincter

Questions 6.5.48 to 6.5.50 relate to the following figure.

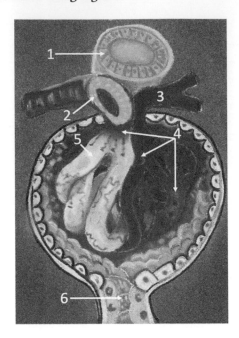

6.5.48 Which of the following cells match structures labelled 1, 2, 4 and 6?

	1	2	4	6
A	Lacis	Juxtaglomerular	Fenestrated epithelial	Macula densa
B	Juxtaglomerular	Lacis	Squamous epithelial	Mesangial
C	Cuboidal epithelial	Juxtaglomerular	Squamous epithelial	Macula densa
D	Macula densa	Juxtaglomerular	Fenestrated epithelial	Cuboidal epithelial
E	Macula densa	Mesangial	Fenestrated epithelial	Cuboidal epithelial

6.5.49 Which of the following corresponds with structure labelled 3?
  A Afferent arteriole
  B Efferent arteriole
  C Vasa recta
  D Renal artery
  E Glomerulus

6.5.50 Which of the following regarding structure labelled 5 is **not** correct?
  A Confers charge selectivity to filtered particles
  B Confers size selectivity through fenestrations
  C Restricts movement of cationic particles into Bowman's space
  D Contains podocytes
  E Contains irregularly shaped contractile cells

6.6   Lower limb

6.6.1 Which of the following muscles of the medial compartment of the thigh is innervated by the sciatic nerve?
A Adductor longus
B Adductor brevis
C Adductor magnus
D Gracilis
E Obturator externus

6.6.2 Which of the following muscles attaches to the ischial spine proximally and the medial surface of the greater trochanter of the femur distally?
A Obturator internus
B Quadratus femoris
C Tensor fasciae latae
D Superior gemellus
E Inferior gemellus

6.6.3 Which of the following regarding boundaries of the femoral triangle is correct?
A The medial border is bound by the medial margin of sartorius
B The floor is formed medially by iliopsoas and laterally by pectineus
C The base is formed by the adductor canal
D The superior border is bound by the inguinal ligament
E The roof is formed by adductor longus

6.6.4 Which of the following arteries supplies most of the femoral head and neck?
A Obturator
B Descending genicular
C Medial circumflex
D Lateral circumflex
E Perforating

6.6.5 Which of the following is **not** contained within Hunter's canal?
A Femoral artery
B Femoral vein
C Femoral nerve
D Saphenous nerve
E Nerve to vastus medialis

6.6.6 Which of the following muscles inserts into quadriceps femoris tendon and the lateral margin of the patella?
A Vastus medialis
B Vastus intermedius
C Adductor longus
D Rectus femoris
E Sartorius

6.6.7 Which of the following muscles inserts onto the posterior surface of the medial tibial condyle?
A Semimembranosus
B Semitendinosus
C Long head of biceps femoris
D Short head of biceps femoris
E Hamstring part of adductor magnus

Questions 6.6.8 to 6.6.12 relate to the following MRI figure of the lower limb.

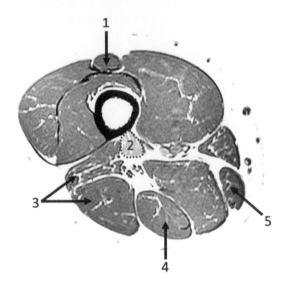

6.6.8 Which of the following is the correct distal attachment of muscle labelled 1?
A   Quadriceps femoris tendon
B   Lesser trochanter of femur
C   Linea aspera
D   Trochanteric fossa
E   Head of fibula

6.6.9 Which of the following is the correct function of muscle labelled 2?
A   Extends the leg at the knee joint and abducts flexed thigh
B   Extends the thigh at the hip joint and abducts the thigh at hip joint
C   Flexes the leg at the knee joint and adducts the thigh at hip joint
D   Medially rotates and adducts the thigh at the hip joint
E   Laterally rotates the thigh at the hip joint and the leg at the knee joint

6.6.10 Which of the following is correct regarding muscle labelled 3?
A   It is innervated by the femoral nerve
B   It laterally rotates the thigh at the hip joint
C   It medially rotates the leg at the knee joint
D   It distally attaches to the medial tibial condyle
E   The long head originates from the inferomedial part of the upper area of the ischial spine

6.6.11 Which of the following nerves innervates muscle labelled 4?
A   Posterior femoral cutaneous
B   Lateral sural cutaneous
C   Obturator
D   Femoral
E   Sciatic

6.6.12 Which of the following corresponds to muscle labelled 5?
A   Sartorius
B   Gracilis
C   Vastus medialis
D   Semimembranosus
E   Semitendinosus

Questions 6.6.13 to 6.6.17 relate to the following MRI figure of the lower limb.

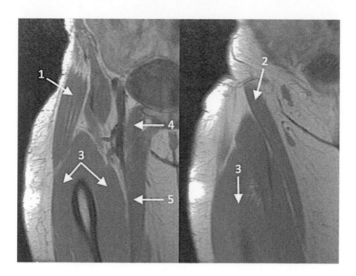

6.6.13 Which of the following muscles corresponds to label 1?
  A Gluteus minimus
  B Gluteus medius
  C Tensor fasciae latae
  D Sartorius
  E Rectus femoris

6.6.14 Which of the following muscles are **not** innervated by the femoral nerve?
  A 1 and 5
  B 1 and 2
  C 2 and 3
  D 2 and 4
  E 4 and 5

6.6.15 Which of the following muscles adducts and flexes the thigh at the hip joint?
  A 1
  B 2
  C 3
  D 4
  E 5

6.6.16 Which of the following muscles does profunda femoris pass between posteriorly?
  A 1 and 2
  B 1 and 3
  C 2 and 3
  D 3 and 5
  E 4 and 5

6.6.17 Which of the following muscles attaches distally to the quadriceps femoris tendon?
  A 1
  B 2
  C 3
  D 4
  E 5

6.6.18 Which of the following is **not** contained within the popliteal fossa?
  A Popliteal vein
  B Small saphenous vein
  C Tibial nerve
  D Posterior cutaneous nerve of the thigh
  E Posterior tibial artery

6.6.19 Which of the following nerves supplies the skin on the posterolateral aspect of the leg and lateral side of the foot?
A Saphenous
B Tibial
C Sural
D Common fibular
E Superficial fibular

6.6.20 Which of the following bones of the foot does tibialis posterior insert into?
A Cuboid and first metatarsal
B Navicular and talus
C Medial cuneiform and fifth metatarsal
D Navicular and medial cuneiform
E Cuboid and talus

6.6.21 Which of the following muscles proximal attachment is the lateral femoral condyle?
A Plantaris
B Popliteus
C Medial head of gastrocnemius
D Fibularis longus
E Soleus

6.6.22 Which of the following arteries branches into the medial and lateral plantar arteries?
A Peroneal
B Posterior tibial
C Anterior tibial
D Fibular
E Dorsalis pedis

6.6.23 Which of the following muscles inverts the foot?
A Tibialis posterior
B Fibularis longus
C Flexor digitorum longus
D Flexor hallucis longus
E Plantaris

6.6.24 Which of the following bones of the foot is associated with the sustentaculum tali?
A Sesamoids
B Cuboid
C Talus
D Calcaneus
E Navicular

6.6.25 Which of the following retinacula extends between the calcaneus and lateral malleolus?
A Inferior fibular
B Superior fibular
C Superior extensor
D Inferior extensor
E Flexor

6.6.26 Which of the following veins is formed by the lateral convergence of the dorsal venous arch?
A Medial marginal
B Lateral marginal
C Great saphenous
D Small saphenous
E Dorsal metatarsal

6.6.27 Which of the following is **not** contained within the tarsal tunnel?
A Tibial nerve
B Posterior tibial artery
C Tibialis posterior tendon
D Flexor hallucis longus tendon
E Flexor digitorum brevis

6.6.28 Which of the following joints of the foot is stabilised by the interosseous talocalcaneal ligament?
A Talocalcaneonavicular
B Calcaneocuboid
C Subtalar
D Interphalangeal
E Metatarsophalangeal

6.6.29 Which of the following muscles is innervated by the lateral plantar nerve?
A Abductor hallucis
B Flexor digitorum brevis
C First lumbrical
D Flexor hallucis brevis
E Flexor digiti minimi brevis

6.6.30 Which of the following regarding dorsal interossei of the feet is **not** correct?
A There are four in the sole of the foot
B All four muscles are bipennate
C The third and fourth toes only have one on their lateral sides
D They adduct toes three to five
E The deep fibular nerve innervates the first and second interossei

6.6.31 Which of the following does **not** form part of the deltoid ligament of the ankle?
A Calcaneofibular
B Tibionavicular
C Tibiocalcaneal
D Posterior tibiotalar
E Anterior tibiotalar

6.6.32 Which of the following is the main action of fibularis tertius?
A Dorsiflexion of the ankle, eversion of the foot
B Plantarflexion of the ankle, eversion of the foot
C Dorsiflexion of the ankle, inversion of the foot
D Plantarflexion of the ankle, inversion of the foot
E Dorsiflexion of the ankle, extension of the lateral four digits

6.6.33 Which of the following muscles are **not** innervated predominantly by S2?
A Plantaris
B Soleus
C Flexor hallucis longus
D Flexor digitorum longus
E Extensor digitorum longus

Questions 6.6.34 to 6.6.36 relate to the following MRI figure of the knee.

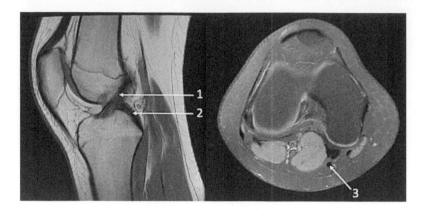

6.6.34 Which of the following ligaments corresponds to label 1?
A Lateral collateral
B Medial collateral
C Oblique popliteal
D Anterior cruciate
E Posterior cruciate

6.6.35 Which of the following is the correct function of structure labelled 2?
A It serves to resist excessive posterior translation of the tibia
B In extension, it is the stabiliser of the femur
C It originates from the lateral femoral condyle
D It has a posteromedial bundle which tightens when the knee is flexed
E It decreases the amount of stress on the knee joint

6.6.36 Which of the following corresponds to label 3?
A Tendon of semimembranosus
B Tendon of semitendinosus
C Great saphenous vein
D Popliteal artery
E Tendon of gracilis

6.6.37 Which of the following is correct regarding muscles labelled 1 and 2?

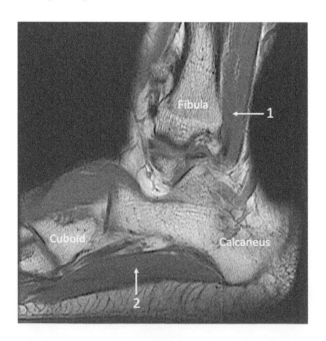

A 1 plantarflexes the foot and 2 corresponds to abductor hallucis
B 1 everts the foot and 2 corresponds to flexor digitorum brevis
C 1 extends the lateral four toes and 2 corresponds to abductor hallucis
D 1 everts the foot and 2 corresponds to abductor digiti minimi
E 1 plantarflexes the foot and 2 corresponds to abductor digiti minimi

Questions 6.6.38 to 6.6.40 relate to the following axial MRI.

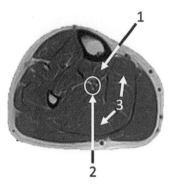

6.6.38 Which of the following muscles corresponds with label 1?
   A Tibialis anterior
   B Tibialis posterior
   C Flexor digitorum longus
   D Flexor hallucis longus
   E Extensor digitorum longus

6.6.39 Which of the following nerves is found within label 2?
   A Tibial
   B Superficial fibular
   C Deep fibular
   D Sural
   E Saphenous

6.6.40 Which of the following is correct regarding muscle labelled 3?
   A It dorsiflexes the foot
   B It is innervated by the sural nerve
   C It is supplied by the anterior tibial artery
   D It originates from the posterior aspect of the fibular head
   E It inserts into the dorsomedial surface of the base of the 5th metatarsal

Questions 6.6.41 to 6.6.43 relate to the following axial MRI figure of the lower limb.

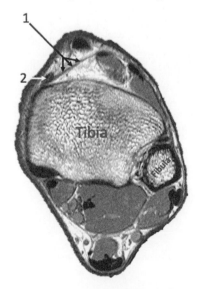

6.6.41 Which of the following muscle tendons is **not** evident?
   A Flexor digitorum longus
   B Tibialis posterior
   C Popliteus
   D Tibialis anterior
   E Extensor digitorum longus

6.6.42 Which of the following structures corresponds with label 1?
   A Superior fibular retinaculum
   B Inferior fibular retinaculum
   C Superior extensor retinaculum
   D Inferior extensor retinaculum
   E Flexor retinaculum

6.6.43 Which of the following structures corresponds with label 2?
   A Small saphenous vein
   B Peroneal vein
   C Posterior tibial artery
   D Sural nerve
   E Great saphenous vein

Questions 6.6.44 to 6.6.46 relate to the following radiograph of the lower limb.

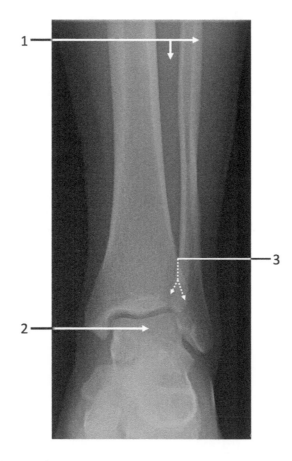

6.6.44 Which of the following muscles attaches proximally at regions labelled 1?
   A Tibialis anterior
   B Extensor hallucis longus
   C Extensor digitorum longus
   D Fibularis tertius
   E Fibularis longus

6.6.45 Which of the following arteries does **not** supply structure labelled 2?
  A Tarsal sinus
  B Anterior tibial
  C Tarsal canal
  D Deltoid
  E Lateral plantar

6.6.46 Which of the following terms describes the fibrous connection found within region labelled 3?
  A Pseudoarthrosis
  B Epiphysiodesis
  C Aponeurosis
  D Syndesmosis
  E Articulation

Questions 6.6.47 to 6.6.50 relate to the following radiograph of the ankle and foot.

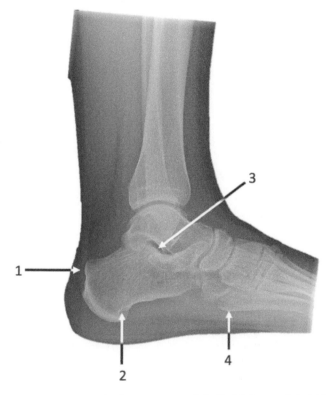

6.6.47 Which of the following nerve roots are tested when structure labelled 1 is struck briskly?
  A L3–L4
  B L4–L5
  C L5–S1
  D S1–S2
  E S2–S3

6.6.48 Which of the following is the correct innervation and action of the muscle that has its proximal attachment on the medial surface and lateral process of region labelled 2?

	Innervation	Action
A	Lateral plantar nerve	Flexion of lateral four toes
B	Lateral plantar nerve	Flexion of great toe
C	Medial plantar nerve	Flexion of lateral four toes
D	Medial plantar nerve	Flexion of great toe
E	Lateral plantar nerve	Abduction of toes 2–4

6.6.49 Which of the following ligaments is found within region labelled 3?
   A Talonavicular
   B Long plantar
   C Plantar calcaneocuboid
   D Calcaneofibular
   E Interosseous talocalcaneal

6.6.50 Which of the following attaches proximally at region labelled 4?
   A Flexor digitorum brevis
   B Abductor digiti minimi
   C Flexor digiti minimi brevis
   D Lumbricals
   E Dorsal interossei

Answers

6.1.1 *E – Stylohyoid*

Stylohyoid is innervated by the facial nerve; hence E is the correct response. Mylohyoid and the anterior belly of digastric are innervated by the mylohyoid nerve, a division of the inferior alveolar nerve which is a branch of the trigeminal nerve (V_3). The posterior belly of digastric is innervated by the facial nerve. Omohyoid, sternohyoid and thyrohyoid are innervated by the anterior rami of C1–C3, carried by a branch of the ansa cervicalis.

6.1.2 *C – posterior border of sternocleidomastoid, anterior border of trapezius and middle third of clavicle*

As shown in the figure below, C is the correct response.

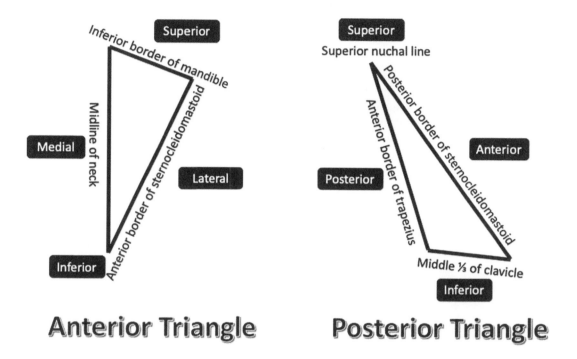

Anterior Triangle   **Posterior Triangle**

6.1.3 *D – Hypoglossal nerve passes medial to internal and external carotid arteries*

The hypoglossal nerve enters the skull via the hypoglossal canal in the occipital bone. It then continues through the nasopharyngeal space, passing medial to the internal carotid artery and internal jugular vein. At the transverse process of C1 it turns and runs on the lateral surface of the internal and external carotid arteries (not medial). It then enters the digastric triangle of the neck, deep to the posterior belly of the digastric muscle. It then descends and joins the cervical rami of C2 and C3 of the ansa cervicalis; hence D is the correct response.

6.1.4 *E – The maxillary division exits the skull through the foramen rotundum*

The middle cranial fossa is composed of the sphenoid and paired temporal bones. The sphenoid bone contains a number of foramina, including the foramen rotundum, foramen ovale, foramen spinosum, foramen lacerum and the optic canal. The foramen rotundum transmits the maxillary division (V_2) of the trigeminal nerve; hence E is the correct response. The sensory nuclei merge at the level of the pons (not the medulla) to form a sensory root which expands into the trigeminal ganglion. The lingual nerve supplies sensory innervation to the anterior two-thirds of the tongue. Taste to the posterior one-third of the tongue is accomplished via innervation from the glossopharyngeal nerve. The zygomatic nerve originates in the pterygopalatine fossa and passes into the orbit via the inferior orbital fissure (not the superior). The pterygopalatine ganglion (or sphenopalatine ganglion) lies in the pterygoid fossa and is the main parasympathetic ganglion of the upper jaw. Preganglionic axons reach the pterygopalatine ganglion from the greater petrosal nerve (a branch of the facial nerve) and the Vidian nerve (nerve of pterygoid canal).

6.1.5 *A – Glossopharyngeal*

The superior orbital fissure transmits the oculomotor, trochlear and abducens nerves, and the ophthalmic division (V_1) of the trigeminal nerve. The glossopharyngeal nerve originates in the medulla oblongata and exits the skull via the jugular foramen; hence A is the correct response.

6.1.6 *C – The caudate nucleus lies in the wall of the lateral ventricle*

The caudate nucleus is a large C-shaped structure with a head, body and tail found within the basal ganglia. It forms the lateral wall of the frontal horn and the body of the lateral ventricle; hence C is the correct response. The precentral gyrus is the location of the primary motor cortex and found on the lateral surface of the frontal lobe (not parietal). The cingulate sulcus is found on the medial surface of the anterior cerebrum (not lateral). The word 'cingulate' is derived from the Latin word for 'belt', which is apt given the fact the cingulate cortex (sulcus and gyrus) surrounds the corpus callosum. The occipital lobe is primarily responsible for visual processing as it contains the primary visual cortex (not auditory). The primary auditory cortex is found within Heschl gyrus, a region of the cerebral cortex in the temporal lobes. The forebrain is composed of the telencephalon, which gives rise to the cerebral hemispheres, and the diencephalon, which gives rise to the thalamus and hypothalamus. The cerebellum is a component of the hindbrain.

6.1.7 *A – Central sulcus*

As shown in the figure below, the central sulcus separates the frontal and parietal lobes; hence A is the correct response. The calcarine sulcus extends from the parieto-occipital sulcus anteriorly to the occipital pole posteriorly. The primary visual cortex is located within and around the calcarine sulcus. The lateral sulcus (Sylvian fissure) separates the frontal and parietal lobes from the temporal lobe. The cingulate sulcus is found on the medial aspect of the anterior cerebral hemispheres, and predominantly in the frontal lobe. It serves to delineate the cingulate gyrus. The lunate sulcus is found in the occipital lobe, and with the inferior occipital sulcus, forms a limit for the boundary between the primary (V1) and secondary (V2) visual cortex.

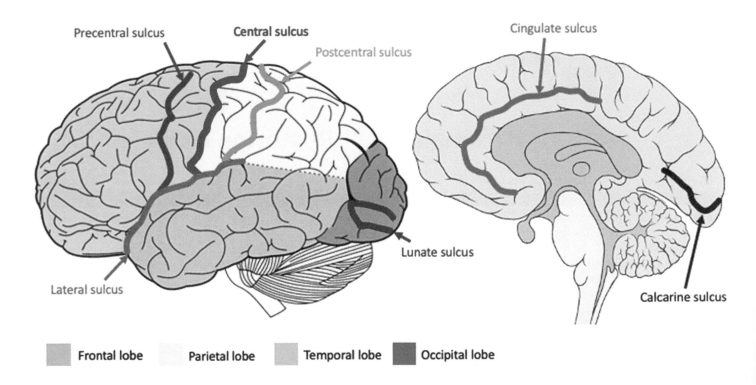

6.1.8 *D – Choroid plexus*

The choroid plexus is a complex network of capillaries located within the pia mater. It has a specialised lining composed of ependymal cells, glial cells which line the ventricles and produce cerebrospinal fluid (CSF); hence D is the correct response. The choroid plexus also serves as a barrier between the blood and the CSF. The superior sagittal sinus is the longest dural sinus which extends along the superior border of the falx cerebri. It receives venous drainage from the superior superficial veins, superior cerebral veins, emissary veins, diploic veins and meningeal veins. It drains into the transverse sinus. The cisterna magna (also known as the cerebellomedullary cistern) is located between the cerebellum and dorsal surface of the medulla oblongata. CSF drains into the cisterna magna from the fourth ventricle via the median (foramen of Magendie) and lateral apertures (foramina of Luschka). The pineal gland lies between the two superior colliculi of the tectum, and functions to secrete melatonin and regulate circadian rhythm. The pontine cistern (prepontine) is located on the anterior surface of the pons and houses the basilar artery within the basilar sulcus, and the abducens nerve. It communicates with the interpeduncular cistern and cisterna magna.

6.1.9 *E – Corpus callosum*

The anterior cerebral artery (ACA) (and middle cerebral artery) is a branch of the internal carotid artery. The two anterior cerebral arteries supply the medial surfaces of the anterior portion of the cerebral hemispheres and the contralateral counterparts anastomose via the anterior communicating artery, forming the anterior components of the circle of Willis. In addition, the ACA supplies the basal forebrain, hypothalamus, corpus callosum, cingulate gyrus and the caudate nucleus. The ACA runs rostromedially towards the interhemispheric (medial longitudinal) cerebral fissure where it curves (posteromedially) around the genu of the corpus callosum. It extends posteriorly along the body of the corpus callosum and eventually anastomoses with the middle and posterior cerebral arteries, beneath the splenium; hence E is the correct response.

6.1.10 *D – Sigmoid*

Venous sinuses of the brain are endothelial-lined spaces between the two layers of the dura mater (endosteal and meningeal layers). The brain is drained by the superficial and deep venous systems and associated with the lateral and medial surfaces of the cerebral cortex, respectively. All cerebral veins typically drain into the nearest sinus, and all sinuses eventually drain into the internal jugular vein. The superior and inferior sagittal sinuses are located in the falx cerebri and drain into the confluence of sinuses and straight sinus, respectively. The superior sagittal and straight, and occipital sinus (in the falx cerebelli) empty into the confluence of sinuses which drain into the left and right transverse sinuses. Each transverse sinus forms an S-shaped sinus anteriorly and inferiorly, the sigmoid sinus, which drains directly into the internal jugular vein; hence D is the correct response. The sigmoid sinuses also receive blood from cerebral, cerebellar, diploic and emissary veins. Emissary veins are clinically significant as they allow passage of infection into the cranial cavity due to their absence of valves. For completeness, the cavernous sinuses are found on the sphenoid bone (lateral to the sella turcica) and drain the ophthalmic veins, the sphenoparietal sinus, cerebral and emissary veins from the pterygoid plexus. The superior petrosal sinuses drain the cavernous sinuses into the transverse sinuses. The inferior petrosal sinuses, which begin at the inferior part of the intercavernous sinus, drain into the internal jugular vein with the sigmoid sinus.

6.1.11 *A – Internal capsule*

As shown in the figure below, the caudate nucleus (head) is partially separated from the putamen by the internal capsule; hence A is the correct response.

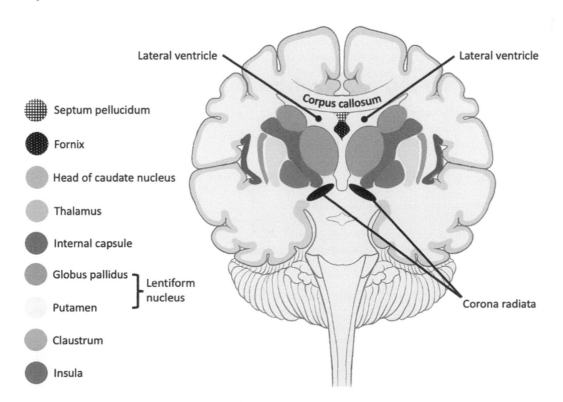

6.1.12 *B – Lateral ventricle – caudate head – claustrum – corona radiata*

As shown in the figure in 6.1.11, most rostrally is the anterior horn of the lateral ventricle, followed by the head of the caudate nucleus, the claustrum and finally, most caudally, is the corona radiata; hence B is the correct response.

6.1.13 *C – 4*

There are four colliculi in the midbrain; hence C is the correct response – the uppermost left and right superior colliculi and below them, the left and right inferior colliculi. Together these four colliculi are known as corpora quadrigemina. The superior and inferior colliculi have roles in visual and auditory processing, respectively.

6.1.14 *D – Red nucleus*

The corticospinal tract passes anterior to the four colliculi and to the red nucleus; hence D is the correct response. The corticospinal tract (pyramidal tract) forms part of the descending tracts of the spinal cord that originate in the cerebral cortex and brain stem. Axons leave the cerebral hemispheres, pass through the corona radiata and posterior limb of the internal capsule and enter the crus cerebri. They then enter the medulla where they form medullary pyramids. The majority of fibres decussate in the caudal medulla (ca. 85%) and form the lateral corticospinal tract (contralateral fibres), which descend in the posterior part of the lateral funiculus. Those that do not decussate (ca. 15%) descend ipsilaterally as the anterior (ventral) corticospinal tract. These fibres decussate near to their termination. These fibres innervate the contralateral side of the spinal cord. The main function of the corticospinal tract is to mediate and control fine, voluntary movements of distal musculature. This tract is important in motor and sensory functions. The majority of the tract (ca. 80%) arises from the primary motor cortex and premotor cortex; the remainder arising from supplementary motor areas and somatosensory areas.

The red nucleus is found at the level of the substantia nigra and occupies the tegmentum of the upper midbrain. It is notably 'red' due to the extensive capillary network and high iron content. The rubrospinal tract originates in the red nucleus which functions to control excitation of the limb flexors and inhibits antagonistic extensors. The dentate nucleus is deep and lateral to the cerebellum and functions to regulate fine, voluntary movements, cognition, language and visuospatial processing. The subthalamic nucleus is found at the boundary between the midbrain and diencephalon, rostrolateral to the red nucleus and ventral to the thalamus. The vestibular nucleus (of which there are four) are located in the pons and medulla, which have roles in processing sensory information such as in eye and head movements, and orientation in space to control these movements. The emboliform nucleus (and the globose nucleus) are found deep within the white matter of the cerebellum and are surrounded laterally by the dentate nucleus. Fibres project from the emboliform nucleus to the contralateral red nucleus. This nucleus has important roles in muscle tone and posture. The corticospinal tract does not run anterior to the dentate, subthalamic, vestibular or emboliform nuclei.

6.1.15 *B – Spinothalamic tract*

Nerve fibres that run between the brain and spinal cord form ascending (sensory) and descending (motor) tracts. Ascending tracts are subdivided into (1) general somatic afferent fibres which carry sensory information such as pain, temperature, touch, vibration, pressure and proprioception, and (2) general visceral afferent fibres which carry sensory information such as pain and pressure from visceral organs. There are three distinct ascending sensory systems:

- anterolateral pathway which includes the
  - spinothalamic tract, which carries pressure and crude touch (anterior), and pain and temperature (lateral)
  - spinoreticulothalamic tract, which consciously transmits impulses of chronic and deep pain to the brain stem reticular formation
  - spinotectal tract which regulates spinovisual reflexes, transmitting pain, thermal and tactile information to the superior colliculus.
- somatosensory pathway to the cerebellum which includes the
  - spinocerebellar tract (dorsal and ventral) which carries unconscious proprioceptive information
- dorsal column-medial lemniscus pathway which includes the
  - fasciculus gracilis (situated medially) and fasciculus cuneatus (situated laterally) which carry impulses concerned with discriminative (fine) touch, vibratory sense and conscious proprioception

The spinothalamic tract is a sensory not motor pathway; hence B is the correct response.

All other options are descending motor tracts of the spinal cord. The tectospinal tract arises from the superior colliculus and mediates reflex postural movements in response to visual stimuli. The reticulospinal tract arises from the pontine reticular formation (medial reticulospinal tract) and the medulla (lateral reticulospinal tract). It facilitates or inhibits voluntary movement and reflex activity by mediating the activity of alpha and gamma motor neurones. Vestibulospinal tracts arise from the vestibular nuclei of the pons and medulla. The lateral vestibulospinal tract mediates excitatory activity of extensor muscles. These muscles function to counteract the force of gravity (antigravity muscles). Fibres are also involved in the control of posture and balance. This tract extends throughout the length of the spinal cord. The medial vestibulospinal tract only projects as far as the cervical or upper thoracic spinal levels and therefore transmits signals to neck extensor muscles. Simultaneously, inhibitory signals are sent to flexors. The rubrospinal tract originates from the red nucleus. It serves to control muscle tone of flexor muscles by being excitatory, and thus inhibiting the activity of extensor/antigravity muscles.

6.1.16   B – *Medial lemniscus*

The medial lemniscus forms part of the dorsal (posterior) column-medial lemniscus pathway; hence B is the correct response. First-order neurones in the fasciculus gracilis and fasciculus cuneatus of the dorsal column sends impulses to second-order neurones in the nucleus gracilis and nucleus cuneatus, respectively. These nuclei send out axons which sensory decussate in the medulla as internal arcuate fibres which become the medial lemniscus. Cell bodies of myelinated axons lie in the contralateral nucleus gracilis and nucleus cuneatus. It ascends rostrally through the medulla, pons and midbrain to terminate in the ventral posterolateral nucleus of the thalamus, where it synapses with third-order neurones. Cells in this nucleus send axons to the postcentral gyrus of the cerebral cortex. Clinically it is important to remember that injury to the dorsal columns (fasciculi gracilis and cuneatus) can result in ipsilateral deficits, whereas injury of the medial lemniscus results in contralateral deficits.

The pyramids are found between the anterior median fissure and the ventrolateral sulcus of the caudal medulla. They contain motor fibres of the corticospinal and corticobulbar tracts. Fibres of the dorsal column are located behind the pyramids. The central canal (ependymal canal) is a CSF-filled space that spans the whole length of the spinal cord from the conus medullaris to the fourth ventricle. Pontine nuclei are found in the ventral pons and serve to relay signals from the cerebral cortex (via corticopontine fibres) to the dentate nucleus of the cerebellum via pontocerebellar fibres. The superior cerebellar peduncles are paired tracts that connect the cerebellum with the midbrain. They are associated with predominantly efferent fibres (cerebellorubral, dentatothalamic and fastigioreticular) and a small number of afferent fibres (anterior spinocerebellar and tectocerebellar).

6.1.17   B – | Lateral corticospinal | Lateral spinothalamic | Anterior spinothalamic | Anterior corticospinal |

As shown in the figure below, B is the correct response. All ascending and descending tracts are present bilaterally. Other important tracts have also been highlighted (in grey).

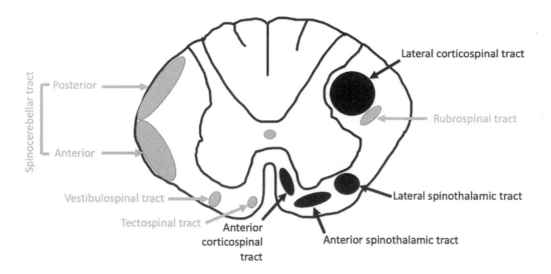

6.1.18   A – *The inferior cerebellar peduncle connects the cerebellum and pons*

The middle (not the inferior) cerebellar peduncle connects the transverse pontocerebellar (afferent) fibres that arise from the pontine nuclei of the pons with the cerebellum; hence A is the correct response.

6.1.19   D – *The lamina terminalis lies anteriorly*

The diencephalon consists of four main subdivisions: the thalamus, subthalamus, hypothalamus and epithalamus. Together with the cerebral hemispheres, it forms the forebrain and the two sides of the diencephalon are separated by the lumen of the third ventricle (whose lateral walls they constitute). It has an anterior and posterior wall, two lateral walls, a roof and a floor. Posteriorly, the floor and roof converge at a point where the third ventricle merges with the cerebral aqueduct. The anterior wall is formed by the lamina terminalis; hence D is the correct response. This is a membrane that stretches from the anterior commissure to the optic chiasm. The third ventricle lies medially (not superiorly), and the lateral ventricle lies superiorly (dorsally). The optic chiasm forms part of the floor, with the infundibulum and mammillary bodies. The pituitary gland (not the pineal gland) is found inferior (ventral) to the hypothalamus in the midline. The pineal gland is a component of the epithalamus, and its stalk, together with the posterior commissure form the posterior wall. The subthalamus and hypothalamus lie inferiorly (ventrally), forming the lower part of the lateral walls and floor. The anterior column of the fornix forms part of the anterior wall (it is not medial). It is important to highlight that the lateral walls of the third ventricle are the medial surface of the diencephalon. Thus, the thalami can be demarcated by the hypothalamic sulcus into a superior (dorsal) portion (thalamus and epithalamus), and inferior (ventral) portion (hypothalamus and subthalamus).

6.1.20 *C – Basilar artery – pons*

The subclavian artery gives rise to two vertebral arteries which unite at the junction of the medulla and pons to form the basilar artery. It is located on the ventral surface of the pons; hence C is the correct response. The fourth ventricle is located anterior to the cerebellum, and posterior to the pons and rostral medulla. It is a CSF-filled cavity within the hindbrain (not midbrain). Olives (olivary bodies) are located on the ventral surface of the medulla, lateral to the pyramids (not the spinal cord). The central canal is a CSF-filled space that extends throughout the entire length of the spinal cord (not the medulla). The anterior median fissure contains the anterior spinal artery that supplies the anterior two-thirds of the spinal cord. It is found in the midline of the medulla (not pons) and is continuous along the entire length of the spinal cord.

6.1.21 *D –* | thalamus | lateral spinothalamic | contralateral |

When secondary axons decussate in the anterior commissure of the cord, they ascend to the thalamus in the lateral spinothalamic tract on the contralateral side; hence D is the correct response.

Remember, peripheral sensation is carried to the brain via an ascending tract from dorsal root ganglia. Somatosensory stimuli from the head, face and mouth are carried via the cranial nerves, namely the trigeminal pathway, whereas stimuli below the neck are transmitted along sensory pathways of the spinal cord. Axons of the dorsal column from the lower limb are located medially within the fasciculus gracilis, whereas axons from the upper limb are located laterally within the fasciculus cuneatus. Axons of the dorsal column synapse with second-order neurones and terminate in either the nucleus gracilis or cuneatus of the medulla. These second-order neurones decussate and continue as the medial lemniscus. They synapse with a third-order neurone in the thalamus, where axons are subsequently projected to the postcentral gyrus.

The dorsal column and spinothalamic tract are similar in many ways. Both systems have contralateral second-order neurones, as they project axons across the midline to the other side of the brain/spinal cord. One of the main differences is the point at which they decussate. In the spinothalamic tract, neurones in the dorsal root ganglion extend their axons to the dorsal horn where they synapse with second-order neurones. The axons of second-order neurones decussate within the spinal cord and ascend towards the thalamus, whereas in the dorsal column, decussation occurs in the brain stem.

6.1.22 *E –*

	III			VII			XI		
	S	B	V	S	B	V	S	B	V
	✓		✓		✓	✓		✓	

The 12 pairs of cranial nerves (CN) may possess motor and/or sensory modalities, or both. There are three types of sensory (afferent) neurones: (1) general somatic (CN V, VII, IX and X), (2) special visceral (CN I, II, VII, VIII, IX and X), and (3) general visceral (CN IX and X). There are also three types of motor (efferent) neurones: (1) somatic motor (III, IV, VI and XII), (2) branchial motor (special visceral, CN V, VII, IX, X and XI), and (3) visceral motor (III, VII, IX and X); hence E is the correct response. The oculomotor nerve (CN III) has somatic motor and visceral motor neurones, the facial nerve (CV VII) has branchial motor and visceral motor neurones, and the accessory nerve (CN XI) has only branchial motor neurones. The table below summaries the afferent and efferent fibres of all 12 cranial nerves.

		Cranial nerve											
		I	II	III	IV	V	VI	VII	VIII	IX	X	XI	XII
Motor	S			✓	✓		✓						✓
	B					✓		✓		✓	✓	✓	
	V			✓				✓		✓	✓		
Sensory	S					✓		✓		✓	✓		
	GV									✓	✓		
	SV	✓	✓					✓	✓	✓	✓		

Key: S: somatic; B: branchial; V: visceral; GV: general visceral; SV: special visceral

6.1.23 *A – Trochlear*

The trochlear nerve, along with the oculomotor and abducens nerves, is responsible for ocular movement. It innervates superior oblique and controls abduction of the eye. It is the smallest of the cranial nerves but has the longest course, as it is the only nerve to have a posterior (dorsal) exit from the brainstem; hence A is the correct response. It originates from paired trochlear nuclei within the midbrain at the level of the inferior colliculus. The nerves decussate before they exit the midbrain and run on contralateral sides. It also is the only nerve to innervate its target contralaterally.

6.1.24 *D – Decreased gastric motility*

The vagus nerve is the longest cranial nerve and represents the parasympathetic nervous system for autonomic regulation of the neck, thorax and abdomen. It originates in the posterior sulcus of the medulla, dorsal to the olive and exits between the medullary pyramid and inferior cerebellar peduncle, coursing out of the skull through the jugular foramen. The vagus nerve functions to regulate heart rate and blood pressure, mediate gastric emptying and influences motility of biliary and intestinal tracts. Therefore, a lesion close to the origin of the vagus nerve would result in decreased gastric motility (not increased), bronchodilation (not bronchoconstriction) and increased heart rate (not decreased); hence D is the correct response. The vagus nerve has no control over pupillary constriction or dilation. Pupillary constriction (pupillary light reflex) results from the actions of the afferent limb of the optic nerve and efferent limb of the oculomotor nerve. In dim light, postganglionic sympathetic fibres from the long ciliary nerve, a branch of the ophthalmic division of the trigeminal nerve innervates the dilator muscle causing pupillary dilation.

6.1.25 *C – VII*

The facial nerve (CN VII) contains a motor, sensory and parasympathetic component. It is preganglionic parasympathetic fibres that synapse with postganglionic neurones via pterygopalatine ganglia, which innervate the lacrimal gland. The corneal reflex uses the efferent limb of the facial nerve; hence C is the correct response. The corneal reflex uses the afferent limb of the trigeminal nerve (V_1).

6.1.26 *E – It is present throughout the length of the spinal cord*

Shaded area X corresponds to the fasciculus cuneatus. It is not present throughout the length of the spinal cord since it contains afferents from the upper limb, in the upper thoracic and cervical spine levels (C1–T6). The more medial fasciculus gracilis is present throughout the length of the spinal cord and contains afferents from the lower limb, below T6; hence E is the correct response, as all other options are correct in relation to shaded area X.

6.1.27 *C –*

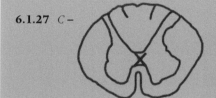

The key to this scenario is the symmetrical nature of the symptoms. The patient did not feel pain in both hands, despite repeatedly touching a hot object. Therefore, the lesion cannot be unilateral, it must reside close to the midline of the spinal cord. It also means that the lateral spinothalamic tract (responsible for transmitting pain and temperature) remained intact bilaterally since pain and temperature sensation were not affected below the arms. The lesion is located in close proximity to the central canal of the spinal cord; hence C is the correct response. This suggests that there is a progressive myelopathy due to cavitation of the spinal cord, known as syringomyelia. It can be caused by cysts, tumours, infection or trauma. It commonly affects the cervical and upper thoracic spinal cord, but it can extend throughout the entire spinal cord. If the condition is left untreated, the cavity can reach the lower brainstem (syringobulbia) and lead to death.

Answers 6.1.28 to 6.1.31 relate to the following annotated figure. Additional structures have also been highlighted.

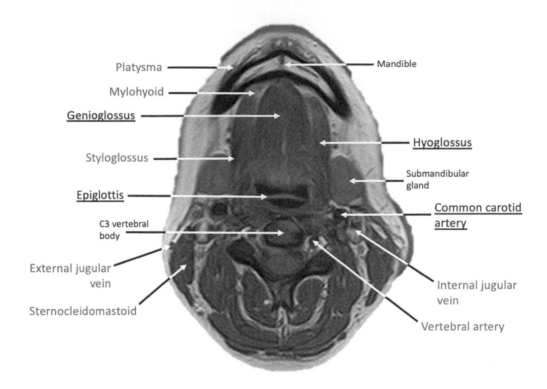

6.1.28	*D – Genioglossus*

6.1.29	*B – Hyoglossus*

6.1.30	*B – Protects the airway and prevents aspiration*

Structure labelled 3 corresponds to the epiglottis. This is a single flap of fibrocartilage that closes the laryngeal inlet during swallowing thus preventing aspiration; hence B is the correct response. It has ligamentous attachments to the thyroid cartilage (via the thyroepiglottic ligament), the hyoid bone (via the hyoepiglottic ligament), the base of the tongue (via median glossoepiglottic folds) and the pharynx (via lateral glossoepiglottic folds). It receives a blood supply via the superior laryngeal artery, and it is innervated by the internal laryngeal branch of the superior laryngeal nerve (a branch of the vagus nerve).

6.1.31	*E – Common carotid artery*

The common carotid artery bifurcates within the carotid triangle into the internal and external carotid arteries between the hyoid bone and thyroid cartilage. This occurs at or between the levels C3 and C4. The carotid triangle is bound by omohyoid, posterior belly of digastric and sternocleidomastoid.

Answers 6.1.32 to 6.1.37 relate to the following annotated figure. Additional structures have also been highlighted.

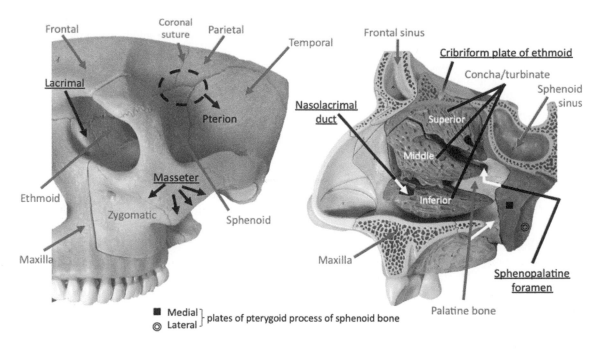

6.1.32 *C – Lacrimal*

The lacrimal bone is the smallest bone of the skull and located at the most anterior aspect of the medial orbital wall; hence C is the correct response. In addition to the lacrimal bone, the bony orbit is composed of six other bones – the maxilla, zygomatic, ethmoid, frontal, sphenoid and palatine bones. The frontal process of the maxilla and the lacrimal bone unite to form the lacrimal groove, which contains the lacrimal sac and borders the anterior and posterior lacrimal crests (parts of the maxilla and lacrimal bones, respectively). The anterior lacrimal crest attaches the anterior portion of the medial canthus and the medial palpebral ligament to the palpebral part of orbicularis oculi. Fibres of the medial canthus and orbicularis oculi also run deep on the medial border and attach to the posterior lacrimal crest. The medial canthus consists of a tendinous attachment of the orbicularis oculi. This muscle is important in closing the eyelids and contraction may lead to drainage of tears from the lacrimal sac into the nasolacrimal canal.

6.1.33 *A – Masseter*

The masseter is an important muscle of mastication (in addition to the temporalis, lateral and medial pterygoid muscles). It originates from the zygomatic arch and maxillary process of the zygomatic bone, and inserts into the coronoid process, ramus and angle of the mandible; hence A is the correct response.

There are two heads to the medial pterygoid: the smaller superficial head originates from the pyramidal process of the palatine bone and maxillary tuberosity, whilst the larger deep head originates from the medial aspect of the lateral pterygoid plate of the sphenoid bone. Both the superficial and deep heads insert onto the medial surface of the ramus and angle of the mandible. There are also two heads to the lateral pterygoid: the superior head originates from the infratemporal surface and crest of the greater wing of the sphenoid bone, whilst the inferior head originates from the lateral surface of the lateral pterygoid plate of the sphenoid bone. The superior head inserts into the anteromedial aspect of the temporomandibular capsule and disc, whilst the inferior head inserts into the pterygoid fovea on the neck of the mandible. Temporalis originates at the temporal fossa up to the inferior temporal line and the zygomatic bone and inserts on to the coronoid process and ramus of the mandible. The middle pharyngeal constrictor contracts to narrow the pharyngeal lumen in order to assist food bolus transport. It originates from the greater and lesser horn of the hyoid bone and stylohyoid ligament and inserts into the medial pharyngeal raphe. This muscle also converges with the superior and inferior pharyngeal constrictors.

6.1.34 *E – Ethmoid*

Region labelled 3 is known as the pterion. It is an H-shaped suture complex which marks the union of four bones – the squamous portion of the temporal bone, parietal bone, frontal bone, and the greater wing of the sphenoid bone; hence E is the correct response, as the ethmoid bone does not contribute to the formation of the pterion. It is the thinnest and weakest part of the calvarium, and this region is clinically significant as fractures can result in damage to the anterior branch of the middle meningeal artery, resulting in an extradural haematoma. In neurosurgery, it provides a vital landmark allowing access to important structures such as the Sylvian fissure, cavernous sinus, circle of Willis and optic nerve.

6.1.35   *B – Nasolacrimal duct*

Structure labelled 4 corresponds to an opening in the inferior nasal concha or turbinate. The nasolacrimal duct is found within the nasolacrimal canal and passes inferiorly to the anterior aspect of the middle nasal concha. It opens into the inferior nasal meatus, under the anterior lip of the inferior nasal concha; hence B is the correct response. It serves to humidify inhaled air and aids in olfaction. The maxillary sinus opens into the semilunar hiatus found in the lateral wall of the middle nasal meatus. The sphenoidal sinus opens into the posterior wall of the sphenoethmoidal recess of the nasal cavity. Middle ethmoidal cells drain into the middle nasal meatus via an opening on or above the ethmoid bulla. For completeness, the anterior ethmoidal cells drain into the ethmoidal infundibulum of the middle nasal meatus, or frontonasal duct and the posterior ethmoidal cells drain into the superior nasal meatus. The frontonasal duct or recess, together with the frontal ostium and frontal infundibulum forms a drainage pathway from the frontal sinus, draining into the middle nasal meatus (predominantly) and ethmoid infundibulum.

6.1.36   *C – Descending palatine artery*

Structure labelled 5 corresponds to the sphenopalatine foramen. It connects the nasal cavity to the pterygopalatine fossa of the skull. It contains the sphenopalatine artery and vein, the nasopalatine nerves and the posterior superior lateral nasal nerve. The descending palatine artery is not found within the sphenopalatine foramen; hence C is the correct response. The descending palatine artery is a branch of the maxillary artery and passes through the greater palatine foramen to supply the hard palate.

6.1.37   *D – Olfactory*

Structure labelled 6 corresponds to the cribriform plate of the ethmoid bone which forms the roof of the nasal cavity. It has a sieve-like structure and it is infiltrated by numerous olfactory nerve fibres; hence D is the correct response. Projecting superiorly in the midline is the crista galli (Latin for 'crest of the rooster'), which is interposed between olfactory bulbs and provides attachment of the falx cerebri. The lateral aspect of the ethmoid bone is the lamina papyracea, which forms part of the medial wall of the orbit. The perpendicular plate of the ethmoid forms a large part of the nasal septum.

The greater petrosal nerve, a branch of the facial nerve (CN VII), arises from the geniculate ganglion. It passes through the facial canal to the foramen lacerum and exits the skull through the stylomastoid foramen. The zygomaticofacial nerve is a terminal branch of the zygomatic nerve which in turn is a branch of the maxillary division of the trigeminal nerve (CN V). It emerges on the face through the zygomaticofacial foramen. The infra-orbital nerve is also a branch of the maxillary nerve which supplies the skin of the lower eyelids, lateral parts of the nose and anterior cheek. This nerve exits through the infra-orbital foramen. The optic nerve (CN II) is transmitted within the optic canal.

Answers 6.1.38 to 6.1.39 relate to the following annotated figure. Additional structures have also been highlighted.

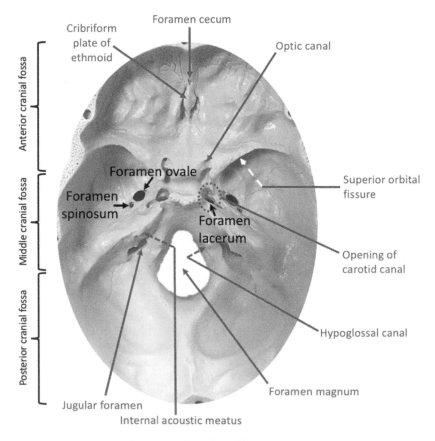

6.1.38 *A – Mandibular division of trigeminal nerve*

Structure labelled 1 corresponds to the foramen ovale. Structures which passes through this foramen include the mandibular division of the trigeminal nerve and the lesser petrosal nerve. Hence A is the correct response.

6.1.39 *C –* | Foramen spinosum | Carotid canal |

Structure labelled 2 corresponds to the foramen spinosum and structure labelled 3 is the foramen lacerum within the carotid canal; hence C is the correct response. The table below shows internal foramina of the cranial cavity and the structures which pass through them. The carotid canal lies posteromedial to the foramen ovale, and inferior to this lies the foramen lacerum. In life, this foramen is closed by a cartilaginous plate and no structures pass through it. However, some meningeal arterial branches and small veins pierce the cartilage, and the internal carotid artery with sympathetic and venous plexuses pass on the superior aspect. Posterolateral to the foramen lacerum lies the groove/hiatus for the greater and lesser petrosal nerves.

Cranial fossa	Foramen	Structures passing through foramen
Anterior	Foramen cecum	Emissary veins to nasal cavity
	Olfactory foramina in cribriform plate	Olfactory nerves
	Optic canal	Optic nerve and ophthalmic artery
Middle	Superior orbital fissure	Oculomotor nerve, trochlear nerve, ophthalmic division of trigeminal nerve, abducent nerve, ophthalmic veins
	Foramen rotundum	Maxillary division of trigeminal nerve
	Foramen ovale	Mandibular division of trigeminal nerve and lesser petrosal nerve
	Foramen spinosum	Middle meningeal artery and vein, and meningeal branch (of mandibular branch) of trigeminal nerve
	Hiatus/groove of greater petrosal nerve	Greater petrosal nerve and petrosal branch of middle meningeal artery
	Hiatus/groove of lesser petrosal nerve	Lesser petrosal nerve
Posterior	Internal acoustic meatus	Facial nerve, vestibulocochlear nerve and labyrinthine artery
	Jugular foramen	Glossopharyngeal nerve, vagus nerve, accessory nerve, inferior petrosal sinus and sigmoid sinus
	Hypoglossal canal	Hypoglossal nerve, meningeal branch of the ascending pharyngeal artery
	Condylar canal	Emissary vein
	Mastoid foramen	Mastoid emissary vein
	Foramen magnum	Vertebral arteries, anterior and posterior spinal arteries, dural veins, spinal roots of accessory nerve, meninges, medulla

Answers 6.1.40 to 6.1.42 relate to the following annotated figure. Additional structures have also been highlighted.

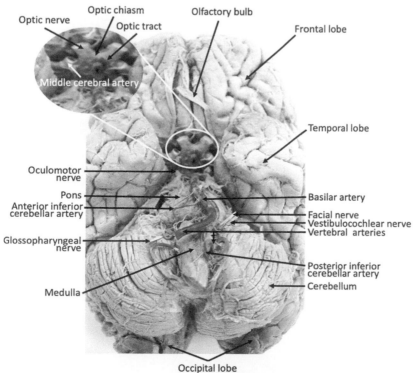

6.1.40 *C – Posterior cerebral arteries*

Structure labelled 4 corresponds to the basilar artery. This artery is formed by union of the vertebral arteries, which have entered the cranial cavity through the foramen magnum. The basilar artery travels in a caudal to rostral direction along the anterior surface of the pons giving rise to several branches including the anterior inferior cerebellar arteries, small pontine arteries, and superior cerebellar arteries. The terminal branch of the basilar artery which ends as a bifurcation are two posterior cerebral arteries; hence C is the correct response.

6.1.41 *A – Superior portion of parietal lobe*

Structure labelled 5 corresponds to the middle cerebral artery. This artery supplies the lateral surface of the cerebral hemispheres of the frontal, parietal and temporal lobes. Small, central branches supply the basal ganglia and internal capsule. The superior division supplies the lateral inferior frontal lobe (Broca's area), and the inferior division supplies the superior temporal gyrus (Wernicke's area). The superior portion of the parietal lobe is not supplied by the middle cerebral artery but by the anterior cerebral artery; hence A is the correct response.

6.1.42 *E – Anticipation*

Lobe labelled 6 corresponds to the temporal lobe. The temporal lobe is important in emotional (and feelings) and visuospatial processing, language, memory, fear, learning, hearing and speech. More specifically, label 6 points to the fusiform gyrus. This is a region of the inferior temporal cortex that plays important roles in reading, and face, object and word recognition. The frontal lobe controls anticipation; hence E is the correct response. The figure below highlights the functions of the four lobes of the brain and the cerebellum.

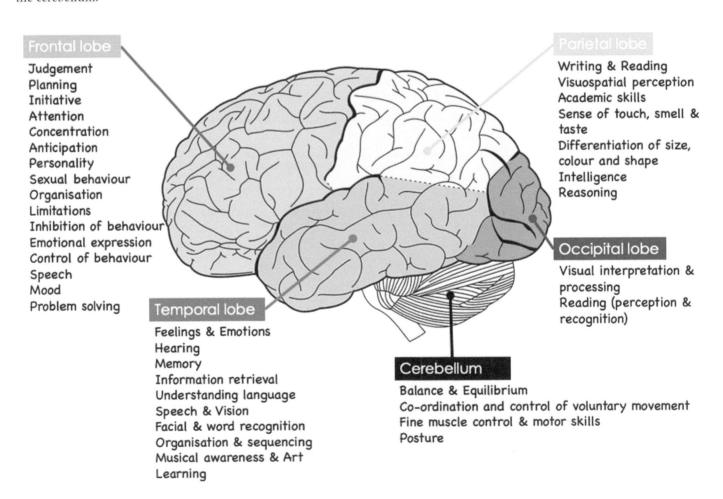

Answers 6.1.43 to 6.1.44 relate to the following annotated figure. Additional structures have also been highlighted.

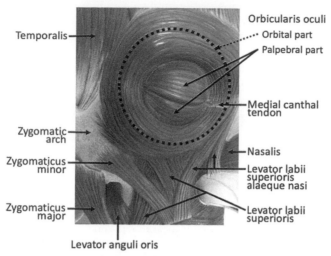

6.1.43 *C – Levator palpebrae superioris*

Structure labelled 7 corresponds to the orbital part of orbicularis oculi. This part is responsible for closing the eyelids tightly, whereas the palpebral part closes the eyelid gently. The major antagonist to this muscle is levator palpebrae superioris; hence C is the correct response. Levator palpebrae superioris serves to elevate the upper eyelid. In addition to the superior, inferior, medial and lateral recti, and superior and inferior oblique muscles, levator palpebrae superioris is an extrinsic (extra-ocular) muscle within the orbit. Antagonists to the superior oblique muscle are the inferior oblique and superior rectus. Antagonists to superior rectus are inferior rectus and superior oblique. Upon contraction, corrugator supercilii serves to elevate the medial portion of the eyebrow, depressing the lateral portion and is responsible for producing vertical frown lines. Antagonists to corrugator supercilii are frontalis for the lateral third of the eyebrow, procerus and the orbital part of orbicularis oculi. Levator labii superioris is involved in facial expression, and elevation (and eversion) of the upper lip. Antagonists to levator labii superioris include depressor anguli oris and orbicularis oris.

6.1.44 *D – Draws the upper lip upward*

Structure labelled 8 corresponds to zygomaticus minor. It is one of the main elevators of the lip, together with levator labii superioris and levator labii superioris alaeque nasi; hence D is the correct response. Protrusion of the lower lip is achieved by the mentalis and depressor labii oris muscles. Protrusion and closure of both lips (as in kissing) are achieved by orbicularis oris. Depressor anguli oris draws the corner (or angle) of the mouth downward and laterally. The platysma is responsible for retracting and depressing the corner of the mouth (as in pouting). Zygomaticus major draws the corner of the mouth upwards and laterally (as in smiling).

Answers 6.1.45 to 6.1.47 relate to the following annotated figure. Additional structures have also been highlighted.

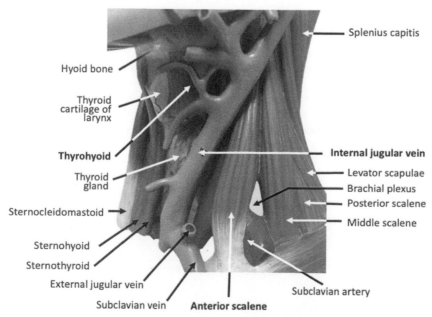

6.1.45 *E – Thyrohyoid*

Structure labelled 1 corresponds to the thyrohyoid muscle; hence E is the correct response. It is one of the four muscles that constitute the infrahyoid muscles; the other three being omohyoid, sternohyoid and sternothyroid. The infrahyoid muscles are separated into superficial and deep layers. Omohyoid and sternohyoid belong to the superficial layer, and thyrohyoid and sternothyroid belong to the deep layer. Thyrohyoid originates on the oblique line of the lamina of the thyroid cartilage and inserts into the inferior border of the body and greater horn of the hyoid bone. Unlike other infrahyoid muscles which are all innervated by the ansa cervicalis, thyrohyoid receives nerve fibres from the anterior rami of the 1ˢᵗ cervical spinal nerve via the hypoglossal nerve. It functions to depress the hyoid and elevate the larynx.

6.1.46 *D –* | *Sigmoid and inferior petrosal sinus* | *Subclavian vein* | *Middle thyroid vein* | *Vagus nerve* |

Vessel labelled 2 corresponds to the internal jugular vein. This paired structure drains blood from the brain, superficial face and neck, and delivers it to the right atrium. It originates in the posterior cranial fossa and exits the cranium through the jugular foramen. It is continuous with the sigmoid sinus and it receives in its course the inferior petrosal sinus, the common facial, lingual, pharyngeal, superior and middle thyroid veins (terminal tributary). It runs parallel in the carotid sheath with the vagus nerve posteriorly and the common carotid artery anteromedially. It unites with the subclavian vein to then form the brachiocephalic vein; hence D is the correct response. The inferior thyroid vein drains directly into the brachiocephalic vein.

6.1.47 *B – Elevation of rib I; anterior rami of C4–C7*

Muscle labelled 3 corresponds to the anterior scalene. It originates from the transverse processes of cervical vertebrae 3 to 6 (C3–C6) and inserts into the scalene tubercle on the inner border of the first rib. It receives a blood supply from the ascending cervical artery (branch of the inferior thyroid artery) and is innervated by the anterior (ventral) rami of cervical nerves C4–C7 from the cervical plexus. It functions as an accessory muscle of inspiration by elevating the first rib. It also flexes the neck with bilateral contraction, and laterally flexes (ipsilateral) and rotates the neck (contralateral) with unilateral contraction; hence B is the correct response.

The middle scalene is the largest and longest of the scalene muscles. It originates from the posterior tubercles of transverse processes C3–C7 and inserts into the superior border of the first rib. It is innervated by the anterior rami of C3–C8. It also elevates the first rib and laterally flexes the neck. The posterior scalene is the smallest of the scalene muscles. It originates from the posterior tubercles of transverse processes C5-C7 and inserts onto the external surface of the second rib. It is innervated by the anterior rami of C6-C8. It elevates the second rib and also laterally flexes the neck.

6.1.48 *B – Cricothyroid*

Cricothyroid is a deep muscle in the anterior compartment of the neck. It is one of the intrinsic laryngeal muscles and the only tensor muscle of the larynx that aids in phonation by tensing and elongating the vocal folds; hence B is the correct response. All intrinsic laryngeal muscles move the vocal cords aiding in phonation. The only abductor muscle in this group is the posterior cricoarytenoid, adductors include lateral cricoarytenoid and transverse arytenoid, and sphincter muscles include oblique and transverse arytenoid and aryepiglottic. Intrinsic laryngeal muscles that are involved in relaxation of the vocal cords are the vocalis muscle and thyroarytenoid. Salpingopharyngeus is a longitudinal pharyngeal muscle that aids in speech by elevating the pharynx, and it assists the tensor veli palatini muscle by opening the Eustachian tube during swallowing.

6.1.49 *D –* | *Nasopharynx* | *Superficial cervical* |

Lymph nodes are small collections of lymphatic tissue located along lymphatic vessels which filter and drain lymph en route to the venous system. Lymph nodes of the head and neck are divided into a superficial ring and a vertical group of deep nodes. Superficial nodes receive lymph from the scalp, face and neck, and drain into the deep nodes. Superficial nodes include occipital, preauricular, posterior auricular (mastoid), parotid, submandibular, submental and superficial cervical. The deep nodes receive all lymph from the head and neck and are arranged in a vertical chain along the internal jugular vein, and under cover of sternocleidomastoid. They include prelaryngeal, pretracheal, paratracheal, retropharyngeal, infrahyoid, tonsillar (jugulodigastric), jugulo-omohyoid and supraclavicular. The nasopharynx drains into the deep (not superficial) cervical lymph nodes, alongside the ear, tongue, trachea, nasal cavities, palate, and oesophagus; hence D is the correct response. All other options correctly match anatomical site to the lymph nodes into which they drain. The figure below highlights important lymph nodes of the head and neck.

In addition, there is a collection of nasal-associated lymphoid tissue (NALT) which forms Waldeyer's ring of the posterior oropharynx. This ring is composed of unpaired nasopharyngeal (adenoids) tonsils which form the antero-inferior part of the ring, and lingual tonsils which form the postero-superior part of the ring. There are also paired tubal and palatine tonsils which form the lateral part of the ring. The ring is a unique site for B and T-cell production.

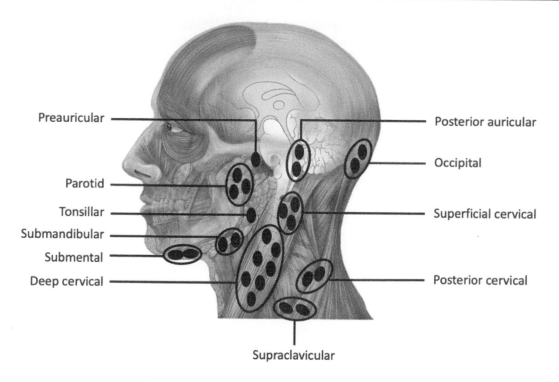

Preauricular

Posterior auricular

Occipital

Parotid

Tonsillar

Superficial cervical

Submandibular

Submental

Deep cervical

Posterior cervical

Supraclavicular

6.1.50 *D – Ophthalmic*

The external carotid artery supplies blood to the scalp, face and neck. It originates at the bifurcation of the common carotid at the level of C3–C4 and the superior border of the thyroid cartilage. It gives off six branches before dividing into two terminal branches. In ascending order, they are superior thyroid, ascending pharyngeal, lingual, facial, occipital and posterior auricular. The two terminal branches are the maxillary and superficial temporal arteries; hence D is the correct response. The ophthalmic artery is the first branch of the internal carotid artery. Several branches of the external carotid artery are important for collateral circulation and anastomoses in the event of occlusion of the internal carotid artery.

6.2   Special senses

6.2.1 *A – The organ of Corti is a specialised receptor organ for hearing supported by Deiter's and Claudius cells*

The organ of Corti is located within scala media of the cochlea and serves in auditory signal transduction. It is composed of sensory epithelium with both inner and outer mechanosensory hair cells and supporting cells. There are four different supporting cells – Corti pillars, and Hensen's, Deiter's and Claudius cells; hence A is the correct response. Architecturally, supporting cells such as Corti pillars and Deiter's (or phalangeal cells) are rich in cytoskeletal proteins (tubulin and actin) and provide mechanical support to the organ of Corti. These cells develop and open spaces around hair cells creating the tunnel of Corti and the spaces of Nuel. Hensen's and Claudius cells are located towards the lateral wall and act as mediators of ion homeostasis and have roles in cell regeneration.

Müller cells are the principal glial cells of the retina, and they form architectural support structures which help stabilize the retina. The cytoplasmic processes of these cells fill the spaces between photoreceptors, bipolar and ganglion cells. They do not relay information from cones to rods. Horizontal cells help synapse and integrate rods and cones from varying parts of the retina. Amacrine cells receive input from bipolar cells and act as interneurons between bipolar and ganglion cells. Cones contain iodopsin (not photopsin) and are less sensitive to light than rods. Rods contain rhodopsin which operates during night vision. Iodopsin discriminates colour (red, green and blue) and is responsible for colour vision.

Type I and II hair cells are supporting cells located along the basal lamina of the macula. Along the apical surface of both cells lie ca. 60 stereocilia and a single kinocilium. There is a larger proportion of type I hair cells at the ridge of the crista ampullaris, whereas type II hair cells predominate at the base. Along with the semilunar canals, the macula of the saccule and utricle are important components of the vestibular system.

The inner two-thirds of the retina is supplied by the central retinal artery. The short posterior ciliary arteries and choriocapillaris supply the external layers of the retina including the pigmented epithelium and outer segments of photoreceptors.

6.2.2   D – The abducens nerve enters the orbit through the superior orbital fissure

The abducens nerve (or cranial nerve VI) enters the orbit through the superior orbital fissure within the tendinous annulus; hence D is the correct response. Venous drainage of the orbit is primarily through the superior ophthalmic vein out of the superior orbital fissure into the cavernous sinus. The pterygoid plexus is a complex of veins located in the infratemporal fossa. The inferior ophthalmic vein exits the orbit through the inferior orbital fissure into the pterygoid plexus behind the maxillary sinus. It is an important drainage system of the nasal cavity, paranasal sinuses and nasopharynx. The ciliary ganglion receives preganglionic parasympathetic fibres from the inferior division of the oculomotor nerve. Postganglionic parasympathetic fibres innervate the ciliary muscles and sphincter pupillae. Clinically, lesions of the ciliary ganglion lead to mydriasis. The tympanic nerve (or nerve of Jacobson) arises from the glossopharyngeal nerve (cranial nerve IX), as does the lesser petrosal nerve. The sphenoid sinus and posterior ethmoid cells drain into the sphenoethmoidal recess. This recess is found above the superior concha, between the ethmoid and sphenoid bones and medial to the nasal septum.

6.2.3   D – Filiform papillae contain no taste buds

Papillae line the superior surface of the oral part of the tongue. There are four types of papillae: filiform, fungiform, circumvallate and foliate. Filiform cover the dorsal anterior two-thirds of the tongue, are the most numerous and contain no taste buds; hence D is the correct response. Foliate are the least numerous. All other papillae contain taste buds. The chorda tympani carries taste from the anterior two-thirds of the tongue and parasympathetic innervation to the salivary glands. It originates from the facial nerve and joins with the lingual nerve (a branch of the mandibular nerve) in the infratemporal fossa. Extrinsic muscles of the tongue include genioglossus, hyoglossus and styloglossus, which are all innervated by the hypoglossal nerve, and palatoglossus, which is innervated by the vagus nerve. The vomer is a small, midline bone that occupies and separates the nasal cavity. The alae (or wings) of the vomer and adjacent sphenoidal processes of the palatine bone form the roof of the nasal cavity. The lateral wall is formed partly by the maxilla, ethmoid bone and perpendicular plate of the palatine bone, the medial plate of the pterygoid process of the sphenoid bone, and the inferior concha. In the ear, the cochlear canal spirals around a hollow bony core called the modiolus. The lamina of modiolus (spiral lamina) is a thin sheet of bone that extends laterally throughout the length of the modiolus and supports the basilar membrane. It is not found in the semicircular canals.

6.2.4   E – Ciliary muscles are innervated by sympathetics from the oculomotor nerve

Ciliary muscles are responsible for accommodation of the lens of the eye for near vision. Neurons of the ciliary ganglion project to the iris and ciliary muscles via short ciliary nerves. This ganglion is the site where parasympathetic preganglionic fibres of the oculomotor nerve synapse with parasympathetic postganglionic fibres; hence E is the correct response. Sympathetics do not innervate ciliary muscles. Postganglionic fibres innervate the dilator pupillae muscle. The ciliary ganglion is also associated with sensory fibres of the nasociliary branch of the ophthalmic nerve.

6.2.5   C – Lymphatic drainage is primarily to the parotid and pre-auricular nodes

There are three groups of lymph nodes to the face: submental, which drain the medial aspect of the lower lip and chin; submandibular, which drain the medial aspect of the orbit, external nose, medial cheek, and the upper and lateral lower lip; and the pre-auricular and parotid, which drain most of the eyelids, external nose and lateral aspect of the cheek; hence C is the correct response. The supra-orbital artery (and supratrochlear) is a branch of the ophthalmic artery which supplies the anterosuperior aspect of the scalp. The superficial temporal artery is a terminal branch of the external carotid artery, which branches into vessels that supply the lateral aspect of the scalp. The infratrochlear nerve is a branch of the ophthalmic nerve and innervates the medial upper eyelid and medial aspect of the nose. Loss of innervation of the orbicularis oculi via the facial nerve causes an inability to close the eyelids (not the superior tarsal muscle, which assists levator palpebrae superioris to elevate the upper eyelid). The superior branch of the oculomotor nerve (not the trochlear nerve) innervates levator palpebrae superioris.

6.2.6   B – Superior oblique – look laterally and downward

There are seven extrinsic muscles of the eye: superior rectus, inferior rectus, medial rectus, lateral rectus, superior oblique, inferior oblique and levator palpebrae superioris. The latter is only involved in elevating the upper eye lid, whereas all others move the eyeball itself. Superior oblique depresses, abducts and medially rotates the eyeball; hence B is the correct response. Medial rectus adducts the eyeball – look medially. Inferior oblique elevates, abducts and laterally rotates the eyeball – look laterally and upward. Superior rectus elevates, adducts and medially rotates the eyeball – look medially and upwards. Inferior rectus depresses, adducts and laterally rotates the eyeball – look medially and downward. Lateral rectus abducts the eyeball – look laterally.

6.2.7   E – Inferior oblique

The inferior oblique originates from the orbital floor, lateral to the nasolacrimal groove and inserts into the posterior inferolateral surface of the eyeball; hence E is the correct response. All four rectus muscles originate from a common tendinous ring (also known as the anulus tendineus communis or annulus of Zinn). This ring encircles the optic canal and parts of the superior orbital fissure, and it transmits the optic nerve, ophthalmic artery and several nerves to the orbit. The superior, inferior, lateral and medial recti insert into the superior, inferior, lateral and medial parts of the eyeball, respectively. The superior oblique muscle originates on the lesser wing of the sphenoid bone, superomedial to the optic canal. It forms a tendon anteriorly that passes through a pulley-like structure called the trochlea and inserts into the superoposterior lateral part of the eyeball.

6.2.8 *D – Posteriorly, the orbital process of the palatine bone contributes to the roof*

Posteriorly, the lesser wing of the sphenoid bone contributes to the roof of the orbit, not the orbital process of the palatine bone; hence D is the correct response. In addition, the zygomatic bone also contributes to the orbital rim inferiorly, and the frontal process of the zygomatic bone and zygomatic process of the frontal bone contribute to it laterally.

6.2.9 *D – Cornea → Aqueous humour → Pupil → Lens → Vitreous humour → Retina*

Light enters the eye through the dome-shaped cornea, through the transparent, fluid-filled aqueous humour, through the black-holed pupil which surrounds the coloured iris, through the crystalline lens which refracts light maintaining visual acuity, through the posterior chamber of the eye (vitreous humour) and is finally focussed accurately on the retina; hence D is the correct response.

6.2.10 *A – Lens*

The lens is designed to be transparent and helps images focus on the retina. Cataracts are opaque regions of the lens which can lead to cloudy vision and reduced visual acuity; hence A is the correct response. Cataracts can develop with advancing age, but also, they can be hereditary, metabolic (galactosaemia, Fabry disease), infectious (rubella, CMV, toxoplasmosis), iatrogenic (steroids) and idiopathic.

6.2.11 *B – Meibomian*

Meibomian glands are holocrine lipid-secreting sebaceous glands that are embedded in the tarsal plate of the eyelids which act as a barrier to dehydration of the cornea; hence B is the correct response. Clinically, dysfunction of these glands leads to decreased secretion and abnormal composition of the tear film layer which can lead to inflammation and ocular surface disease. Glands of Krause and Wolfring are accessory lacrimal glands located in the stroma of the conjunctival fornix and along the orbital border of the tarsal plate, respectively. Similar to the main lacrimal gland, these contribute to the aqueous layer of the tear film. Glands of Moll are modified apocrine sweat glands located on the lid margins that secrete IgA, lysozyme and other antibacterial agents to the tear film. Glands of Zeis are sebaceous glands which secrete sebum into the hair follicle, coating the eyelash shaft ensuring it remains supple and does not become brittle. Blockage of the glands of Moll and/or Zeis can lead to a stye.

6.2.12 *E – Nasociliary and abducens*

The annulus of Zinn (or tendinous ring) encircles the superior orbital fissure and optic canal. This region is called the oculomotor foramen. The optic canal transmits the optic nerve and the ophthalmic artery. The superior orbital fissure transmits the superior and inferior division of the oculomotor nerve, nasociliary nerve and abducens nerve; hence E is the correct response.

6.2.13 *D – The largest proportion of blood flow in the eye passes through the choroid*

The choroid is a dense network of pigmented, vascular tissue between the retina and sclera forming the posterior uvea. It supplies nutrients, maintains temperature and volume of the eye. The choroidal circulation is a high-flow system with relatively low oxygen content and is the largest proportion of blood flow in the eye (ca. 85%); hence D is the correct response. The ophthalmic artery enters the orbit through the optic canal and runs inferolaterally (below not above) to the optic nerve. It is the first branch of the internal (not external) carotid artery. The lacrimal artery (not the central retinal artery) is the second and the largest branch of the ophthalmic artery. The lacrimal artery runs along the upper border of the lateral (not medial) rectus muscle.

6.2.14 *E – In dim light, pupils dilate as circular muscles relax*

In dim light, pupils dilate (sympathetic control) so more light enters the eye as the circular muscles of the iris relax and the radial muscles contract; hence E is the correct response. In bright light, pupils constrict (parasympathetic control) and less light enters the eye as the circular muscles contract and the radial muscles relax. The optic nerve and oculomotor nerves mediate the afferent and efferent limbs of the pupillary reflex, respectively. The pupillary light reflex lies at the level of the midbrain-diencephalic junction, and it is mediated by projections from the retina to the pretectal nucleus, which lies anterolateral to the superior pole of the superior (not inferior) colliculus.

6.2.15 *A – Ptosis*

The superior tarsal muscle is a unique structural muscle as it consists of thin smooth muscle fibres, and it originates and adjoins from underneath the levator palpebrate superioris (skeletal muscle) to insert on the superior tarsal plate of the upper eyelid. It has sympathetic innervation derived from the cervical sympathetic chain and its function is to maintain the elevation of the upper eyelid. Damage to this muscle can lead to ptosis, as seen in Horner's syndrome; hence A is the correct response. Miosis or pupillary constriction results from parasympathetic innervation of the iris sphincter muscle via the short ciliary nerves. Mydriasis or pupillary dilation results from sympathetic innervation of the iris dilator (pupillae) muscle. Diplopia or double vision causes are myriad. Monocular diplopia is often a result of ocular abnormalities when there are issues with light transmission to the retina, as seen with a dislocated lens or irregularities in refraction in the lens which can be seen in early cataract, or corneal irregularities. Patients with monocular diplopia lose their diplopia when the affected eye is covered but regain it when their unaffected eye is covered. Binocular diplopia can be caused by trauma, vascular lesions, endocrinopathies, neuromuscular disorders, neoplasms and autoimmune disorders. Patients with binocular diplopia often experience it upon certain directions of gaze and will lose it when covering either eye. Proptosis or eyeball protrusion causes are also myriad. It is also referred to as exophthalmos, commonly seen in thyroid eye disease where the superior tarsal muscle is hyperactive (not paralysed).

6.2.16 *C – Parasympathetic preganglionic fibres enter the greater petrosal nerve*

The lacrimal gland is a bilobed gland with the predominant function of secreting the aqueous portion of the tear film in response to sympathetic and parasympathetic stimulation. The gland receives parasympathetic innervation from the lacrimatory nucleus located in the dorsal pons medial to the motor nucleus of the facial nerve. Presynaptic fibres travel with the facial nerve to the geniculate ganglion and enter the greater petrosal nerve (a branch of the facial nerve); hence C is the correct response. The nerve passes through the foramen lacerum where it is joined by the deep petrosal nerve to form the nerve of the pterygoid canal (Vidian nerve), and eventually joining the pterygopalatine ganglion. Postganglionic sympathetic (not parasympathetic) fibres originating in the superior cervical ganglion travel with the internal carotid artery and leave this plexus as the deep petrosal nerve. They then join and course with parasympathetic fibres in the nerve of the pterygoid canal. The pterygopalatine ganglion contains both sympathetic and parasympathetic fibres. Postganglionic fibres leaving the pterygopalatine ganglion form the zygomatic and zygomaticotemporal (not zygomaticofacial) nerves, which join the lacrimal nerve. The pterygoid canal runs through the base of the pterygoid process of the sphenoid bone, inferomedial to the foramen rotundum. The canal transmits the nerve, artery and vein to the pterygoid canal towards the pterygopalatine fossa. The foramen rotundum transmits the maxillary nerve.

6.2.17 *C – It appears yellow due to high concentrations of lutein and zeaxanthin*

The macula lutea (from the Latin meaning yellow spot) of the retina is a yellowish spot at the posterior pole (fundus) of the eye which contains a central depression called the fovea centralis. The yellow hue is due to the xanthophyll pigments, lutein and zeaxanthin which are found in high concentrations in the macula but are also found throughout the retina; hence C is the correct response. The macula is approximately 5–6 mm in diameter (not 50 μm). The central fovea of the macula is a region where cone (not rod) photoreceptor density is the highest and visual acuity is maximal. The blind spot, or scotoma, is a retinal region devoid of photoreceptors, where the optic nerve joins the retina. It does not involve the macula.

6.2.18 *D – Sensory innervation of the tympanic membrane inner surface is carried entirely by the glossopharyngeal nerve*

Sensory innervation of the inner (medial) surface of the tympanic membrane is carried entirely by the tympanic branch of the glossopharyngeal nerve; hence D is the correct response. The fleshy lobule is the only part of the auricle that is non-cartilaginous and hence not supported by cartilage. The tragus is an elevated structure in front of the concha located at the entrance of the external acoustic meatus. The superficial part of the auricle is supplied by (1) the great auricular nerve (from C2 and C3) which innervates the anterior and posteroinferior portion, (2) the lesser occipital nerve (from C2) which innervates the posterosuperior portion, and (3) the auriculotemporal branch of the mandibular nerve which innervates the anterosuperior portion. The external carotid artery branches into six vessels that supply the face and neck: superior thyroid, ascending pharyngeal, lingual, facial, occipital, and posterior (not anterior) auricular. It terminates by dividing into the superficial temporal and maxillary arteries. Sensory innervation of the external acoustic meatus is carried by nervus intermedius (a branch of the facial nerve), the auriculotemporal nerve (a branch of the mandibular nerve) and the auricular branch of the vagus nerve.

6.2.19 *E – The tympanic nerve forms the tympanic plexus, of which, the lesser petrosal nerve is a major branch*

The tympanic nerve arises from the inferior ganglion projecting towards the tympanic cavity via the tympanic canaliculus. It forms the tympanic plexus and divides into two routes: one which supplies the mucous membranes of the tympanic cavity, auditory tube and mastoid air cells; and another which forms the lesser petrosal nerve that goes on to supply the parotid gland; hence E is the correct response. The middle ear has six boundaries: the tegmental wall (roof), the jugular wall (floor), the membranous wall (lateral), the mastoid wall (posterior), the labyrinthine wall (medial) and anterior wall. The stapes (not oval window) is attached to the oval window. Tensor tympani is innervated by a branch from the mandibular nerve (not facial). Stapedius is innervated by a branch of the facial nerve. The malleus (not the stapes) is the largest of the auditory ossicles.

6.2.20 *A – There are three semicircular canals*

The bony labyrinth consists of three semicircular canals, the vestibule and the cochlea; hence A is the correct response. The coch-lear canaliculus (aqueduct) connects the osseous vestibule and perilymph containing cochlea to the subarachnoid space. The heli-cotrema is the connecting channel between the scala vestibuli and scala tympani. The membranous labyrinth is a collection of ducts and chambers filled with endolymphatic fluid within the bony labyrinth. It consists of two sacs – the utricle and saccule, and four ducts (not two) – three semicircular canals and the cochlear duct. The vestibulocochlear nerve exits the temporal bone and brainstem through the cerebellopontine angle passing into the internal acoustic meatus. The stylomastoid foramen transmits the facial nerve and the stylomastoid artery. The greater petrosal nerve carries preganglionic parasympathetic fibres to the pterygo-palatine ganglion (not the geniculate). The geniculate ganglion is the point at which the facial nerve branches into the greater petrosal nerve.

6.2.21 *D – Malleus Incus Stapes Utricle*

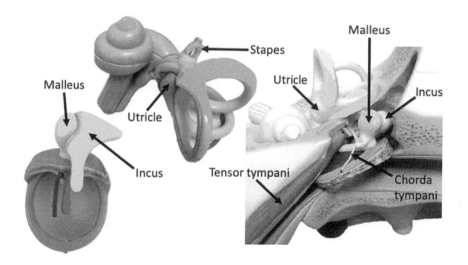

6.2.22 *E – It inserts into the base of structure labelled 3*

Structure labelled 3 corresponds to the stapes, and the stapedius attaches to it. The stapedius is the smallest skeletal muscle in the body. It arises from the pyramidal eminence in the tympanic cavity and inserts into the neck (not the base) of the stapes; hence E is the correct response.

6.2.23 *E – Semicircular ducts*

Structure labelled 4 corresponds to the utricle, a component of the vestibular labyrinth, which receives endolymph from the semi-circular ducts; hence E is the correct response. The saccule communicates with the cochlear duct via the ductus reuniens, and it communicates with the utricle via the utriculosaccular duct. The endolymphatic duct passes from the saccule to the petrous part of the temporal bone via the vestibular aqueduct. The utricle is most sensitive to sideways head tilts and rapid lateral displacements in the horizontal plane, whereas the saccule is most sensitive to up-down and forward-backward movements in the vertical plane.

6.2.24 *B – Branch of mandibular nerve*

Muscle labelled 5 corresponds to the tensor tympani, a tendon of which attaches to the neck of malleus. The tensor tympani nerve supplies the tensor tympani muscle, which is a branch of the mandibular nerve (a branch of the trigeminal nerve); hence B is the correct response. In addition, the mandibular nerve provides sensory and motor innervation to the masseter muscle.

6.2.25 *E – Facial nerve | Lingual nerve | Petrotympanic fissure*

Structure labelled 6 corresponds to the chorda tympani. It arises from the facial nerve superior to the stylomastoid foramen. It enters the tympanic cavity anterosuperiorly, passes medial to the tympanic membrane and the handle of the malleus, and enters the temporal bone. It exits the skull through the petrotympanic fissure. It merges with the lingual nerve, a branch of the maxillary nerve, medial to the lateral pterygoid muscle; hence E is the correct response.

6.2.26 *D – Cochlear duct*

The organs of vestibular function i.e., balance are the semicircular canals (and ducts), the saccule and the utricle. The cochlea (and duct) is the organ of hearing; hence D is the correct response. The saccule and utricle have areas of hair cells called the macula, and an otolithic membrane which is composed of calcium carbonate crystals (otoconia) embedded in a gelatinous matrix. These organs are extremely sensitive to linear head acceleration and head tilt. Clinically, otolith dysfunction is seen in benign paroxysmal positional vertigo where otoconia are displaced from the utricle.

6.2.27 *C – Anterior inferior cerebellar and basilar*

The labyrinthine artery supplies the entire arterial circulation of the inner ear. It is most often a branch of the anterior inferior cerebellar artery, but it can also be a direct branch of the basilar artery; hence C is the correct response. The labyrinthine artery enters the inner ear dividing into the anterior vestibular artery which supplies the vestibular nerve, and the common cochlear artery, which further divides into the cochlear artery and vestibulocochlear artery, both of which supply the cochlea. Clinically, the labyrinthine artery has no anastomoses and is therefore susceptible to ischaemia – complete occlusion can lead to sudden profound loss of auditory and vestibular function.

6.2.28 *E – Sigmoid or inferior petrosal sinus*

Venous drainage of the cochlear duct occurs via the vestibular and cochlear veins which merge to form the labyrinthine vein. This drains into the sigmoid or inferior petrosal sinus; hence E is the correct response.

6.2.29 *A – Tensor veli palatini*

The tensor veli palatini originates from the inferior surface of the cartilage of the Eustachian tube, and the scaphoid fossa and spine of the sphenoid bone. It then fans out, becoming tendinous and attaching to the palatine aponeurosis. It functions by tensing the soft palate and opening the Eustachian tube. It is innervated by the motor part of the mandibular nerve; hence A is the correct response. Clinically, this muscle, as well as the levator veli palatini, is important in otitis media since it controls dilation of the Eustachian tube. All other muscles of the soft palate – levator veli palatini, palatopharyngeus, palatoglossus and musculus uvulae are innervated by the vagus nerve via the pharyngeal branch of the pharyngeal plexus.

6.2.30 *B – Maxillary branch of trigeminal*

All nerves that innervate the teeth and gingivae are branches of the trigeminal nerve. All the upper oral cavity and upper teeth are innervated by the anterior, middle, and posterior superior alveolar nerves, which originate from the maxillary nerve; hence B is the correct response. The anterior superior alveolar nerve innervates the canine and incisor teeth. The middle superior alveolar nerve supplies the premolar teeth. The posterior superior alveolar nerve supplies the molar teeth. The lower teeth are all innervated by branches of the inferior alveolar nerve.

6.2.31 *D – The deep and dorsal lingual veins drain into the external jugular vein*

The tongue is drained by the dorsal inguinal and deep inguinal veins which both drain into the internal (not external) jugular vein; hence D is the correct response.

6.2.32 *C – Deep cervical*

All lymphatic vessels from the tongue drain into the deep cervical nodes along the internal jugular vein; hence C is the correct response. The pharyngeal part of the tongue drains into the jugulodigastric node of the deep cervical chain. The oral part of the tongue drains directly into the deep cervical nodes, and indirectly into the submental and submandibular nodes. The tip of the tongue drains into the jugulo-omohyoid nodes of the deep cervical chain.

6.2.33 *D – Superior longitudinal*

The superior longitudinal muscle is one of the four intrinsic muscles of the tongue which shortens the tongue and elevates or curls it upward (dorsiflexes) the tip; hence D is the correct response. The other intrinsic muscles include the vertical, transverse and inferior longitudinal. There are also four extrinsic muscles of the tongue – genioglossus, styloglossus, hyoglossus and palatoglossus.

6.2.34 *C – Bitterness*

Circumvallate papillae are located at the base (posterior) of the tongue in a V-shaped pattern and are sensitive to bitter substances; hence C is the correct response. Fungiform papillae are located at the tip of the tongue and are more sensitive to sweet taste. Fungiform and filiform papillae are also found at the lateral border of the tongue and are more sensitive to saltiness and sourness, respectively.

6.2.35 *A – Foramen caecum*

The thyroid gland originates from the foramen caecum, a midline depression positioned at the pharyngeal part or posterior one-third of the tongue; hence A is the correct response. The thyroglossal duct marks the path of migration of the thyroid gland, and it maintains the connection of the thyroid gland to the base of the tongue until involution. Embryologically, by the seventh week the thyroid gland has reached its final destination in the neck and by the tenth week, the thyroglossal duct has degenerated. The sulcus terminalis is the V-shaped shallow groove that divides the anterior two-thirds and posterior one-third of the tongue. Not to be confused with the sulcus terminalis of the right atrium, an adipose-filled groove, and the crista terminalis, a C-shaped muscular ridge on the lateral endocardium of the right atrium. The median (pharyngeal) raphe serves as the origin and insertion for pharyngeal constrictor muscles. The epiglottis (and the posterior one-third of the tongue) develops from the caudal half of the hypobranchial eminence (copula of His), a derivative of the third and fourth pharyngeal arches. The tuberculum impar is the region of the first pharyngeal arch that gives rise to the medial part of the tongue. The anterior two-thirds of the tongue is formed from the lateral lingual swellings and the tuberculum impar. The second pharyngeal arch makes no contribution to development of the tongue.

6.2.36 *C – It arises from the greater cornu of the hyoid*

Structure labelled 1 corresponds to the styloglossus muscle, one of the four extrinsic muscles of the tongue. It arises from the apex of the styloid process of the temporal bone and inserts into the lateral aspect of the tongue; hence C is the correct response. The hyoglossus muscle arises from the hyoid bone – anterior part from the body of the hyoid and the posterior part from the greater cornu of the hyoid. All muscles of the tongue are innervated by the hypoglossal nerve, apart from the palatoglossus which is innervated by the pharyngeal branch of the vagus nerve.

6.2.37 *D – It is supplied by the dorsal lingual artery*

Region labelled 2 corresponds to the lingual tonsil, an area posterior to the V-shaped sulcus terminalis. The blood supply to this region is provided by the dorsal lingual artery, a branch of the lingual artery which branches from the external carotid artery; hence D is the correct response. In addition, the tonsillar branch of the facial artery and ascending pharyngeal branch of the external carotid artery are also known to supply this region. Filiform (not fungiform) papillae are the most abundant in this region. In addition to the adenoid and palatine tonsils, the lingual tonsil constitutes a major part of Waldeyer's ring – nasal-associated lymphoid tissue. The lingual tonsil is covered by stratified squamous epithelium and forms a single crypt. Whereas the palatine tonsils consist of approximately 15–20 crypts, which help to increase the surface area. This region is covered with non-keratinised stratified squamous epithelium and plays a key role in the immunological function of the mucosa-associated lymphoid tissue (MALT). The adenoids are covered with ciliated pseudostratified columnar epithelium.

6.2.38 *B – Median glossoepiglottic fold*

Structure labelled 3 corresponds to the epiglottis. The mucosa of lingual part of the tongue is reflected solely on the pharyngeal part of the tongue as the median glossoepiglottic fold and forms the attachment between the epiglottis and base of the tongue; hence B is the correct response. The mucosa is also reflected on to the lateral pharyngeal walls (and lateral parts of the tongue) as two lateral glossoepiglottic folds. These give rise to two vallecula, a depression between the pharynx and larynx which helps trap saliva and preventing the swallowing reflex when a person is supine. The sides of the epiglottis are attached to the arytenoid cartilages by aryepiglottic folds. Aryepiglotticus is a continuation of the oblique arytenoid muscle which arises from the apex of the arytenoid cartilage and inserts into the lateral border of the epiglottis. This muscle aids in closure of the laryngeal inlet.

6.2.39 *A – Mandibular division of trigeminal*

The mandibular division of the trigeminal nerve provides no innervation to the nasal cavities; hence A is the correct response. The maxillary division of the trigeminal nerve provides innervation to the alae and lateral dorsum of the nose. The anterior aspect of the nasal cavity, frontal sinus and the lateral mucosa are innervated by the anterior ethmoidal nerve which branches from the nasociliary nerve (as does the posterior ethmoidal nerve). The posterior aspect is innervated by the nasopalatine nerve. The facial nerve innervates the nasal musculature, mucous glands and paranasal sinuses. The olfactory nerve is responsible for the sense of smell.

6.2.40 *D – Uncinate process*

The ethmoid bone (and sphenoid and frontal bones, and vomer) is an unpaired bone of the nasal cavity. It is a small, cuboidal bone composed of two ethmoidal labyrinths which unite superiorly across the midline by the cribriform plate, and the perpendicular plate which descends vertically to form the nasal septum. The uncinate process is a superior extension of the medial maxillary wall which articulates with the inferior concha; hence D is the correct response. The cribriform plate is enclosed between two medial orbital walls, with the midline crista galli – a triangular process that anchors the falx cerebri of the dura mater in the cranial cavity, to the planum sphenoidale. Clinically, this is a common site for meningiomas.

6.2.41 *E – Sphenoidal sinus*

The sphenoidal sinus is the most posterior paranasal sinus. They open into the nasal cavity via the sphenoethmoidal recess super-oposteriorly to the superior concha, and not onto the lateral wall of the nasal cavity; hence E is the correct response.

6.2.42 *E – Laterally by the vaginal process of the pterygoid process*

The choanae are posterior nasal apertures between the nasal cavity and nasopharynx. Their lateral margins are by the posterior margin of the medial plate (not the vaginal process) of the pterygoid process; hence E is the correct response. The roof is formed anteriorly by the ala of the vomer and the vaginal process of the medial plate of the pterygoid process, and posteriorly by the body of the sphenoid bone. Their inferior margins are by the posterior border of the horizontal plate of the palatine bone, and medial borders are by the posterior aspect of the vomer.

6.2.43 *C – Superior nasal branches of the maxillary nerve*

The sphenopalatine foramen connects the nasal cavity to the pterygopalatine fossa. It is found at the superoposterior corner of the maxillary sinus, deep to middle nasal concha. Contents of this foramen include the sphenopalatine artery (branch of the maxillary artery) and vein, the nasopalatine branch of the maxillary nerve and the superior nasal branches of the maxillary nerve; hence C is the correct response.

6.2.44 *B – Tendon of masseter*

The infratemporal fossa is an irregularly wedge-shaped cavity deep to the masseter and ramus of the mandible that serves to house and protect neurovasculature that transmit through it. The contents of the fossa include the lateral and medial pterygoid, the tendon of temporalis, the mandibular nerve, chorda tympani, parts of the maxillary artery and vein, the pterygoid plexus of veins and the sphenomandibular ligament. The tendon of masseter is not a content of the fossa; hence B is the correct response.

Answers 6.2.45 to 6.2.48 relate to the following annotated coronal CT of the sinuses.

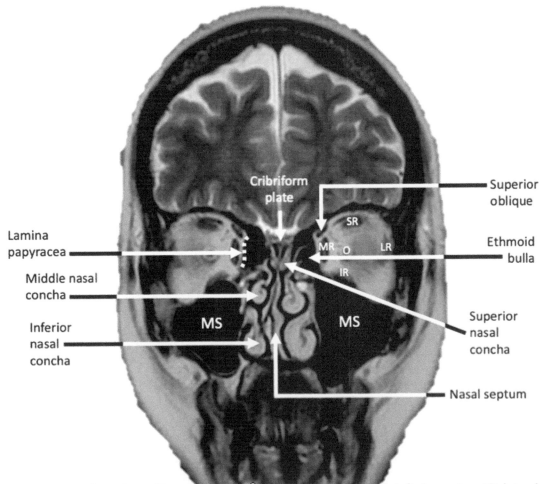

Key: MS: maxillary sinus; SR: superior rectus; MR: medial rectus; IR: inferior rectus; LR: lateral rectus; O: optic nerve;

6.2.45 *E – Medially with the maxilla*

Structure labelled 1 corresponds to the lamina papyracea of the ethmoid bone. This is the weakest aspect of the medial orbital wall, which forms a connection between the paranasal sinuses and the orbit. It articulates anteriorly with the lacrimal bone, posteriorly with the sphenoid bone, superiorly with the orbital plate of the frontal bone, and inferiorly with orbital process of the palatine bone and maxilla (not medially); hence E is the correct response.

6.2.46 *A – Inferior concha*

Structure labelled 2 corresponds to the inferior concha; hence A is the correct response.

6.2.47 *D – It receives its blood supply from the ophthalmic artery*

Structure labelled 3 corresponds to the superior oblique muscle. The blood supply to structures of the orbit is via the ophthalmic artery, a branch of the internal carotid artery; hence D is the correct response. It is innervated by the trochlear nerve. Lateral rectus is innervated by the abducens nerve. Superior oblique elevates, abducts and laterally rotates the eyeball. It originates from the body of the sphenoid bone.

6.2.48 *B – Ethmoid bulla*

Structure labelled 4 corresponds to the ethmoid bulla; hence B is the correct response. This is the largest anterior ethmoid air cell which forms the superoposterior walls of the ethmoid infundibulum and hiatus semilunaris.

6.2.49 *D – The pituitary gland can be surgically approached via the frontal sinuses*

The pituitary gland (hypophysis) is found in a depression within the body of the sphenoid bone – the sella turcica (from the Latin meaning *Turkish saddle*). The floor of the sella forms the roof of the sphenoid sinuses posteriorly. Due to partial or complete aeration of the sphenoid sinus and pneumatisation, a transsphenoidal hypophysectomy allows passage of an endoscope between the nasal septum and middle concha towards the pituitary. It is an indicated procedure for pituitary adenomas; hence D is the correct response. The cavernous sinuses lie lateral to the sella.

6.2.50 *D – Depressor supercilii*

The nares or nostrils are oval apertures on the inferior aspect of the external nose which act as a vestibule through the nasal cavities anteroposteriorally. Although the nares remain open, they can be opened further via muscles of facial expression – nasalis, procerus, depressor septi nasi and levator labii superioris alaeque nasi. Compressor naris and dilator naris form the transverse and alar component of the nasalis muscle, respectively. Depressor supercilii acts as a depressor of the eyebrow; hence D is the correct response.

6.3   Upper limb

6.3.1 *E – Musculocutaneous*

The musculocutaneous nerve is a terminal branch of the lateral cord of the brachial plexus, as shown in the figure below; hence E is the correct response. This nerve innervates the flexor muscles of the arm. Clinically, damage to C5 and C6 leads to Erb's palsy or 'waiter's tip' where the elbow is extended, and the arm is internally rotated and adducted. This results from functional loss of (1) brachialis and biceps due to damage of the musculocutaneous nerve, (2) supraspinatus and infraspinatus due to damage of the suprascapular nerve, and (3) deltoid due to damage of the axillary nerve.

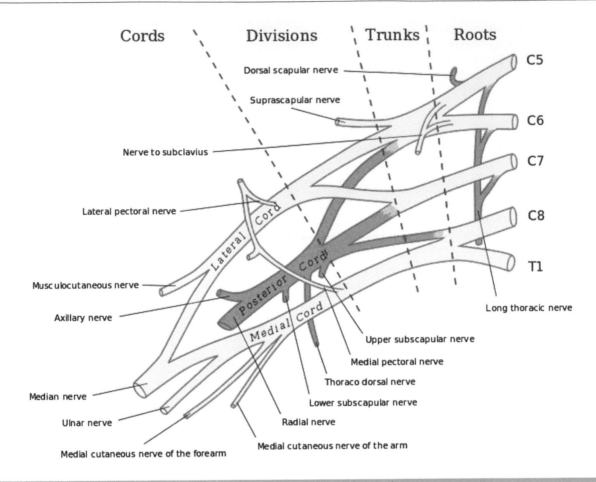

Cords   Divisions   Trunks   Roots

C5
C6
C7
C8
T1

Dorsal scapular nerve
Suprascapular nerve
Nerve to subclavius
Lateral pectoral nerve
Musculocutaneous nerve
Axillary nerve
Median nerve
Ulnar nerve
Medial cutaneous nerve of the forearm
Medial cutaneous nerve of the arm
Radial nerve
Lower subscapular nerve
Thoraco dorsal nerve
Medial pectoral nerve
Upper subscapular nerve
Long thoracic nerve
Lateral Cord
Posterior Cord
Medial Cord

6.3.2 D – The medial cord is a continuation of the anterior division of the inferior trunk

The medial cord is a continuation of the anterior division of the inferior trunk, as shown in Q 6.3.1; hence D is the correct response. C5 and C6 unite to form the superior/upper trunk. The roots and trunks can be found within the posterior triangle of the neck, between the anterior and middle scalene muscles. The posterior cord is formed by the posterior division of the superior, middle and inferior trunks. The long thoracic nerve originates from the rami of C5, C6 and C7. This nerve, like the dorsal scapular nerve which originates from the rami of C5, completely originates from the roots of the brachial plexus, and often pierce the middle scalene muscle.

6.3.3 A – The lateral wall is formed by the intertubercular sulcus of the humerus

There are five anatomic borders of the axilla: the superior (apex or inlet), anterior, posterior, medial and lateral walls. The lateral wall is formed by the intertubercular sulcus of humerus, the short head of the biceps and the coracobrachialis; hence A is the correct response. The medial wall is formed by the first four ribs and serratus anterior. The anterior wall is formed by pectoralis major and minor muscles (not supraspinatus). The posterior wall is formed by the latissimus dorsi, subscapularis, and teres major muscles. The apex is formed by the superior border of the scapula, the lateral border of the first rib, and the posterior border of the clavicle. The axilla has no floor.

6.3.4 C – Circumflex scapular

In the shoulder, the triangular space lies between the supraspinatus and subscapularis tendons. The base of the triangle is at the coracoid process, and the tip/apex is at the transverse humeral ligament which forms the roof of the bicipital groove. The subscapular artery divides into the circumflex scapular and the thoracodorsal artery. The circumflex scapular travels through the triangular space into the infraspinatus fossa where it anastomoses; hence C is the correct response. The circumflex scapular artery supplies the teres minor muscle.

6.3.5 C – Intercostobrachial

The intercostobrachial nerve originates from the lateral cutaneous branch of the second intercostal nerve (which originates from the anterior ramus of T2), and supplies the axilla, lateral chest, and medial surface of the arm; hence C is the correct response. Clinically, left-sided chest pain which radiates down the left arm in patients with myocardial infarction is mediated by the intercostobrachial nerve.

Answers 6.3.6 to 6.3.8 relate to the following annotated figure.

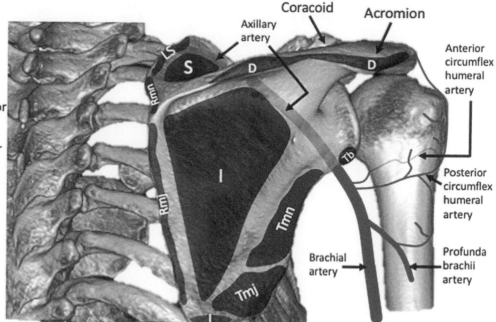

Scapula muscle attachments

LS: Levator scapulae

S: Supraspinatus

Rmn: Rhomboid minor

D: Deltoid

Rmj: Rhomboid major

I: Infraspinatus

L: Latissimus dorsi

Tmj: Teres major

Tmn: Teres minor

Tb: Long head of triceps brachii

6.3.6 *C – Inferior subscapular*

The muscle which originates in region labelled 1 is teres major. This muscle is innervated by the inferior/lower subscapular nerve, derived from C5 to C7 nerve roots; hence C is the correct response. The thoracodorsal nerve innervates latissimus dorsi. The axillary nerve innervates teres minor. The superior/upper subscapular nerve innervates subscapularis. The rhomboid muscles are innervated by the dorsal scapular nerve.

6.3.7 *B – Profunda brachii*

Label 2, as shown in the figure, corresponds to the profunda brachii artery; hence B is the correct response. Also referred to as the deep brachial artery, it is the first and largest of the brachial artery. Within the posterior compartment of the arm, it gives off a branch that anastomoses with the posterior circumflex humeral artery, and then proceeds inferiorly along the radial groove.

6.3.8 *E – It is an accessory abductor at the glenohumeral joint*

The muscle that originates at region labelled 3, the infraglenoid tubercle, corresponds to the long head of triceps brachii. The primary function of the triceps is forearm extension at the elbow joint. The long head ensures that the humeral head remains in the glenoid cavity when the arm is adducted (not abducted), in addition to extending and adducting the arm at the shoulder joint; hence E is the correct response.

6.3.9 *E – Skin on lateral aspect of the elbow tests for T1*

Dermatomes are areas of skin which are supplied by a single nerve root. The dermatomes of the upper portions of the brachial plexus (C5 and C6) are on the lateral aspect of the upper limb, the lower portions (C8 and T1) are on the medial aspect and C7 is in the middle. There is however overlap across adjoining dermatomes. Skin on the medial (not lateral) aspect of the elbow tests for T1; hence E is the correct response.

6.3.10 *A – Coracoclavicular*

The acromioclavicular joint is stabilised by the coracoclavicular and acromioclavicular ligaments. The coracoclavicular ligament is composed of two other ligaments: the conoid and trapezoid. These ligaments are continuous inferiorly at the coracoid process attachment but become separate before they attach to the inferior aspect of the clavicle superiorly. The conoid ligament attaches to the conoid tubercle of the clavicle, whereas the more anterolateral trapezoid ligament attaches to the trapezoid line of the clavicle; hence A is the correct response.

Answers 6.3.11 to 6.3.16 relate to the following annotated sagittal MRI figure of the shoulder.

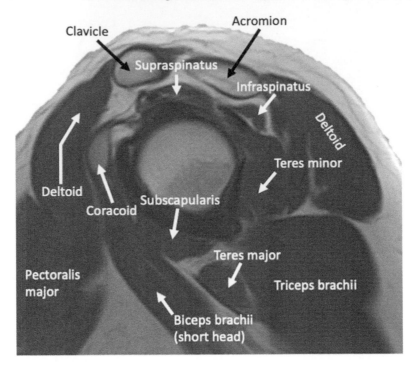

6.3.11   *B – 2*

The rotator cuff muscles include supraspinatus, infraspinatus, subscapularis and teres minor. They help maintain the stability of the glenohumeral joint. Muscle labelled 2 corresponds to deltoid which is not a rotator cuff muscle; hence B is the correct response.

6.3.12   *E – Coracoid process*

6.3.13   *E – 7*

Muscle labelled 7 corresponds to infraspinatus, which is innervated by the suprascapular nerve; hence E is the correct response. Muscle labelled 1, supraspinatus, is also innervated by the suprascapular nerve.

6.3.14   *A – 1*

Muscle labelled 1 corresponds to supraspinatus, which initiates shoulder abduction from 0 to 15 degrees, beyond which deltoid becomes the shoulder abductor; hence A is the correct response. Infraspinatus and teres minor are external rotators of the shoulder, and subscapularis is an internal rotator. Clinically, Jobe's test evaluates supraspinatus function which is positive i.e., painful, or weak when downwards force is applied to the arm when it is at 90 degrees abduction and internally rotated.

6.3.15   *C – Coracobrachialis and short head of biceps brachii*

Label 3 corresponds to the coracoid. The short head of biceps brachii attaches at the apex of the coracoid and inserts onto the radial tuberosity via the bicipital aponeurosis. Coracobrachialis, as the name suggest, also originates at the coracoid (apex) and inserts into the middle of the medial humerus; hence C is the correct response. The long head of biceps brachii originates from the supraglenoid tubercle of the glenoid. The triceps muscle has three attachment sites: the long head – infraglenoid tubercle, lateral head – above the spiral groove of the posterior humeral shaft (upper half), and medial head – below the spiral groove of the posterior humeral shaft (lower half). Brachialis attaches to the lower half of the humerus and inserts into the coronoid process of the ulna.

6.3.16   *D – Posterior humeral circumflex*

The deltoid muscle receives its main blood supply from the thoracoacromial branch of the axillary artery. It also receives a minor blood supply from the posterior humeral circumflex artery; hence D is the correct response. This artery also supplies teres minor and teres major, alongside the subscapular and circumflex scapular arteries.

6.3.17 *D – The profunda brachii artery passes through the triangular interval*

There are several gateways to the posterior scapular. The triangular interval serves as a passageway between the anterior and posterior compartments of the arm. It is formed by the shaft of the humerus laterally, the lateral border of the long head of triceps brachii medially, and the inferior border of teres major. The profunda brachii traverses the triangular interval with the radial nerve into the posterior compartment of the arm; hence D is the correct response. The triangular space is formed from teres major superiorly, teres minor inferiorly and the long head of triceps brachii medially. The circumflex scapular artery and vein traverse this space. The quadrangular space is located along the posterolateral shoulder and serves as a passageway for the axillary nerve and posterior humeral circumflex artery. Teres minor is a superior boundary (not inferior) of the quadrangular space. Teres major is an inferior boundary, the surgical neck of the humerus is a lateral boundary and the long head of triceps brachii is a medial boundary. The triangular space is medial to the quadrangular space. The final passageway is the suprascapular foramen formed by the suprascapular notch and the suprascapular ligament. It contains the suprascapular nerve and artery which course below and above the ligament respectively.

6.3.18 *A – Radial*

The radial nerve passes through the triangular interval; hence A is the correct response.

Answers 6.3.19 to 6.3.22 relate to the following annotated figure.

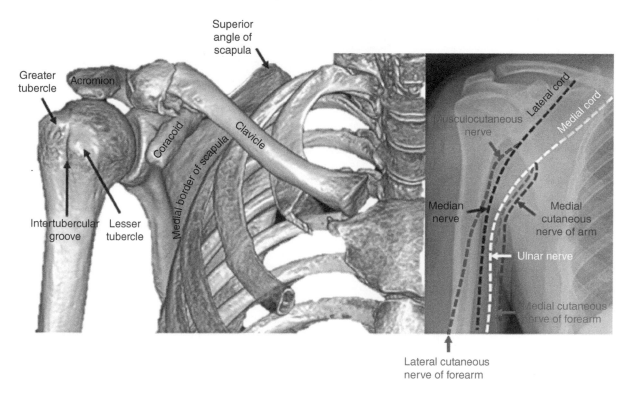

6.3.19 *D – Subscapularis*

Region labelled 1 corresponds to the lesser tubercle of the humerus. Subscapularis inserts into this region; hence D is the correct response.

6.3.20 *B – Long thoracic*

The asterisks denote the medial border of the scapula. Serratus anterior inserts into the costal surface of the medial border of the scapula. Serratus anterior is innervated by the long thoracic nerve; hence B is the correct response. Clinically, damage to this nerve leads to a winged scapula and elevation of the arm is prevented.

6.3.21 *E – Radial tuberosity | Musculocutaneous nerve | Flexion of forearm at elbow*

The long head of biceps brachii originates as a tendon from the supraglenoid tubercle of the scapula, passing over the humeral head where it enters the intertubercular sulcus or groove. It is held in position by the transverse humeral ligament. It then forms a muscle belly in the arm. Both long and short heads insert into the radial tuberosity. It is innervated by the musculocutaneous nerve, and it functions to flex the forearm at the elbow and supinate the forearm; hence E is the correct response.

6.3.22 *D – Lateral cutaneous nerve of arm*

The lateral cutaneous nerve of the forearm is a termination of the musculocutaneous nerve, a branch of the lateral cord of the brachial plexus. It courses distally between biceps brachii and brachialis to penetrate coracobrachialis. It supplies the skin of the anterolateral surface of the forearm and distal arm. The nerve(s) depicted by the line labelled 3 would not represent this nerve; hence D is the correct response.

Answers 6.3.23 to 6.3.25 relate to the following annotated CT figure of the shoulder.

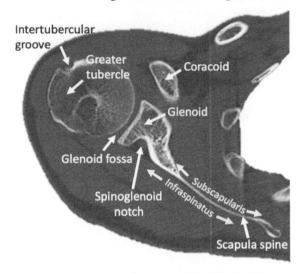

6.3.23 *C – Glenoid fossa*

6.3.24 *C – Infraspinatus*

Infraspinatus originates in the infraspinous fossa (medial two-thirds). In this axial CT scan, and as the name suggests, this is located inferior to the scapula spine; hence C is the correct response. Subscapularis originates in the subscapular fossa (medial two-thirds), which lies at the anterior surface of the scapula.

6.3.25 *E – Greater tubercle*

Facets are difficult to appreciate in this axial CT scan. There are three facets to the greater tubercle – the superior, middle and inferior, where supraspinatus, infraspinatus and teres minor attach respectively. Separating the greater tubercle from the lesser tubercle is the intertubercular groove (sulcus), or bicipital groove where the long head of bicep brachii runs in the groove to attach to the supraglenoid tubercle. The spinoglenoid notch is also highlighted. This is a connection between the infraspinous and supraspinous fossa. The suprascapular nerve and artery traverse the notch. Clinically, ganglion cysts can form in this notch, compressing the nerve which results in posterior shoulder discomfort with pain on external rotation and abduction.

Answers 6.3.26 to 6.3.31 relate to the following annotated MRI figures of the elbow.

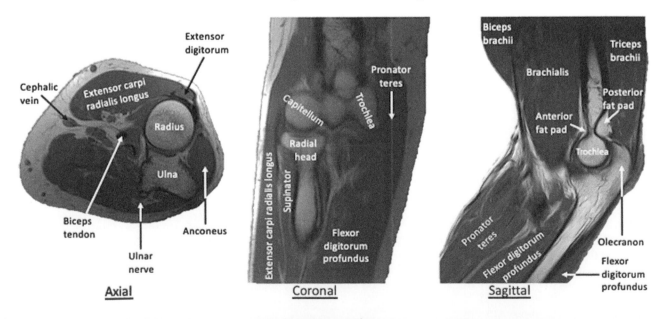

6.3.26 *B – Extensor carpi radialis longus*

6.3.27 *A – Ulnar nerve*

6.3.28 *A – Posterior interosseous recurrent artery and radial nerve*

Muscle labelled 3 corresponds to anconeus. This triangular-shaped muscle originates posterior to the lateral epicondyle of the humerus and fans out to insert into the proximal posterolateral ulna. The primary blood supply comes from the interosseous recurrent artery when the muscle is more distally based, but there is also a small contribution from the medial collateral artery (from the deep brachial artery) when the muscle is more proximally based. Anconeus is innervated by the radial nerve (C7, C8 and T1); hence A is the correct response. The muscle helps stabilise the elbow and abducts the ulna during pronation. It is also a weak extensor of the elbow.

6.3.29 *E – 4 is innervated by the deep branch of the radial nerve and 5 receives a blood supply from the ulnar artery*

Muscles labelled 4 and 5 correspond to supinator and pronator teres, respectively. Supinator's broad origins include the lateral epicondyle of the humerus, the supinator crest and fossa of the ulna, the radial collateral ligament and annual radial ligament, and inserts into the lateral, anterior and posterior surfaces of the proximal third of the radius. It is innervated by the deep branch of the radial nerve (C5, C6). Supinator supinates the forearm. Pronator teres originates at the medial epicondyle of the humerus and coronoid process of the ulna and inserts into the lateral surface (midshaft) of the radius. It is innervated by the median nerve (C6, C7) and receives a blood supply from the ulnar artery and anterior recurrent ulnar artery; hence E is the correct response. Pronator teres pronates the forearm. Pronator teres pronates the forearm; hence E is the correct response.

6.3.30 *D – Olecranon*

6.3.31 *C – Flexes distal phalanges at distal interphalangeal joints of medial four digits*

Muscle labelled 7 corresponds to flexor digitorum profundus. This extrinsic hand muscle flexes the MCP and DIP joints of the medial four digits (index, middle, ring and little fingers); hence C is the correct response. This muscle lies in the deep volar compartment of the forearm; the tendons originating at the medial epicondyle of the humerus, ulnar collateral ligament and coronoid process of the ulnar, and the radial head, and inserting into the bases of the distal phalanges of the medial four digits. The lateral part of the muscle (digits 2 and 3) is innervated by the anterior interosseous branch of the median nerve, and the medial part (digits 4 and 5) is innervated by the ulnar nerve (C8 and T1). It receives a blood supply from the anterior interosseous artery, a branch of the common interosseous artery, which is a proximal branch of the ulnar artery.

6.3.32 *E – Median cubital vein*

The antecubital fossa marks the transition between the arm and forearm. It is triangular and has three borders: superior – a horizontal line between the epicondyles of the humerus, lateral – medial border of brachioradialis, medial – lateral border of pronator teres; a roof – bicipital aponeurosis, fascia, and fat; and a floor – brachialis (proximally) and supinator (distally). Contents include the radial nerve, biceps tendon, brachial artery, and the median nerve. The brachial artery bifurcates into the radial and ulnar arteries at the apex of the fossa. The median cubital vein is not found within the fossa, but within the roof; hence E is the correct response. Clinically, this vein is often accessed for venepuncture.

6.3.33 *E – Ulnar collateral*

Elbow ligaments are complex. The elbow contains two collateral ligaments: the medial (ulnar) collateral (MCL) and lateral (radial) collateral ligaments (LCL). MCL has three ligamentous portions – (1) anterior and (2) posterior which originate from the medial epicondyle of the humerus and attach to the coronoid process of the ulna and medial olecranon of the ulna respectively; and (3) transverse (Cooper's ligament) which originates from the olecranon process and inserts into the sublime tubercle of the ulna; hence E is the correct response. LCL has four ligamentous portions – (1) lateral ulnar collateral and (2) radial collateral which originate between the trochlea and capitellum of the lateral epicondyle of the humerus and courses distally inserting into the annular ligament; (3) annular and (4) accessory collateral. The annular ligament plays an important role in elbow stabilisation by supporting articulation of the radial head with the radial notch of the ulna during supination and pronation. This ligament attaches to the anterior and posterior aspect of the radial notch of the ulna, and it begins to taper and then attach to the neck of the radius. The accessory ligament originates at the supinator crest of the ulna and attaches to the annular ligament. The quadrate ligament attaches the radial neck to the inferior aspect of the radial notch, thus limiting rotation of the radial head and maintaining tension.

6.3.34 *E – Extensor carpi radialis longus*

The posterior interosseous nerve is a deep branch of the radial nerve which supplies motor innervation to common extensors – extensor carpi ulnaris, extensor digitorum communis, extensor digit minimi and extensor carpi radialis brevis; and deep extensors – extensor pollicis longus, extensor pollicis brevis, extensor indicis, abductor pollicis longus and supinator. Extensor carpi radialis longus is innervated directly by the radial nerve (C6, C7); hence E is the correct response.

6.3.35 *C – Palmaris longus*

The table below shows superficial and deep flexor and extensor forearm muscles. Palmaris longus is an anterior forearm flexor which attaches proximally to the medial humeral epicondyle and distally to the palmar aponeurosis and flexor retinaculum; hence C is the correct response. It is a weak flexor at the wrist. Clinically, this is one of the most anatomically variable muscles and can often be absent uni- or bilaterally. Interestingly this absence has no effect on grip strength. It is a common tendon used in harvesting for autologous tendon grafting.

Forearm muscles	Flexors	Extensors
Superficial	• Flexor digitorum superficialis • Flexor carpi ulnaris • Flexor carpi radialis longus • Pronator teres • Palmaris longus	• Extensor digitorum • Extensor digiti minimi • Extensor carpi radialis longus • Extensor carpi radialis brevis • Extensor carpi ulnaris • Brachioradialis • Anconeus
Deep	• Flexor digitorum profundus • Flexor pollicis longus • Pronator quadratus	• Extensor pollicis longus • Extensor pollicis brevis • Extensor indicis • Abductor pollicis longus • Supinator

6.3.36 *B – Flexor pollicis brevis*

The carpal tunnel contains the median nerve and nine tendons – four flexor digitorum profundus and four flexor digitorum superficialis tendons, and the flexor pollicis longus tendon. As the median nerve exits the carpal tunnel, it gives off the recurrent thenar branch which supplies the thenar muscles of the hands – flexor pollicis brevis, abductor pollicis brevis and opponens pollicis; hence B is the correct response. Flexor pollicis longus is supplied by the anterior interosseous nerve, which is outside of the tunnel. Opponens digiti minimi is supplied by the deep branch of the ulnar nerve. Flexor carpi radialis is supplied by the median nerve (C6, C7). Dorsal interossei are supplied by the deep branch of the ulnar nerve (C8, T1). Remember Guyon's (ulnar) canal contains the ulnar nerve and artery, venae comitantes of the ulnar artery and lymphatic vessels.

Answers 6.3.37 to 6.3.41 relate to the following annotated MRI figures of the forearm, wrist, and hand.

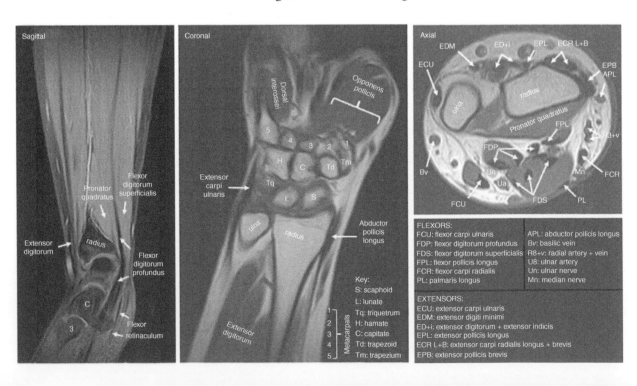

6.3.37 *B – Capitate*

6.3.38 *E – Opponens pollicis*

Together with adductor pollicis, abductor pollicis brevis and flexor pollicis brevis, opponens pollicis is located within the thenar eminence of the hand. It originates from tubercle of trapezium and the flexor retinaculum and inserts into the first metacarpal; hence E is the correct response. As the name suggests, it actions to oppose the thumb to the fingertips. In this MRI slice, there is only a marginal appearance of the first metacarpal and trapezium. Moving towards the dorsal surface, the first metacarpal and trapezium emerge with abductor pollicis longus, adductor pollicis brevis and extensor pollicis brevis and longus. The pisometacarpal ligament joins pisiform to the base of the fifth metacarpal and is a continuation of the flexor carpi ulnaris tendon. Guyon's canal is a space at the ulnar border of the volar aspect of the wrist. The hook of hamate is a volar projection that serves as the lateral border of Guyon's canal and protects the ulnar nerve. Opponens digiti minimi is a hypothenar eminence, intrinsic muscle of the hand. It originates from the hook of hamate and flexor retinaculum and inserts onto the medial aspect of the fifth metacarpal.

6.3.39 *C – Extends and adducts the wrist*

Muscle labelled 3 corresponds to extensor carpi radialis. It is located within the posterior compartment of the forearm and functions to extend and adduct the wrist; hence C is the correct response. It originates at the lateral epicondyle of the distal humerus and inserts onto the dorsal base of the fifth metacarpal after traversing through the extensor retinaculum.

6.3.40 *A – Posterior interosseous*

Muscles labelled 4 correspond to tendons of extensor pollicis brevis and abductor pollicis longus. Both muscles are supplied by the posterior interosseus artery, a branch of the common interosseous artery; hence A is the correct response. This artery also supplies the ulna, supinator and other extensors of the forearm. Most distally it anastomoses with the anterior interosseous artery, ultimately joining the dorsal carpal arch.

6.3.41 *B – Palmaris longus*

6.3.42 *E – Flexor carpi radialis tendon*

The carpal tunnel contains the median nerve and nine tendons – one flexor pollicis longus, four flexor digitorum profundus and four flexor digitorum superficialis. Flexor carpi radialis, the most powerful wrist flexor, is not found within the carpal tunnel; hence E is the correct response.

6.3.43 *C – Adductor digiti minimi forms the lateral (radial) wall and floor*

The anatomic boundaries of Guyon's canal include pisiform, flexor carpi ulnaris tendon and abductor digiti minimi which form the medial (ulnar) wall, the hook of hamate which forms the lateral (radial) wall, the volar (palmar) carpal ligament which forms the roof, and the pisohamate ligament, flexor digitorum profundus tendons, abductor digiti minimi muscle and the flexor retinaculum which forms the floor; hence C is the correct response. The flexor retinaculum also forms part of the roof and lateral wall of the canal.

6.3.44 *D – Palmar interossei*

The palmar interossei adduct the first, second, fourth and fifth digits at the MCP joints; hence D is the correct response. They also flex at the MCP joints and extend at the PIP and DIP joints. The dorsal interossei are involved in abduction and flexion of the second, third and fourth digits at the MCP joints, and extension of the PIP and DIP joints. The lumbricals, named after the earthworm genus *Lumbricus* – hence 'worm-like', are involved in flexion of the MCP joints and extension of the PIP and DIP joints. Palmaris brevis functions to wrinkle the skin of the palm, tightening the palmar aponeurosis and increasing grip strength. Adductor pollicis functions to adduct the thumb.

6.3.45 *D – There are seven extensor compartments of the wrist*

There are six (not seven) extensor compartments of the wrist:

1) Extensor pollicis brevis and abductor pollicis longus
2) Extensor carpi radialis longus and brevis
3) Extensor pollicis longus
4) Extensor digitorum and indicis
5) Extensor digiti minimi
6) Extensor carpi ulnaris

Hence D is the correct response.

6.3.46 *B – Flexor digiti minimi*

Flexor digiti minimi originates at the hook of hamate and flexor retinaculum and inserts onto the medial side of the base of the proximal phalanx of the fifth digit; hence B is the correct response. Abductor digiti minimi originates at pisiform and inserts onto the medial side of the base of the proximal phalanx of the fifth digit. Adductor pollicis has two heads: the oblique head originates at the base of the second and third metacarpals and capitate, and the transverse head originates at the anterior surface of the third metacarpal. The heads then taper inserting onto the medial side of the base of the proximal phalanx of the thumb. Opponens pollicis originates at the flexor retinaculum and scaphoid and trapezium tubercles and insert onto the lateral side of the first metacarpal. The lumbricals are four small intrinsic muscles of the hand and are unique in that they have both tendinous origins and insertions. Lumbricals 1–2 are unipennate and are innervated by the median nerve, whereas lumbricals 3–4 are bipennate and are innervated by the ulnar nerve.

6.3.47 *A – Biceps brachii*

Biceps brachii is a strong forearm supinator and weak elbow flexor; it has no role in extension; hence A is the correct response. Acting antagonistically to biceps, triceps brachii is the primary extensor of the forearm at the elbow. Together with teres major and pectoralis major, latissimus dorsi adduct, medially rotate, and extend the arm at the glenohumeral joint. Interossei extend at the PIP and DIP joints.

6.3.48 *C – Anastomoses occur in the shoulder, elbow and hand*

There are anastomoses in the scapular and shoulder, elbow, wrist and hand; hence C is the correct response. The aortic arch gives off the brachiocephalic trunk, the left common carotid artery, and the left (not right) subclavian artery. The brachial artery usually bifurcates to form the radial and ulnar artery in the cubital fossa at the level of the radial neck (not usually superior to the trochlea of the humerus). Cephalic and basilic veins are major superficial (not deep) veins of the upper limb. The ulnar artery branches into the anterior and posterior ulnar recurrent arteries, the common interosseous artery, the palmar and dorsal carpal arch, and superficial palmar arch. The radial artery terminates as the deep palmar branch which is the primary blood supply to the deep palmar arch.

6.3.49 *E – Median nerve and ulnar artery*

This is a dorsal view of the hand. The median nerve and its branches provide cutaneous innervation to the dorsal surface of the distal phalanx of the lateral 3½ digits including the thumb and nails, and the palmar surface and lateral two-thirds of the palm. The ulnar nerve and its branches provide cutaneous innervation to the medial one-third of the dorsal surface including the palmar and dorsal surfaces of the medial 1½ digits, and the medial one-third of the palm. The radial nerve provides innervation to the lateral two-thirds of the dorsal surface including the dorsal surface of the proximal and middle phalanges of the lateral 3½ digits. The first digit and half of the second digit are supplied mainly by the radial artery. The ulnar artery supplies the other half of the second digit and the remaining three digits; hence E is the correct response.

6.3.50 *A – Palmar branch of median nerve*

Region labelled 2 corresponds to the anatomical snuffbox, a triangular depression on the dorsum of the hand at the base of the thumb. Boundaries to this region include tendons of extensor pollicis longus medially, tendons of extensor pollicis brevis and abductor pollicis longus laterally, the floor being formed by scaphoid and trapezium, and tendons of extensor carpi radialis longus and brevis. Both the cephalic vein and radial artery lie within the anatomical snuffbox. The palmar branch of the median nerve is not located within this region; hence A is the correct response.

6.4 Thorax, mediastinum and back

6.4.1 *C – T4*

The table below shows common landmarks associated with vertebral levels. The azygos vein curves anteriorly over the hilum of the right lung and drains into the superior vena cava; hence C is the correct response.

Vertebral level	Landmark
C3	Hyoid bone
C4	Superior border of thyroid cartilage Bifurcation of common carotid artery
C6	Cricoid cartilage End of larynx and pharynx Start of trachea and oesophagus
C7	Vertebral prominence Isthmus of thyroid gland
T2/T3	Suprasternal notch
T4	Sternal angle Tracheal bifurcation Start and end of aortic arch Start of thoracic aorta Division between superior and inferior mediastinum Azygos vein arches over hilum of right lung and drains into SVC
T7	Inferior angle of scapula
T8	IVC passes into diaphragm
T10	Xiphoid process of sternum Oesophagus opens into diaphragm
T12	Aorta, thoracic duct and azygos vein open into diaphragm
L1	Transpyloric plane Origin of superior mesenteric artery Hilum of kidneys Coeliac artery above plane Renal arteries below plane
L2	Thoracic duct begins Azygos and hemiazygos veins begin
L4/L5	Iliac crest Bifurcation of aorta into right and left common iliac arteries Start of IVC

6.4.2 *C – Pectoralis minor*

Pectoralis minor originates from ribs 3 to 5 close to their costal cartilages and inserts onto the coracoid process of the scapula; hence C is the correct response.

6.4.3 *D – The oesophagus passes through the oesophageal hiatus at T12*

The oesophagus passes through the oesophageal hiatus at T10 (not T12), as shown in the table in 6.4.1; hence D is the correct response.

6.4.4 *A – Great cardiac vein*

The coronary sulcus or atrioventricular groove separates the atria and ventricles, running transversely around the heart. It contains the right coronary artery, the small cardiac vein, the coronary sinus and the circumflex artery (a branch of the left coronary artery). It does not contain the great cardiac vein; hence A is the correct response. The two ventricles are separated by the anterior and posterior interventricular sulci or grooves. The great cardiac vein, with the anterior interventricular artery, runs in the anterior interventricular sulcus. The middle cardiac vein and posterior interventricular artery run in the posterior interventricular sulcus.

6.4.5 C – The septomarginal trabecula is found in the right ventricle

The septomarginal trabecula or moderator band is a muscular band which extends from the interventricular septum to the base of the anterior papillary muscle. Anatomically, this acts as a marker which helps differentiate between the left and right ventricle. The band crosses to the lateral wall of the right ventricle; hence C is the correct response. It carries a portion of neuronal fibres from the right bundle branch of the atrioventricular conduction system to the anterior wall of the right ventricle. Crista terminalis is smooth myocardium found near the opening of the superior vena cava and extends down the lateral wall of the right atrium (not left) to the inferior vena cava. Pectinate muscles project from the crista and are found on the inner walls of the right atrium (and right auricle). Papillary muscles or trabeculae carneae are found in the ventricles, with those found in the left ventricle being far more delicate than the right. Most of these structures have their entire length attached to the ventricular walls, whilst others have one end attached to the walls and the other end attached to fibrous cords (chordae tendineae). These attach to the free edges of the cusps of the tricuspid valve and mitral valve in the right and left ventricle, respectively. The septal papillary muscle is only found in the right ventricle and is the smallest, and sometimes can even be absent. Two other papillary muscles are found in both the left and right ventricles – the anterior and posterior papillary muscles. The anterior is the larger of the two. The conus arteriosus or infundibulum derives from the embryonic bulbus cordis and is the cone-shaped outflow tract of the right ventricle which leads to the pulmonary valve. It has smooth walls which lack trabeculae. The primitive ventricle becomes the trabeculated parts of the left and right ventricles in adulthood.

6.4.6 B – Marginal

The right coronary artery emerges from the right sinus of Valsalva, through the atrioventricular groove before curving posteriorly, and making a bend at the crux of the heart and continuing in the posterior interventricular sulcus. The right coronary artery gives off two branches: the conus (arteriosus) artery which supplies the right ventricle, and the sinoatrial nodal artery which supplies the sinoatrial node and right atrium. Other branches of the right coronary artery include the right acute marginal artery, posterior descending artery and the atrioventricular nodal artery; hence B is the correct response. All other arteries listed are branches of the left coronary artery – the anterior interventricular artery commonly being referred to as the left anterior descending artery (LAD).

6.4.7 E – Oesophageal plexus

Contents of the superior and inferior (anterior, middle, and posterior) mediastinum include:
Superior

- Oesophagus
- Trachea
- Thymus
- Arch of aorta (and branches)
- Brachiocephalic veins
- Upper half of SVC
- Phrenic nerves
- Vagus nerves
- Left recurrent laryngeal nerve

Inferior

Anterior

- Internal thoracic vessels
- Parasternal lymph nodes

Middle

- Heart
- Pericardium
- Tracheal bifurcation
- Bronchi
- Ascending aorta
- Pulmonary trunk
- Lower half of SVC
- Cardiac plexus
- Phrenic nerves

Posterior

- Descending aorta
- Oesophagus
- Oesophageal plexus with vagus nerves
- Thoracic duct
- Azygos vein
- Hemiazygos vein
- Sympathetic trunks

Hence E is the correct response.

6.4.8 *E – Xiphoid process T12*

The xiphoid process is the most inferior part of the sternum, with its tip located at the level of T10 (not T12); hence E is the correct response.

6.4.9 *A – Manubriosternal*

A symphysis is the joining of cartilaginous joints by fibrocartilage. In comparison, a synchondrosis is the joining of cartilaginous joints by hyaline cartilage. Synchondroses are primary cartilaginous joints, whereas symphyses are secondary cartilaginous joints. Examples of symphyses include the manubriosternal joint between the body of the sternum and the manubrium, the pubic symphysis between the left and right pubic bones, intervertebral discs and sacrococcygeal symphysis; hence A is the correct response. Synchondroses are ossification sites of the developing skeleton and do not exist in the mature skeleton. Examples include the xiphisternal joint, costochondral joint, the first sternocostal joint between the first rib and the manubrium (all others are synovial joints), growth plates, ischiopubic synchondroses of the pelvis and petro-occipital synchondroses of the skull (sutures). Interchondral joints are synovial joints.

6.4.10 *D – Brachial*

The arterial supply to the breast is via branches of the axillary artery – superior thoracic, thoracoacromial, lateral thoracic and subscapular arteries, mamillary branches of the internal thoracic artery (a branch of the subclavian artery), and perforating branches of the second to fourth intercostal arteries. The brachial artery and its branches do not supply the breast; hence D is the correct response.

6.4.11 *B – Supraclavicular*

Supraclavicular lymph nodes are not axillary; hence B is the correct response. These are cervical lymph nodes found in the posterior triangle. They are anatomically bound by the scalene muscles posteriorly, sternocleidomastoid muscle anteriorly, the common carotid artery and internal jugular vein medially, and the lateral edge of sternocleidomastoid laterally.

6.4.12 *D – Serratus posterior superior*

The thoracic wall is composed of five muscles: external intercostal, internal intercostal and innermost intercostal muscles, subcostalis, and transversus thoracis. Muscles which do not make up the thoracic wall but instead attach to it include subclavius, pectoralis major and minor, serratus anterior, and posterior thoracic muscles – levatores costarum, serratus posterior superior and serratus posterior inferior. The table below shows the origin and insertion of these muscles; hence D is the correct response.

Muscle	Origin	Insertion
External intercostal	Inferior border of rib above	Superior border of immediate rib below
Internal intercostal	Lateral edge of costal groove of rib above	Superior border of immediate rib below
Innermost intercostal	Medial edge of costal groove of rib above	Superior border of immediate rib below
Subcostalis	Internal surface of lower ribs	Internal surface of 2nd or 3rd rib below
Transversus thoracis	Lower 3rd of posterior surface of sternal body; posterior surface of xiphoid process and sternal ends of costal cartilages of 4th–7th ribs	Inner surfaces of 2nd–6th costal cartilages
Levatores costarum	Transverse processes of C7–T11	Ribs 1–12 below
Serratus posterior superior	Lower part of nuchal ligament and spinous processes of C7–T3	Superior border of ribs 2–5
Serratus posterior inferior	Spinous processes of T11–L2	Inferior border of ribs 9–12

6.4.13 *C – Left main bronchus passes superior to the aortic arch and posterior to the oesophagus*

The left main bronchus passes inferior (not superior) to the aortic arch and anterior (not posterior) to the oesophagus (with the thoracic aorta); hence C is the correct response.

6.4.14 *B – Sternopericardial ligaments attach fibrous pericardium to the posterior surface of the sternum*

Weak sternopericardial ligaments attach the anterior aspect of the fibrous pericardium to the posterior surface of the sternum; hence B is the correct response. The fibrous pericardium (not serous) is continuous with the central tendon of the diaphragm. The apex is fused with roots of the great vessels of the base of the heart. Weak sterno pericardial ligaments connect the anterior aspect of the fibrous pericardium to the sternum. The inner surface of the fibrous pericardium is lined with an outer layer (parietal) of serous pericardium. The inner layer (visceral) lines the surface of the heart. The pericardiacophrenic artery supplies blood to the pericardium, diaphragm, and phrenic nerve. It is a branch of the internal thoracic artery (which branches from the subclavian artery). The epicardium (not myocardium) is the outermost layer of the heart composed of visceral serous pericardium, which adheres to the myocardium (muscular layer). The pericardium is innervated by the phrenic nerve (not the vagus).

6.4.15 *D – The ligamentum nuchae extends from the external occipital protuberance to the foramen magnum, and then extends inferiorly, where the apex is attached to the spinous process of C4*

The ligamentum nuchae is a thick, fibrous ligament located between the posterior muscles of the neck, and limits hyperflexion. It extends from the inion of the occipital bone (or external occipital protuberance) to the spinous processes in between, and apically attaches to the spinous process of C7 (not C4); hence D is the correct response.

6.4.16 *A – Latissimus dorsi*

Latissimus dorsi is innervated by the thoracodorsal nerve; hence A is the correct response. Trapezius is innervated by the accessory nerve (CN XI). Rhomboid major and minor are innervated by the dorsal scapular nerve. Levator scapulae is innervated by direct branches from anterior rami of C3 and C4 spinal nerves and C5 branches from the dorsal scapular nerve.

6.4.17 *E – Levator scapulae*

Levator scapulae elevates the scapula; hence E is the correct response. Latissimus dorsi is involved in adduction, internal rotation, and extension of the arm at the glenohumeral joint. Trapezius elevates and depresses the scapula, and medially rotates the arm. Middle fibres adduct (retract) the scapula. The rhomboid muscles help support the shoulder girdle. They both elevate, retract (adduct) and rotate the scapula, and also protract the medial aspect of the scapula within the posterior thoracic wall.

6.4.18 *A – C6*

An uncinate process is a hook-shaped projection from a bone or organ. These structures are found in the head of the pancreas, the ribs, the ethmoid bone, and lower cervical vertebrae; hence A is the correct response. They are found on the posterolateral margin of the superior surface of C3–C7.

6.4.19 *C – Superior radicular*

The spinal cord is supplied by three main arteries: the anterior two-thirds by the anterior spinal artery and the posterior third by the pair of posterior (posterolateral) spinal arteries. These arteries are supplied with additional feeding vessels throughout the entire spinal cord at each spinal level – segmental spinal arteries. These bifurcate into anterior and posterior radicular arteries (not superior); hence C is the correct response. Sometimes, the segmental spinal arteries branch into segmental medullary arteries which also feed the anterior and posterior spinal arteries. The largest segmental medullary artery is also known as the artery of Adamkiewicz or the greater anterior radiculomedullary artery, which supplies the thoracolumbar region. Segmental arteries supplying the mid-thoracic region can sometimes branch from the posterior intercostal artery.

Answers 6.4.20 to 6.4.23 relate to the following annotated figure.

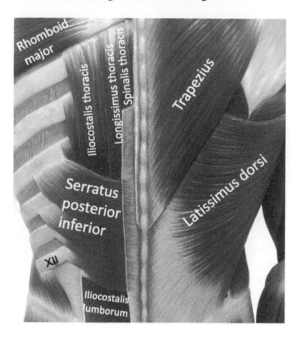

6.4.20   *D – Dorsal scapular*

Muscle labelled 1 corresponds to rhomboid major. It attaches to the spinous processes of T2 – T5 vertebrae and inserts onto the medial border of the scapula near the base of the scapula spine. It is innervated by the dorsal scapular nerve; hence D is the correct response.

6.4.21   *C – Longissimus*

Muscle labelled 2 corresponds to longissimus; hence C is the correct response. This muscle belongs to the erector spinae muscles which are the intermediate layer of deep back muscles. They are divided into three groups from medial to lateral: spinalis, longissimus and iliocostalis. From superior to inferior, these are subdivided into three: spinalis capitis, spinous cervicis, and spinalis thoracis; longissimus capitis, longissimus cervicis, and longissimus thoracic; and iliocostalis cervicis, iliocostalis thoracis, and iliocostalis lumborum. These muscles are all involved in bilateral flexion and ipsilateral lateral flexion of the spine. Splenius cervicis, together with splenius capitis, is a superficial muscle group layer of the deep (intrinsic) back muscles. It aids in bilateral extension of the neck, and ipsilateral lateral flexion and rotation of the neck. Multifidus, together with semispinalis and rotatores, belong to the transversospinales deep back muscles. This group help extend the spine bilaterally, and aid in ipsilateral lateral flexion and contralateral rotation of the spine.

6.4.22   *E – Lumbar*

Muscle labelled 3 corresponds to iliocostalis. More specifically, iliocostalis lumborum as the muscle inserts into the angle of ribs 5–12, and the transverse processes of L1–L4 vertebrae. It originates on the lateral crest of the sacrum, the medial end of the iliac crest and the thoracolumbar fascia. There is a mixed blood supply to this muscle – the dorsal branches of the lumbar arteries from the abdominal aorta at L1–L4, and the dorsal branches of the lateral sacral artery which branches from the posterior division of the internal iliac artery; hence E is the correct response. It is innervated by dorsal rami of thoracic and lumbar spinal nerves (T7– L3). Iliocostalis thoracis receives a blood supply from the dorsal branches of the posterior intercostal and subcostal arteries. Iliocostalis cervicis receives a blood supply from the vertebral, deep cervical and occipital arteries.

6.4.23   *A – Depresses ribs*

Muscle labelled 4 corresponds to serratus posterior inferior. This muscle functions to depresses the ribs; hence A is the correct response. It attaches to the spinous processes of T11–L2 vertebrae and inserts onto the inferior borders of ribs 9–12. Serratus posterior superior elevates the ribs.

Answers 6.4.24 to 6.4.29 relate to the following annotated figure.

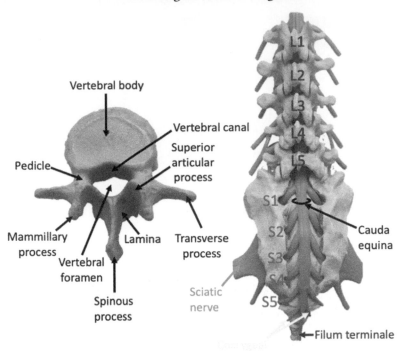

6.4.24 B – |Pedicle|Spinous process|Lamina|Transverse process|

6.4.25 C – *Posterior longitudinal ligament*

The posterior longitudinal ligament runs along the posterior surface of the vertebral body inside the vertebral canal from the body of the axis to the sacrum and provides stability in the spine; hence C is the correct response. Its purpose is to limit flexion of the vertebral column. The anterior longitudinal ligament is attached to the upper and lower edges of the vertebral bodies and limits extension of the vertebral column. The ligamentum flavum connects the laminae of adjacent vertebrae from C2 to S1. The ligament is extremely elastic and hence preserves upright posture. The supraspinous ligament is a fibrous connection between the apices of the spinous processes from C7 to L3/4. This ligamentum is known as the ligamentum nuchae as it ascends from C7 towards the cranium. The interspinous ligament connects adjacent spinous processes from C1 to S1 (from the roots to apices). The fibres connect with the ligamentum flavum anteriorly and the supraspinous ligament posteriorly.

6.4.26 A – *Genitofemoral*

Nerve labelled 6 corresponds to the L3 spinal nerve. The genitofemoral nerve is not a branch of L3; it branches from L1 to L2; hence A is the correct response. The lumbosacral plexus is formed by ventral rami of the lumbar and sacral nerves – T12 to S4. The lumbar component is formed by roots from T12 to L4, and the sacral component formed by roots of L4 to S4. These divide into anterior and posterior divisions/branches: Anterior branches of the lumbar plexus include – iliohypogastric (L1), ilioinguinal (L1), genitofemoral (L1, L2), obturator (L2–L4) and accessory obturator nerves (L2–L3). Posterior branches of the lumbar plexus include – lateral femoral cutaneous (L2, L3) and femoral nerves (L2–L4). Anterior branches of the sacral plexus include sciatic (tibial), posterior femoral cutaneous and pudendal nerves. Posterior branches of the sacral plexus include – sciatic (peroneal), superior and inferior gluteal, and piriformis nerves.

6.4.27 D – *Diminished ankle plantarflexion*

Nerve root labelled 7 corresponds to S1. Compression of this nerve root results in diminished ankle (and toe) plantarflexion, in addition to ankle eversion and hip extension; hence D is the correct response. It is important to note that there can be overlap between myotomes and their actions. Generally, L1 and L2 control hip flexion. L3 controls knee extension and L4 controls ankle dorsiflexion. L5 and S2 control knee flexion. S2 and S3 control adduction of the toes. S5 controls great toe extension.

6.4.28 C – *Pia mater*

Structure labelled 8 corresponds to the filum terminale. This is a fibrous cord that extends from the conus medullaris to the periosteum of the coccyx. It is continuous with the pia mater; hence C is the correct response.

6.4.29 *E – L3*

A typical vertebra consists of a vertebral body and posterior vertebral arch. The vertebral arch forms the posterior and lateral aspects of the vertebral foramen and consists of pedicles and laminae. The transverse process projects from the junction between the lamina and pedicle and is a site for thoracic rib articulation. The spinous process projects posteroinferiorly from the junction of the two laminae and is a site for muscle/ligament attachments. There are five lumbar vertebrae, and they are the largest. They have cylindrical vertebral bodies and a triangular-shaped vertebral foramen. They also lack facets for rib articulation; hence E is the correct response. There are seven cervical vertebrae which have a short, square-shaped vertebral body, a transverse process with a piercing foramen transversarium (which transmits the vertebral artery and vein, and sympathetic fibres), a bifid spinous process and a triangular-shaped vertebral foramen. There are twelve thoracic vertebrae which have two facets (superior and inferior costal) on the sides of the vertebral bodies (which is more heart-shaped), a transverse costal facet which articulates with the tubercle of the rib, and a circular vertebral foramen. The sacrum is a single-fused vertebrae of which there are five, and it is triangular in shape. It articulates with L5 and the coccyx. The coccyx is a small triangular bone of which there are 3–5 fused bones, which have no vertebral arches or a vertebral canal.

Answers 6.4.30 to 6.4.36 relate to the following annotated CT figure.

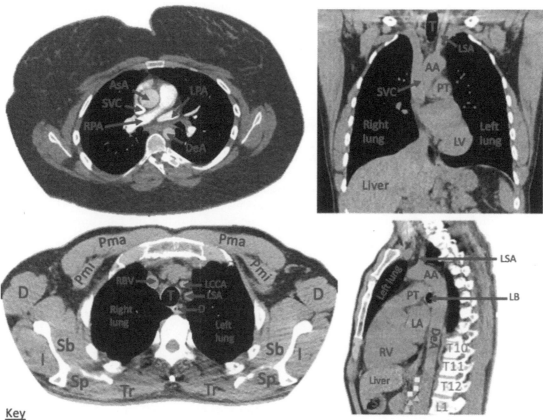

Key

AsA: ascending aorta; SVC: superior vena cava; RPA: right pulmonary artery; LPA: left pulmonary artery; DeA: descending aorta; AA: aortic arch; PT: pulmonary trunk; LSA: left subclavian artery; T: trachea; LV: left ventricle; RV: right ventricle; LA: left atrium; LB: left main bronchus; LCCA: left common carotid artery; RBV: right brachiocephalic vein; O: oesophagus; S: stomach; Pma: pectoralis major; Pmi: pectoralis minor; D: deltoid; Sb: subscapularis; Sp: supraspinatus; I: infraspinatus; Tr: trapezius; ES: erector spinae; ▢: coeliac trunk; ▲: superior mesenteric artery

6.4.30 *C – Ascending aorta*

6.4.31 *B – Pulmonary artery*

More specifically this corresponds to the left pulmonary artery.

6.4.32 *A – Pectoralis minor*

6.4.33 D – Left subclavian artery|Left atrium|Trachea|Deltoid

This is tricky! Remember – the whiter it appears, the denser the tissue (e.g., bone); air and fat appear dark grey or black; and soft tissue, blood or fluids appear as various shades of grey. Structure labelled 4 is a branch of the aortic arch, which has three branches – the brachiocephalic artery which branches into the right common carotid and right subclavian arteries; the left common carotid artery and the left subclavian artery. Structure labelled 4 is in very close proximity to the oesophagus which can be appreciated more in the bottom axial figure. It lies most posterior of the vessels and therefore must correspond to the left subclavian artery. Structure labelled 5 corresponds to the left atrium. The left atrium is the most posterior of all the heart chambers. Structures which lie behind it include the descending aorta, oesophagus and tracheal bifurcation. Structure labelled 6 has an air-filled lumen (which appears black). It could be the trachea or oesophagus; however, in the bottom axial figure it appears more anterior; hence corresponds to the trachea. Structure labelled 7 corresponds to deltoid. Deltoid is an intrinsic triangular-shaped muscle of the shoulder composed of an anterior (clavicular), lateral (acromial) and posterior (spinal) – its name is derived from the Greek letter delta (Δ).

6.4.34 B – T6

Again, this is tricky! The best way to tackle this is to comment on what you can and cannot see. Remember anatomy is about orientation. In the top axial figure, the sternal body is evident anteriorly; the manubrium is not evident. The manubrium is located between T3 and T4 and the sternal body lies between T5 and T9. The tip of the xiphoid process is located at T10. There is no evidence of the liver, duodenum, transverse colon, or spleen which are normally evident at T12. Bifurcation of the trachea, or carina occurs at T4 – T5. The trachea is not evident in this axial figure so from the options available, this leaves levels T6 or T8. At vertebral level T8, the hemiazygos vein crosses the midline posterior to the aorta and oesophagus. This is not evident in this axial figure; hence it must be at a more superior vertebral level. At T6, the SVC is evident which is draining into the right atrium; hence B is the correct response.

6.4.35 E – Perimysial tendons increase in diameter in the hypertrophied heart

Structure labelled 8 corresponds to the left ventricle. In normal cardiac muscle, the collagen matrix consists of thin perimysial tendons or coils that run parallel to the cardiomyocytes. In hypertrophic cardiac muscle, as seen in hypertrophic cardiomyopathy, there is increase in number and thickness of collagen fibres, with perimysial tendons becoming thicker and straighter with a loss in their spring-like coiled configuration; hence E is the correct response. The trabecular network of the left ventricle is much finer and more delicate compared to the right, which has numerous muscular, coarse trabeculae carneae. There are three papillary muscles of the right ventricle (there are normally two in the left). The right ventricle is the most anterior of the four chambers. Bachmann's bundle is a muscular bundle of myocardial strands connecting the left and right atrial walls and the main pathway of interatrial conduction. This is an anterior tract which extends from the sinoatrial node and delivers impulses to the left atrium. There are also two other tracts which extend from the sinoatrial node: Wenckebach's tract which extends from the superior part of the sinoatrial node, runs within the atrial septum and merges with the anterior bundle where it enters the atrioventricular node; and Thorel's tract which extends from the inferior part of the sinoatrial node, penetrates the crista terminalis, and enters the posterior portion of the atrioventricular node.

6.4.36 D – Apical upper lobe

There are three lobes in the right lung and two lobes in the left lung as shown below:

Right	Left
Upper lobe • Apical • Anterior • Posterior	Upper lobe • Apicoposterior • Anterior • Superior lingular • Inferior lingular
Middle lobe • Lateral • Medial	
Lower lobe • Superior • Medial • Anterior • Lateral • Posterior	Lower lobe • Superior • Anteromedial • Lateral • Posterior

This vertebral level is T3 as the medial end and base of the scapula are evident, and the trachea has not bifurcated so it must be more superior than T4. It is inferior to T2 as the coracoid process of the scapula is not evident. T3 is known as the 'five-vessel level' as all five vessels are evident at this level – the left and right brachiocephalic veins, the brachiocephalic artery, the left common carotid artery, and the left subclavian artery. Therefore, segment labelled 9 corresponds to the apical upper lobe of the right lung; hence D is the correct response.

6.4.37 *E – The left phrenic nerve descends between the left common carotid and left subclavian arteries*

The left phrenic nerve runs laterally to the aortic arch, and initially descends between the left common carotid and left subclavian arteries; hence E is the correct response. It is derived from the cervical plexus and receives innervation from C3 to C5 nerve roots. The phrenic nerves provide exclusive motor innervation to the diaphragm. However, they also provide sensory fibres to the fibrous pericardium, mediastinal pleura and parietal peritoneum. It is the longest branch of the cervical plexus. The left phrenic nerve is longer than the right due to the asymmetry of the heart position and the lower lying left hemidiaphragm. The oesophageal hiatus transmits the oesophagus, vagus nerves and small oesophageal arteries. The right phrenic nerve enters the diaphragm at T8 through the vena cava hiatus.

Answers 6.4.38 to 6.4.40 relate to the following annotated figure.

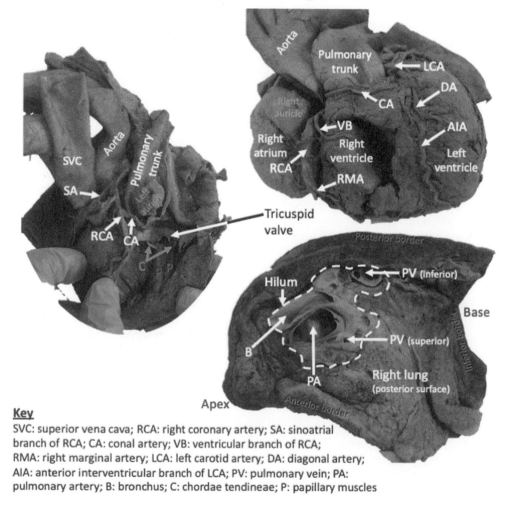

Key
SVC: superior vena cava; RCA: right coronary artery; SA: sinoatrial branch of RCA; CA: conal artery; VB: ventricular branch of RCA; RMA: right marginal artery; LCA: left carotid artery; DA: diagonal artery; AIA: anterior interventricular branch of LCA; PV: pulmonary vein; PA: pulmonary artery; B: bronchus; C: chordae tendineae; P: papillary muscles

6.4.38 *C – Tricuspid valve | Anterior interventricular artery | Right coronary artery | Right bronchus*

The left figure shows a dissected heart in which the walls have been reflected. The question is which wall? The only way to tackle this is to identify structures which are evident and orientate the anatomy. There are several clues: the muscular wall is thin and chordae tendineae and papillary muscles are present (which only extend from cusps of the atrioventricular valve - tricuspid and mitral) to the papillary muscles within the ventricles – the dissection has therefore occurred through the right ventricle since the muscular wall of the left ventricle is far thicker. Therefore, structure labelled 1 corresponds to the tricuspid valve. The orientation is focussed on the right side of the heart since the three great vessels are evident – from left to right – superior vena cava, aorta, and pulmonary trunk. The left auricle or left atrial appendage is also evident which is a small, ear-shaped muscular pouch located at the upper aspect of the left atrium close to the root of the pulmonary trunk. The right coronary artery (structure labelled 3) is also evident emerging from the ascending aorta which branches into the conus artery – the first branch which runs anteriorly, the sinoatrial artery, right (acute) marginal artery and the ventricular branch (VB) which supplies the right ventricle. Structure labelled 2 corresponds to the anterior interventricular artery or left anterior descending artery. This is the largest coronary artery which runs anterior to the interventricular septum in the anterior interventricular groove. It branches into septal and diagonal arteries. The bottom right prosection corresponds to a lung, but is this the left or right lung? This is the medial view of the lung with the pointed apex to the left of the prosection and the base (diaphragmatic surface) to the right. The horizontal and oblique fissures are evident. The main bronchus is posteriorly related to the pulmonary artery, and the upper pulmonary vein is anteroinferior to the pulmonary artery and anterosuperior to the lower pulmonary vein. Hence this is the right lung. The left lung only has one fissure – the oblique fissure. The pulmonary artery is the most superior structure within the left hilum (root). Therefore, structure labelled 4 corresponds to the right bronchus.

6.4.39   *A – Crista terminalis*

Structure labelled 5 corresponds to the right atrium. More anteriorly, the right auricle can also be seen. The right coronary artery can be seen below the right atrium which emerges from the aortic sinus and runs in the coronary sulcus (atrioventricular sulcus). This separates the atria from the ventricles. The crista terminalis is a fibromuscular ridge formed by the junction of the sinus venosus and primitive right atrium within the posterolateral right atrial wall; hence A is the correct response. Chordae tendineae and trabeculae carneae are found in the ventricles. The right ventricle tapers superiorly to become a funnel-shaped outflow tract known as the conus arteriosus or infundibulum. The moderator band or septomarginal trabecula is located in the right ventricular apex and connects the interventricular septum to the anterior papillary muscle.

6.4.40   *B – Lead III*

Structure labelled 6 corresponds to the right (acute) marginal artery, a branch of the right coronary artery. It provides blood supply to the lateral portion of the right ventricle. Occlusion of the right coronary artery (and its branches) causes inferior wall infarction, right ventricular infarction (if occlusion is more proximal – rare) and posterior wall infarction. Inferior wall infarction causes ST-segment elevation in leads II, III and aVF with reciprocal ST-segment depressions in lead I and aVL; hence B is the correct response. ST-segment elevations in leads I and aVL, and II, III and aVF affect the lateral and inferior myocardium, which results from occlusion of the left circumflex artery and right coronary artery respectively. ST-segment elevations in leads V1–V2, V3–V4 and V5–V6 affect the septal, anterior, and apical myocardium, which results from occlusion of the proximal LAD, LAD, and distal LAD (or left circumflex or right coronary artery), respectively. ST-segment elevations in leads V7–V9 with reciprocal ST-depression in V1–V3 affect the posterolateral myocardium, which results from occlusion of the right coronary artery or left circumflex artery. NB: None of the standard leads in the 12-lead ECG truly capture right ventricular infarction. Leads V1 and V2 may capture some dysfunction by displaying ST-segment elevations but to verify infarction in the right ventricle, right-sided chest leads should be connected (V3R-V6R) which will show ST-segment elevation.

6.4.41   *C – Internal intercostal muscle fibres extend anteroinferiorly*

Internal intercostal muscles fibres are more prominent near the midline at the inferior aspect of thoracic cage. They run superomedially to inferolaterally in a posteroinferior (not anteroinferior) direction; hence C is the correct response. In contrast, external intercostal muscle fibres run superolaterally to inferomedially in an anteroinferior direction. External intercostal muscles contract during forced inspiration and elevate the ribs, whereas internal and innermost intercostal muscles contract during forced expiration and depress the ribs.

6.4.42   *A – Venous drainage is usually via the right brachiocephalic vein*

The thymus is a bilobed lymphoid organ located in the superior mediastinum, anterior to the great vessels and posterior to the manubrium. It can in fact also extend superiorly into the neck and inferiorly into the anterior mediastinum. Venous drainage is via the left (not right) brachiocephalic, internal thoracic and inferior thyroid veins; hence A is the correct response. The arterial supply is via the internal thoracic and inferior thyroid arteries. Lymphatic drainage is via parasternal, brachiocephalic and tracheobronchial lymph nodes.

6.4.43   *B – It is the level at which the left recurrent laryngeal nerve curves behind and below the aortic arch*

The left recurrent laryngeal nerve branches off from the vagus nerve, descends along the trachea dorsal to the common carotid artery, and curves below and behind the aortic arch at the level of the ligamentum arteriosum; hence B is the correct response. It is an embryological remnant of the ductus arteriosus, which serves to shunt blood away from the lungs during foetal development and typically closes at birth. Patent ductus arteriosus results in blood flowing from the descending aorta across the ductus arteriosus into the pulmonary circulation (left to right shunt). The patency is promoted by prostaglandin E2, hence in symptomatic newborns treatment with pharmacological agents such as NSAIDs (indomethacin, ibuprofen) – inhibitors of prostaglandin synthesis may be considered. Truncus arteriosus is a rare congenital heart defect which results if a single truncal root does not divide into separate aortic and pulmonary outflow tracts, thereby forming a single truncal valve as opposed to the two aortic and pulmonary valves. The ligamentum venosum is a fibrous remnant of the ductus venosus of the foetal circulation which travels superiorly from the porta hepatis of the liver to the inferior vena cava. It is often obliterated in adults. The ligamentum arteriosum is located at the level of the horizontal (trans)thoracic plane of Ludwig which is used to separate the superior and inferior mediastinum. It connects the left pulmonary artery to the aortic arch/descending aorta at the aortic isthmus (not the ascending aorta).

Answers 6.4.44 to 6.4.46 relate to the following annotated mammary gland.

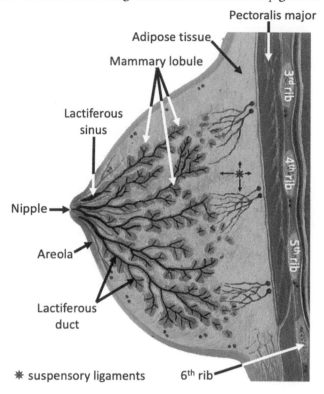

6.4.44 *C – Lactiferous sinus*

6.4.45 *C – Milk*

The mammary gland is divided into three components: skin, parenchyma and stroma. The skin consists of the nipple with ca. 20 lactiferous ducts, rich in smooth muscle fibres and nerves but devoid of sweat glands, fat, or hair; and the areola which encircles the nipple, rich in sebaceous glands that secrete oily substances and devoid of fat and hair. The parenchyma is composed of branching ducts and terminal lobules with ca. 20 lobes. The lactiferous ducts swell to form lactiferous sinuses where the milk is collected; hence C is the correct response. The fibrous stroma provides support to the breast via suspensory ligaments of Cooper which separates the lobes and anchors the breast from the underlying pectoral fascia. The fatty stroma makes up the bulk of the breast tissue.

6.4.46 *C – Sixth rib*

Hopefully it is obvious that label 3 corresponds to a rib, but the question is which one? The pectoralis major muscle forms the base of the breast. It extends from the 2nd to the 6th rib. The nipple is present in the 4th intercostal space between the 4th and 5th ribs, along the midclavicular line; hence label 3 corresponds to the 6th rib.

6.4.47 *D – There are ten bronchopulmonary segments in the right lung*

The right lung is composed of ten bronchopulmonary segments – three in the upper lobe (apical, anterior, and posterior), two in the middle lobe (medial and lateral), and five in the lower lobe (anterior, apicoposterior, inferior and superior lingula); hence D is the correct response. In the thorax, the left and right phrenic nerves descend anteriorly to the lung root, whereas the vagus nerve (and pulmonary plexus) are more posterior. The lingula, meaning 'little tongue' in Latin, is found in the upper lobe of the left lung. The right lung weighs more than the left lung since the left lung must accommodate the hearts position. This leads to the cardiac impression of the left lung. There are three (not four) surfaces of each lung – costal, medial and diaphragmatic. There are also three borders – anterior, posterior and inferior.

6.4.48 *D – 10th rib*

Locations within the thorax where the parietal pleura abruptly changes direction as it passes from one surface to another are called pleural reflections. These are asymmetric in each lung due to the presence of the heart. The parietal pleura is divided into four parts: cervical or cupola, costal, mediastinal and diaphragmatic. The sternal line of pleural reflection is where the costal pleura becomes the mediastinal pleura anteriorly. The costal line of pleural reflection is where the costal pleura becomes the diaphragmatic pleura inferiorly. The vertebral line of pleural reflection is where the costal pleura becomes the mediastinal pleura posteriorly. The lines of pleural reflections are outlined in the figure below. Both the left and right pleural lines pass the midaxillary line at the 10th rib; hence D is the correct response. Both the left and right pleural lines travel posteriorly around the chest wall at the 12th rib. NB: The visceral pleura remains approximately two ribs higher than the lines of pleural reflection in the lower part of the thorax.

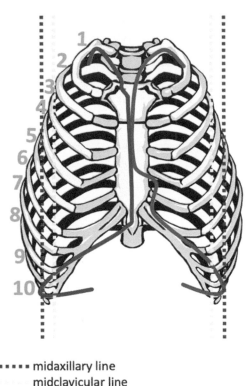

■ ■ ■ ■ ■ ■ midaxillary line
midclavicular line

6.4.49 *E – It lies posterior to the left atrium*

The oesophagus lies posteriorly to the left atrium, left main bronchus, trachea (to T4–T5) and the recurrent laryngeal nerves; hence E is the correct response. It lies anterior to the descending aorta, thoracic duct, vertebral column, hemiazygos and accessory hemiazygos veins. Lying laterally to the left are the thoracic duct, left subclavian artery, aorta, lung and pleura. Lying laterally to the right are the azygos vein, lung and pleura. The cervical oesophagus begins at the inferior margin of the cricoid cartilage at C6 (not C8). The inferior vena cava passes through the diaphragm at the vena caval foramen which is located in the central tendon at T8. The oesophagus passes through the diaphragm through the oesophageal hiatus at T10, along with the anterior and posterior vagus nerves. The innervation of the oesophagus is via sympathetic and parasympathetic fibres of the vagus nerve, and segmental spinal nerves via the cervical and thoracic sympathetic trunk. The phrenic nerve does not contribute to the innervation.

6.4.50 *B – The anterior cardiac vein enters the right atrium*

Cardiac veins that drain into the coronary sinus which subsequently empties directly into the right atrium include the great cardiac vein, middle cardiac vein, small cardiac vein, anterior cardiac vein, left posterior ventricular vein and the oblique cardiac vein; hence B is the correct response. The middle cardiac vein originates from the posterior aspect of the apex of the heart and travels in the posterior interventricular sulcus with the posterior interventricular artery. The small cardiac vein is located in the coronary sulcus between the right atrium and right ventricle. It runs parallel to the right marginal artery. The posterior cardiac vein is more commonly known as the inferior vein of the left ventricle since it drains deoxygenated blood from the inferior and lateral walls of the left ventricle into the coronary sinus. Venae cordis minimae or Thebesian veins are smaller cardiac veins of the heart which drain deoxygenated blood from all aspects of the myocardium, not one chamber, but they are thought to drain the right side of the heart more than the left.

6.5   Abdomen, pelvis and reproductive organs

6.5.1 *C – Kocher Maylard Rutherford-Morison Lanz Pfannenstiel*

Unfortunately, there are several eponyms used in medicine. They tend to offer no clues to the learner. In relation to this question, it is therefore far more practical to understand the incision site and how this relates to the underlying anatomy and surgical procedure. These incisions are summarised below; hence C is the correct response.

- *Kocher* – a right-sided subcostal incision of the abdomen used for open exposure of the gallbladder and biliary tree.
- *Maylard* – a transverse, lower abdominal wall incision, performed approximately 3–8 cm above the pubic symphysis which allows access to the peritoneum in a transverse fashion, giving excellent exposure to the pelvic organs.
- *Rutherford-Morison* – an oblique, curvilinear muscle-cutting incision which begins approximately 2 cm above the anterior superior iliac spine. It can be performed on the left or right and is used for colonic resections and kidney transplants.
- *Lanz* – a transverse incision along Langer's lines (gives maximal wound strength with minimal scarring) in the right lower quadrant of the abdomen used for open appendicectomy. The Gridiron incision (also known as McBurney's incision) is also used in open appendicectomy, but this is oblique. The Lanz incision gives more aesthetically pleasing results with reduced scarring.
- *Pfannenstiel* – a transverse, curved incision two fingers' breadths above the pubic symphysis which extends towards the anterior superior iliac spine and terminates 2–3 cm medial to it on both sides. It is a lower transverse incision than Maylard. It is commonly used for caesarean sections.
- *Chevron* – an extension of Kocher's whereby the incision is also performed on the other side of the abdomen and often used for oesophagectomy, gastrectomy, bilateral adrenalectomy and liver transplantation.
- *Mercedes-Benz* – an extension of the Chevron incision with a vertical incision and break through the xiphisternum which is predominantly seen in liver transplantation.
- *Vertical incisions* – most commonly a midline incision used for various abdominal surgeries as it allows access to the abdominal viscera, often in the form of a midline laparotomy.

6.5.2 *D – Ascending colon*

The GI tract has three divisions: the foregut – oral cavity to first part of the duodenum, the midgut – mid-duodenum to the proximal two-thirds of the transverse: and the hindgut – distal one-third of the transverse colon to the anus. These sections have a different blood supply – the foregut receives vascular supply from the coeliac artery, the midgut from the superior mesenteric artery, and the hindgut from the inferior mesenteric artery. The lymphatic drainage of the GI tract is via collections of pre-aortic lymph nodes, and hence lymph from the viscera supplied by these three arteries drain to pre-aortic lymph nodes near their origins. Since the ascending colon is a midgut structure, it drains into superior mesenteric lymph nodes; hence D is the correct response.

6.5.3 *B – Left gastric*

The coeliac trunk is the anterior branch of the abdominal aorta which supplies the foregut. It immediately divides into the left gastric, splenic and common hepatic arteries; hence B is the correct response. The gastroduodenal artery is a terminal branch of the common hepatic artery. The right gastric artery is a branch of one of the hepatic arteries (common, proper or left hepatic). The short gastric arteries are a group of arteries arising from the terminal splenic artery and the left gastroepiploic artery. The dorsal pancreatic artery is a branch of the proximal splenic artery.

6.5.4 *D – Ilioinguinal nerve*

The spermatic cord originates from the deep inguinal ring, passes through the superficial inguinal ring, descends into the scrotum, and terminates in the testes. It suspends the testes and provides a blood and nerve supply to the vas deferens, testes and epididymis. It consists of the ductus deferens (vas deferens), cremaster muscle, testicular artery, artery of the ductus deferens, cremasteric artery, pampiniform plexus, tunica vaginalis, lymphatic vessels and the genital branch of the genitofemoral nerve. The ilioinguinal nerve runs along the outside of the cord, not within it; hence D is the correct response.

6.5.6 *C – Conjoint tendon*

The boundaries and borders of the superficial and deep inguinal rings, and inguinal canal are highlighted in the table below; hence C is the correct response. The inguinal canal serves as a passageway from the abdomen to both the lower limb and perineum. The spermatic cord in males and the round ligament of the uterus in females passes through the inguinal canal to reach the perineum. The deep inguinal ring is the starting point to the inguinal canal, arising superiorly at the midpoint of the inguinal ligament and at the midpoint between the anterior superior iliac spine and pubic symphysis. It is formed by an invagination of the transversalis fascia. The superficial inguinal ring is the exit point to the inguinal canal and lies superior to the pubic tubercle. It is formed within the external oblique aponeurosis. Hesselbach's triangle is a triangular region on the inferior interior aspect of the anterior abdominal wall. It has three boundaries – inguinal ligament (base), inferior epigastric vessels (lateral) and rectus abdominus (medial). Clinically, direct inguinal hernias occur through this triangular region.

	Superficial ring	**Deep ring**	**Inguinal canal**
Roof	External oblique aponeurosis	Transversalis fascia	Transversus abdominus Internal oblique Conjoint tendon
Floor	Lacunar ligament	Iliopubic tract	Inguinal ligament Lacunar ligament
Anterior	Lateral border: External oblique aponeurosis and fascia External spermatic fascia	Lateral border: Transversus abdominus Internal oblique aponeurosis	External oblique aponeurosis and laterally by internal oblique
Posterior	Medial border: Conjoint tendon	Medial border: Transversalis fascia Inferior epigastric vessels	Transversalis fascia, and medially by the conjoint tendon

6.5.7 *E – Genitofemoral nerve*

The genital branch of the genitofemoral nerve (L1, L2) innervates the cremaster muscle; hence E is the correct response. In males, the cremasteric muscle contracts, pulling the scrotum and testis superiorly when the medial part of the thigh is stroked in an inferior direction – the cremasteric reflex. The female counterpart is the Geigel reflex which involves the contraction of the muscle fibres along the upper part of the inguinal ligament.

6.5.8 *A – Piriformis*

Piriformis and obturator internus are muscles of the pelvic walls. Both muscles aid in lateral rotation of the hip joint in extension and abduction of the hip when flexed. Piriformis originates from the anterior surface of the sacrum between the anterior sacral foramina and attaches to the superior border of the greater trochanter of the femur (medially). It is innervated by branches of L5 (S1, S2); hence A is the correct response. Obturator internus originates from the anterolateral wall of the pelvis and attaches to the medial surface of the greater trochanter. It is innervated by the nerve to obturator internus (L5, S1). Coccygeus, pubococcygeus and iliococcygeus are muscles of the pelvic diaphragm. They contribute to the formation of the pelvic floor. Coccygeus originates from the ischial spine and sacrospinous ligament and attaches to the lateral border of the coccyx and sacrum. It is innervated by branches from the anterior rami of S3 and S4. Pubococcygeus, iliococcygeus and puborectalis are levator ani muscles. They originate on the posterior aspect of the pubic bone and extend across obturator internus to the ischial spine. They attach to the superior surface of the perineal membrane, perineal body, anal canal and the anococcygeal ligament. The primary nerve supply is from S2 to S4. The nerve to levator ani is part of the pudendal plexus which originates from S4. These muscles also receive fibres from the inferior rectal nerve and coccygeal plexus.

6.5.9 *C – Transversus abdominis*

The five muscles of the abdominal wall are divided into two groups: three flat muscles – external oblique, internal oblique, and transversus abdominis; and two vertical muscles – rectus abdominis and pyramidalis.

Flat muscles

External oblique – the most superficial and the largest flat muscle. It runs in an inferomedial direction, and its fibres form an aponeurosis at the midline, which entwine forming the linea alba. This extends from the xiphoid process to the pubic symphysis.

Origin: outer surfaces of the shafts of the lower eight ribs (5–12)

Insertion: lateral lip of iliac crest, and aponeurosis ending in the linea alba

Internal oblique – deep to external oblique is internal oblique which is smaller and thinner, and fibres run in a superomedial direction. Its lateral muscular component ends anteriorly as an aponeurosis which merges into the linea alba.

Origin: thoracolumbar fascia, anterior two-thirds of iliac crest, and lateral two-thirds of inguinal ligament

Insertion: inferior border of lower three ribs (10–12), aponeurosis ending in linea alba, pubic crest and pectineal line

Transversus abdominis – the deepest of the flat muscles and as the name suggests, fibres run transversely. It ends in an anterior aponeurosis, which also merges with the linea alba. Beneath this muscle is the transversalis fascia which lines the abdominal cavity and continues into the pelvic cavity.

Origin: thoracolumbar fascia, medial lip of iliac crest, lateral one-third of inguinal ligament (hence C is the correct response), and costal cartilages of lower six ribs (7–12)
Insertion: aponeurosis ending in linea alba, pubic crest, and pectineal line

Vertical muscles

Rectus abdominis – long paired muscle which extends the entire length of the anterior abdominal wall. It is divided into two segments by the linea alba, and the lateral border is known as the linea semilunaris.
Origin: pubic crest, tubercle and symphysis
Insertion: costal cartilages of ribs 5–7, and xiphoid process
Pyramidalis – small, triangular shaped muscle (which may be absent) is anterior to the rectus abdominis.
Origin: pubic symphysis and pubic crest
Insertion: apex attached superiorly and medially to the linea alba

6.5.10 B – Musculophrenic

The internal thoracic (mammary) artery, a branch of the subclavian artery, gives off branches as it descends along the inner surface of the anterior thorax. These include anterior intercostal arteries, perforating cutaneous branches, pericardiophrenic artery, musculophrenic artery and superior epigastric artery. The musculophrenic artery supplies the superior part of the anterior abdominal wall, not the deeper structures of the anterolateral abdominal wall; hence B is the correct response.

6.5.11 C – External iliac

The external iliac artery branches into the inferior epigastric artery and deep circumflex iliac artery; hence C is the correct response. The inferior epigastric artery supplies the rectus abdominis, whereas the deep circumflex iliac artery supplies the transversus abdominis and internal oblique muscles.

6.5.12 D – Superior phrenic

The branches of the abdominal aorta include:

- Paired branches – the middle suprarenal, renal, gonadal (testicular or ovarian), inferior phrenic and lumbar arteries
- Unpaired branches – the coeliac, superior mesenteric, inferior mesenteric, and median sacral arteries
- Terminal branches – the common iliac arteries

The superior phrenic artery is not a branch of the abdominal aorta; hence D is the correct response. This branches from the lower part of the thoracic aorta.

6.5.13 C – (3) unites with the common bile duct via the ampulla of Vater

Structure labelled (3) corresponds to the main pancreatic duct or duct of Wirsung which drains most of the pancreas (as shown below). It typically joins the common bile duct before draining into the ampulla of Vater via the sphincter of Oddi; hence C is the correct response. Structure labelled (2) corresponds to the accessory pancreatic duct or the duct of Santorini which drains the uncinate process and lower part of the pancreatic head and typically communicates with the main pancreatic duct or the duct of Wirsung. It drains into to duodenum above the major duodenal papilla at the minor duodenal papilla. Structure labelled (1) corresponds to the gastroduodenal artery from the common hepatic artery (a branch of the coeliac trunk). This vessel arises approximately at the level of the lower part of T12 (not L1), and it courses anteroinferiorly. The gastroduodenal artery branches into the anterior and posterior superior pancreaticoduodenal artery. Structure labelled (4) corresponds to the anterior superior pancreaticoduodenal artery. Terminal branches of this artery anastomose with the anterior inferior pancreaticoduodenal artery (a branch of the superior mesenteric artery). Structure labelled (5) corresponds to the superior mesenteric artery, the first branch of which is the inferior pancreaticoduodenal artery. The middle colic artery is the second branch of the superior mesenteric artery. The splenic artery, a branch of the coeliac trunk, lies along the superior border of the pancreas and forms arcades with the pancreatic branches of the gastroduodenal and superior mesenteric arteries. These supply the body and tail of the pancreas. Branches of the splenic artery include pancreatic branches – dorsal, transverse (inferior) and greater pancreatic arteries, short gastric arteries, and the left gastroepiploic artery (which anastomoses with the right gastroepiploic artery along the greater curvature of the stomach).

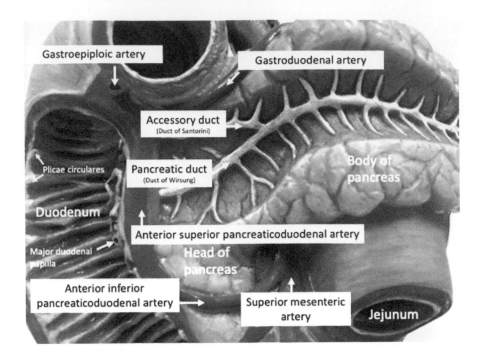

6.5.14 *D – Genitofemoral nerve – L3*

The term plexus refers to a 'web' of nerves. The nerves arising from the lumbar plexus from superior to inferior are:

- Iliohypogastric – from T12 and L1
- Ilioinguinal – from L1
- Genitofemoral – from L1 and L2
- Lateral femoral cutaneous – from L2 and L3
- Femoral – from L2 to L4
- Obturator – from L2 to L4

The genitofemoral nerve arises from the superior aspects of L1 and L2 spinal nerves (not L3); hence D is the correct response.

6.5.15 *C – Obturator nerve*

The obturator nerve travels along the iliopectineal line and descends through psoas major, where it emerges from the medial border close to the pelvic brim; hence C is the correct response. It provides motor innervation to the medial compartment of the thigh and aids in adduction.

6.5.16 *D – L1*

As shown in 6.4.1, the transpyloric plane is located at L1; hence D is the correct response. This is an axial, imaginary line that is located halfway between the suprasternal notch and the upper border of the pubic symphysis. There are several structures which cross this line, including the pylorus of the stomach, neck of the pancreas, second part of the duodenum, hilum of each kidney, fundus of the gall bladder, sphincter of Oddi, duodenojejunal flexure, and the 9th costal cartilages. It is also the origin of the portal vein and superior mesenteric artery, and termination of the spinal cord.

6.5.17 *B – The right gastric artery is a branch of the hepatic artery proper*

The common hepatic arteries branch into the hepatic artery proper and gastroduodenal artery. The hepatic artery proper ascends through the lesser omentum and branches into the right gastric, right and left hepatic, and cystic arteries; hence B is the correct response. The left and right gastric artery supply the lesser curvature of the stomach since they anastomose. The splenic artery travels posterior to the stomach and branches into the left gastroepiploic artery which supplies the greater curvature. Short gastric arteries which also branch from the splenic artery supply the fundus (not pylorus). These arteries are not involved in anastomosis with other arteries, which can lead to ischaemia in the event of arterial obstruction. The posterior gastric artery is a branch of the splenic artery (not right gastric artery).

6.5.18 *B – Pouch of Morison*

The peritoneal cavity is divided by transverse mesocolon into two compartments: supramesocolic and inframesocolic. The supramesocolic compartment is subdivided into left and right by the falciform ligament. The left supramesocolic space is further subdivided into the left subhepatic and left subphrenic space (anterior and posterior). The right supramesocolic space is further subdivided into the right subphrenic and right subhepatic space, and omental bursa. The right subhepatic space, also called the hepatorenal pouch or pouch of Morison, lies between the upper pole of the right kidney and inferior surface of the right lobe of the liver. It is the most gravity-dependent space within the supramesocolic compartment, and it directly communicates with the omental bursa; hence B is the correct response. The omental bursa or lesser sac is a peritoneal space between the stomach and pancreas which is formed by the lesser and greater omentum. Importantly, although extending to the left of the midline, it is a right-sided peritoneal space. The right medial side of the omental bursa is continuous with the greater sac through the epiploic foramen (foramen of Winslow) only, which is located posterior to the free edge of the lesser omentum (hepatoduodenal ligament).

The inframesocolic compartment is further subdivided into the left and right inframesocolic space and left and right paracolic gutters. The right paracolic gutter communicates freely with the supramesocolic compartment, and clinically, this is important when considering spread of infection and malignancy. Passage of peritoneal fluid is far more restricted from the supramesocolic compartment to the left paracolic gutter due to the phrenicocolic ligament. The left subphrenic space is restricted posteriorly by the left triangular ligament. It is also restricted inferomedially by the phrenicocolic, lienogastric and lienorenal ligaments which limit passage between this space and the left paracolic gutter. Various peritoneal spaces within the peritoneal cavity are shown in the figure below.

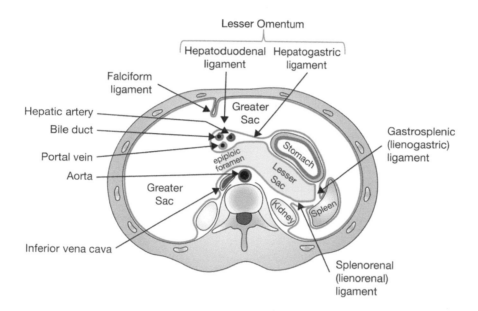

6.5.19 *B – Anterior and posterior caecal arteries supply the caecum and ascending colon*

The anterior and posterior caecal arteries are branches of the inferior division of the ileocolic artery which supplies the corresponding aspects of the caecum, and parts of the ascending colon; hence B is the correct response. Along with the middle colic and right colic arteries, the ileocolic artery is a branch from the right side of the superior mesenteric artery. Branches from the left side include the jejunal and ileal arteries. The left colic artery is the first branch of the inferior mesenteric artery. The middle rectal arteries are branches of the internal iliac arteries (not the internal pudendal artery which is also a branch of the internal iliac artery). The superior rectal artery is a direct terminal branch of the inferior mesenteric artery (not the internal iliac artery).

6.5.20 *A – Oesophagus*

The peritoneum consists of two continuous layers – the parietal and visceral peritoneum. The parietal peritoneum lines the inner surface of the abdominal wall and embryologically it is derived from somatic mesoderm. The visceral peritoneum covers suspended organs and embryologically it is derived from splanchnic mesoderm. Abdominal viscera are either intraperitoneal – suspended from the abdominal wall by mesenteries, or retroperitoneal – lie between the abdominal wall and parietal peritoneum. Retroperitoneal structures include the suprarenal (adrenal) glands, aorta, inferior vena cava, duodenum (except first part), pancreas (except tail), ureters, bladder, ascending and descending colon, kidneys, oesophagus and rectum; hence A is the correct response.

6.5.21 *D – Triangular*

The liver is almost completely surrounded by visceral peritoneum except for the bare area. The anterior and posterior boundaries of this area are enclosed by reflections of peritoneum – the anterior and posterior coronary ligaments, respectively. Anteriorly, the coronary ligament is continuous with the left and right layers of the falciform ligament. On the posteroinferior border and superior border, the layers of the coronary ligament converge as the right and left triangular ligaments, respectively; hence D is the correct response. The hepatogastric ligament connects the liver with the stomach. The hepatoduodenal ligament connects the liver with the duodenum. Ligamentum teres or round ligament of the liver forms the free edge of the falciform ligament and connects the liver to the umbilicus.

6.5.22 *B – Hepatic artery proper*

The porta hepatis (transverse hepatic fissure), located on the visceral inferior surface of the liver, separates the caudate and quadrate lobes, and is where vessels and ducts enter and exit the liver. It runs in the hepatoduodenal ligament. The common hepatic artery, a branch of the coeliac trunk branches into the hepatic artery proper and gastroduodenal artery. The hepatic artery proper then branches into the right gastric and left and right hepatic arteries close to the porta hepatis; hence B is the correct response. The cystic artery is a branch of the right hepatic artery (occasionally it can also be a branch of the left gastric artery).

6.5.23 *E – Transverse colon*

The inferior mesenteric vein joins the splenic vein, which then merges into the portal vein. It drains the descending colon via the left colic vein, the sigmoid colon via the sigmoid vein, and the rectum via the superior rectal vein, and the splenic flexure. It does not drain the transverse colon; hence E is the correct response. The superior mesenteric vein drains the small intestine, caecum, ascending and transverse colon via the jejunal, ileal, ileocolic, right colic and middle colic veins.

6.5.24 *D – Superior mesenteric – ileocolic – appendicular*

The correct sequence of artery branches from the abdominal aorta include:

- Paired branches – inferior phrenic, middle adrenal, renal, gonadal and lumbar
- Unpaired branches – coeliac, superior mesenteric, inferior mesenteric and median sacral
- Terminal branches – common iliac

The coeliac artery/trunk divides into three major branches:

- Left gastric artery which anastomoses with the right gastric artery
- Common hepatic artery
- Splenic artery

The superior mesenteric artery branches include:

- Inferior pancreaticoduodenal artery
- Left-sided – jejunal and ileal branches
- Right sided – ileocolic (which branches into the appendicular artery, and hence D is the correct response), right colic and middle colic arteries

The inferior mesenteric artery branches include:

- Left colic artery
- Sigmoid arteries
- Superior rectal artery (terminal branch)

The superior and inferior mesenteric arteries are linked by an arcade along the mesenteric border called the marginal artery of Drummond, from which extensive vasa recta supply the colon.

6.5.25 *E – Left renal vein*

Similar to the gonadal veins, each side of the suprarenal (adrenal) glands venous drainage is different. The left suprarenal vein drains into the left renal vein; hence E is the correct response. The right suprarenal vein drains directly into the inferior vena cava. The suprarenal veins can sometimes anastomose with the inferior phrenic veins.

6.5.26 *B –* Inferior suprarenal | Superior mesenteric | Gonadal | Quadratus lumborum

Structure labelled 1 corresponds to the inferior suprarenal artery which supplies the adrenal glands (as shown below). At L1/L2, the renal arteries emerge from the lateral aspect of the abdominal aorta. The left renal artery arises more superior to the right and courses more horizontally, whereas the right courses more inferior and obliquely. Both arteries branch into the much smaller inferior adrenal, ureteric and capsular arteries. Upon reaching the hilum of the kidneys, the renal arteries further divide into segmental arteries. In addition, the superior suprarenal artery is a smaller branch of the inferior phrenic artery, and the middle suprarenal artery is a direct branch of the abdominal aorta. Structure labelled 2 corresponds to the superior mesenteric artery. It originates from the anterior surface of the abdominal aorta at L1, superior to the renal arteries. The left renal vein lies posterior to the superior mesenteric artery. Structure labelled 3 corresponds to the gonadal vein. They course along the psoas muscle and ascend anterior to the ureters. The left gonadal vein (not evident in this figure) drains into the left renal vein, and the right drains directly into the inferior vena cava. Structure labelled 4 corresponds to the lumbar artery, of which there are four pairs originating as posterolateral branches of the abdominal aorta at levels L1 to L4. The lumbar arteries and a lumbar branch of the iliolumbar artery (a branch of the internal iliac artery) supply quadratus lumborum, and psoas major and minor. In addition, the psoas muscles are supplied by muscular branches of the common iliac artery and the deep circumflex iliac artery which branches from the external iliac artery.

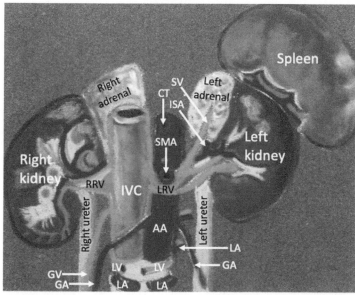

Key: AA: abdominal aorta; IVC: inferior vena cava; SMA: superior mesenteric artery; CT: coeliac trunk; LRV: left renal vein; RRV: right renal vein; ISA: inferior suprarenal artery; SV: suprarenal vein; LA: lumbar arteries; LV: lumbar veins; GA: gonadal artery; GV: gonadal vein

6.5.27 *C – Least*

The splanchnic nerves are paired autonomic nerves that supply the abdominal and pelvic viscera. They provide visceral efferent fibres to internal organs and visceral afferent fibres leaving these organs. They include thoracic splanchnic (greater, lesser, and least), lumbar splanchnic, sacral splanchnic and pelvic splanchnic. The greater splanchnic nerve arises from the 5th to 9th thoracic ganglia and synapses in the coeliac ganglion. The lesser splanchnic nerve arises from the 10th and 11th thoracic ganglia and synapses in the aorticorenal ganglion. The least splanchnic nerve arises from the 12th thoracic ganglion and synapses within the ganglia of the renal plexus; hence C is the correct response. All splanchnic nerves carry preganglionic sympathetic fibres, except for the pelvic splanchnic nerves which carry preganglionic parasympathetic fibres.

6.5.28 *D – Sacrospinous ligament Quadratus lumborum Piriformis Sartorius*

The sacrospinous ligament is triangular with its apex attaching to the ischial spine and base attaching to the borders of the sacrum and coccyx (blue region). Quadratus lumborum is a posterior abdominal wall muscle (alongside psoas major and minor, and iliacus) which attaches to the transverse processes of lumbar vertebrae, the iliolumbar ligament and the iliac crest (red region). Piriformis is a muscle of the pelvic wall (alongside obturator internus) which attaches to the anterior surface of the sacrum between the anterior sacral foramina (green region). Sartorius is a muscle of the anterior compartment of the thigh (discussed more in 6.6) which attaches to the anterior superior iliac spine (yellow region).

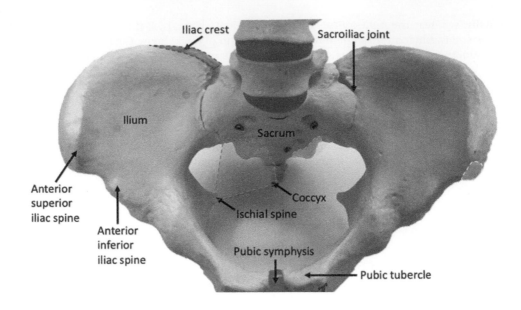

Iliac crest

Sacroiliac joint

Ilium

Sacrum

Anterior
superior
iliac spine

Coccyx

Ischial spine

Anterior
inferior
iliac spine

Pubic symphysis

Pubic tubercle

6.5.29 *E – In females, the acetabulum is smaller, and the greater sciatic notch is wider*

The acetabulum is smaller, wider apart and more medially placed in females than males. The greater sciatic notch is wider in females and narrower in males; hence E is the correct response. The female pelvis is larger and broader than the male pelvis, which is taller and narrower. The pelvic inlet is more circular or oval in shape in females since the distances between the ischium bones is larger, whereas in males the inlet is more heart-shaped. The angle between the inferior pubic rami is larger in females (80–90°) than it is in men (50–60°). The ischial spines project farther into the pelvic cavity in males than they do in females. In males, the pubic arch is narrower, and the obturator foramen is oval-shaped, whereas in females it is triangular. The pubis forms the anterior and inferior part of the pelvic bone, and is composed of a body, superior and inferior pubic rami. The superior pubic ramus projects posterolaterally from the body and joins with the ilium and ischium at the base. The narrow ridge running along the superior border (not posterior) of the superior pubic ramus is the pectineal line which forms part of the linea terminalis. The pelvic outlet is bound by the sacrotuberous ligament posteromedially (not anteriorly). The pubic symphysis defines the anterior boundary in the midline of the pelvic outlet. The pelvic inlet separates the true pelvis inferiorly and the false pelvis superiorly. The false pelvis provides support for lower abdominal viscera (ileum and sigmoid colon). The true pelvis contains the pelvic colon, rectum, bladder and some reproductive organs.

6.5.30 *B – Obturator internus*

The pelvis has four walls – anterior, posterior, lateral and inferior (floor). The anterior wall is formed by the posterior surfaces of the pubic bone bodies, the pubic rami and the pubic symphysis. The posterior wall is formed by the sacrum, coccyx, part of piriformis and pelvic fascia. The lateral wall is formed by the sacrospinous and sacrotuberous ligaments, part of the hip bone inferior to the pelvic inlet, and obturator internus and fascia (anterolateral boundary); hence B is the correct response. Piriformis also forms a large part of the posterolateral walls. The pelvic floor is formed by the pelvic diaphragm, perineal membrane, and muscles in the deep perineal pouch. The pelvic diaphragm is made up of the levator ani muscles (iliococcygeus, pubococcygeus and pubo-rectalis), and coccygeus.

6.5.31 *C – Lateral femoral cutaneous*

The sacral plexus is formed by the anterior rami of S1 to S4, and the lumbosacral trunk (L4 and L5) over the anterior surface of piriformis. All options are branches of the sacral plexus except the lateral femoral cutaneous nerve which is a branch of the lumbar plexus; hence C is the correct response.

6.5.32 *D – The internal pudendal artery enters the ischioanal fossa through the greater sciatic foramen*

The internal pudendal artery is a branch of the anterior trunk of the internal iliac artery and supplies the perineum. It courses through the greater sciatic foramen inferior to piriformis to enter the gluteal region and then curves around the ischial spine and sacrospinous ligament to re-enter the pelvis through the lesser sciatic foramen into the ischioanal fossa; hence D is the correct response. It then branches further to supply erectile tissues of the clitoris and penis.

6.5.33 A – Epididymis – external iliac lymph nodes

The epididymis (and testes) drains into the para-aortic lymph nodes close to the region where the testes developed in the foetus; hence A is the correct response. The scrotum drains into the superficial inguinal lymph nodes.

6.5.34 D – Inferiorly, nerve to obturator internus

The tendon and nerve to obturator internus, and the pudendal vessels and nerve pass through the lesser sciatic foramen, rather than them being boundaries to it; hence D is the correct response.

6.5.35 B – Inferior vesical

In men, the inferior vesical artery supplies the seminal vesicles, prostate, bladder and ureter; hence B is the correct response. The superior vesical artery supplies the superior aspect of the bladder and distal ureter. The obturator artery supplies the adductor region of the thigh. The superior rectal artery supplies the whole of the rectum and the upper part of the anal canal up to the dentate line. The inferior gluteal artery supplies the gluteal region and thigh.

6.5.36 C – External pudendal

The venous drainage of the external female genitalia and scrotum is via the external and internal pudendal veins. The anterior aspect of the labia majora and scrotum drain into anterior labial and scrotal veins, respectively, which ultimately drain into the inferior vena cava via directly draining into the external pudendal vein, then the great saphenous vein, femoral vein and then the external iliac vein; hence C is the correct response. The posterior aspect of the labia major and scrotum drain into posterior labial and scrotal veins, respectively, which ultimately drain into the inferior vena cava via the internal pudendal vein and then the internal iliac vein. Both the external and internal iliac veins ascend and merge to form the common iliac veins, which drain venous blood back into the inferior vena cava.

6.5.37 D – Lymphatics from skin of the penis drain into superficial inguinal nodes

Lymphatic vessels from superficial tissues and skin of the penis and clitoris drain predominantly into the superficial inguinal nodes; hence D is the correct response. Deeper structures drain mostly into internal iliac nodes. The superficial perineal pouch, in males and females, contain erectile tissue and skeletal muscles. The perineum is bound by the pubic symphysis anteriorly, the tip of the coccyx posteriorly and the ischial tuberosities (not spines) laterally. The dorsal nerve of the clitoris (and penis) is a branch of the pudendal nerve. The perineal nerve and inferior rectal nerves are also branches of the pudendal nerve. Cremasteric arteries are present in both male and females. They originate from the inferior epigastric artery which branches from the external iliac artery and course with the spermatic cord into the scrotum in males and accompany the round ligament of the uterus in females.

6.5.38 A – Anterior

The bladder is divided into four parts – the apex (dome) is the anterosuperior part which faces the abdominal wall; the fundus (base) is the posteroinferior part; the body is the part between the apex and fundus; and the neck is the constricted part that continues to the urethra. It is situated posterior to the pubic symphysis and anterior to the vagina in females and rectum in males; hence A is the correct response.

6.5.39 A – The vesicouterine pouch separates the body of the uterus and bladder

In females, the uterus lies between the bladder and rectum. The uterine tubes extend from the superior part of the uterus to the lateral pelvic walls and as a result form two pouches – a shallower anterior vesicouterine pouch between the bladder and uterus, and a deeper posterior rectouterine pouch (pouch of Douglas) between the rectum and uterus; hence A is the correct response. The pouch of Douglas lies in close proximity to the posterior (not anterior) fornix of the vagina. The broad ligament is a remnant of the Müllerian ducts which fuse during development. The round ligaments are remnants of the gubernaculum. The largest part of the broad ligament is the mesometrium. The mesosalpinx and mesovarium are the most superior and posterior parts of the broad ligament respectively. A normal uterus rests in an anteverted and anteflexed position. Flexion relates to the axis of the uterine body relative to the cervix. Version relates to the axis of the cervix relative to the vagina.

6.5.40 E – Dentate

The anal canal is divided into superior and inferior segments by the dentate or pectinate line which demarcates the visceral-parietal transition point; hence E is the correct response. Shenton's line is an imaginary line drawn along the inferior border of the superior pubic ramus along the inferomedial border of the neck of femur. Clinically, interruption of this line can indicate fractured neck of femur and developmental dysplasia of the hip. The arcuate line is the demarcation where the aponeurosis of the rectus sheath of internal oblique and transversus abdominis pass anteriorly to rectus abdominis, leaving behind transversalis fascia only. It is located approximately halfway between the umbilicus and pubic crest. Hilton's (white) line or anocutaneous line or inter-sphincteric groove marks the transition point from non-keratinised stratified squamous epithelium to keratinised stratified squa-mous epithelium of the anal canal. It also marks the border between the internal and external anal sphincter. The pectineal (not to be confused with pectinate) line is a ridge on the superior ramus of the pubic bone and forms part of the pelvic rim. It forms the iliopectineal line with the arcuate line. It is also a ridge located on the posterior surface of the femur which continues to the base of the lesser trochanter where the pectineus muscle attaches.

6.5.41 *C – Skene's glands open into the vulvar vestibule*

The perineum divides into an anterior urogenital triangle and a posterior anal triangle. The urogenital triangle contains the roots of the external genitalia and the openings of the urogenital system. The vulvar vestibule encircles the labia minora into which the urethra and vagina exit the perineum. The ducts of para-urethral glands (Skene's glands) open into this vestibule on either side of the lateral margin of the urethra; hence C is the correct response. Bartholin's glands (greater vestibular glands) are pea-sized mucous glands that lie posterior to the vestibular bulb of the vagina and found only in females. Homologues to these in males are bulbourethral glands. The urogenital triangle is bound laterally (not posteriorly) by the ischiopubic rami, posteriorly by an imagi-nary line between the ischial tuberosities and anteriorly by the pubic symphysis. Muscle development is greater in males since the corpus spongiosum expands over the body of the penis as the proximal end is not attached to the perineal membrane (forming the glans penis). In contrast, the structurally equivalent bulbs of the vestibule are located on either side of the vaginal opening and anchored to the perineal membrane in females. Corpora cavernosa are located on either side of the urogenital triangle and attached to the pubic arch via crura. Corpus spongiosum is a single, erectile mass.

Answers to 6.5.42 and 6.4.43 relate to the following annotated figure of the pelvic diaphragm.

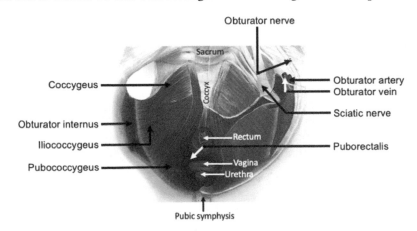

6.5.42 *A – Coccygeus Obturator internus Iliococcygeus Pubococcygeus Puborectalis*

6.5.43 *C – (8) arises from the anterior rami of S2–S4, and accompanies (6–7) to supply the medial compartment of the thigh*

Labels 6, 7 and 8 correspond to the obturator vein, artery and nerve, respectively. The obturator nerve descends in psoas major, emerges near the pelvic brim, and passes across the lateral wall of the pelvic cavity. It arises from the anterior rami of L2–L4 and accompanies the obturator vein and artery through the obturator canal to supply the medial compartment of the thigh; hence C is the correct response. The pudendal nerve arises from the anterior rami of S2–S4 and accompanies the internal pudendal vessels through Alcock's (pudendal) canal (formed by obturator fascia), where it gives off its first branch, the perineal nerve. The terminal branch of the pudendal nerve is the dorsal nerve of the penis/clitoris which provides sensory innervation to the skin. The internal pudendal vein (and artery) exits the pelvis via the lesser sciatic foramen and curves around the sacrospinous ligament to re-enter the pelvis via the greater sciatic foramen. Terminal branches of the internal pudendal artery (not obturator), and external puden-dal artery supply tissues in the deep perineal pouch, erectile tissues and external genitalia. The internal pudendal artery and vein (not obturator) leave the pelvis through the greater sciatic foramen inferior to piriformis.

6.5.44 *E – Base, inferior pubic rami*

The anal triangle is the posterior half of the perineum. It is defined laterally by the medial margins of the sacrotuberous ligaments, anteriorly by the posterior margin of the perineal membrane and a horizontal line between the ischial tuberosities, and posteriorly by the tip of the coccyx. The roof or ceiling of the anal triangle is the pelvic diaphragm which is formed by the levator ani muscles. There is no base to the anal triangle; hence E is the correct response.

6.5.45 *B – In the female pelvis, the uterine artery crosses the ureter*

In the female pelvis, the uterine artery crosses the ureter; hence B is the correct response. In males, the ductus deferens crosses the ureter. The seminal colliculus is an enlarged section located halfway along the length of the prostatic urethra. Medial to the infundibulum of the uterine tubes is the expanded ampulla which then narrows to form the isthmus. The prostate lies inferior to the bladder, anterior to the rectum, and posterior to the pubic symphysis. The neck of the bladder is anchored into position by a pair of tough fibromuscular ligaments – the pubovesical ligaments in females, and the puboprostatic ligaments in males.

6.5.46 *B – Corpus spongiosum*

The corpus spongiosum is the most ventral structure in the penis; hence B is the correct response, and it encloses the urethra. The most dorsal structure is the superficial dorsal vein as shown in the figure below.

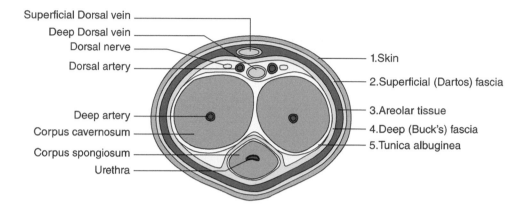

6.5.47 *D – External anal sphincter*

The external anal sphincter is innervated by the inferior rectal branches of the pudendal nerve (not the perineal branch); hence D is the correct response.

Answers 6.5.48 to 6.5.50 relate to the following annotated figure.

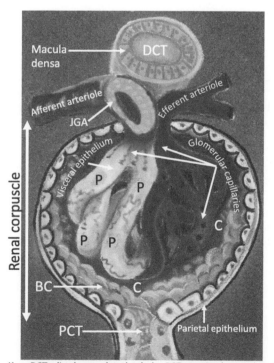

Key: DCT: distal convoluted tubule; PCT: proximal convoluted tubule; JGA: juxtaglomerular apparatus; BC: Bowman's capsule; C: capsular space; P: podocytes

6.5.48 *D –* Macula densa Juxtaglomerular Fenestrated epithelial Cuboidal epithelial

Structure labelled 1 corresponds to the macula densa. These are specialised epithelial cells of the distal convoluted tubule and thick ascending limb of the loop of Henlé which are found in close proximity to the vascular pole of the glomerulus. Collectively with the extraglomerular matrix (secreted by mesangial cells of the glomerulus) and juxtaglomerular granular cells (label 2) of the afferent arterioles (which produce and release renin), they make up the juxtaglomerular apparatus. This tubuloglomerular feedback region regulates sodium homeostasis, glomerular filtration rate and renal blood flow. Since the juxtaglomerular cells are specialised smooth muscle cells, they have the capacity to alter glomerular perfusion. Baroreceptors in the arterioles trigger renin release when blood pressure falls. This catalyses the conversion of angiotensinogen to angiotensin I. Angiotensin I is converted to angiotensin II by angiotensin converting enzyme (ACE) found in the kidneys and lungs. Angiotensin II exerts negative feedback on renin production by the juxtaglomerular cells. Structures labelled 4 and 5 correspond to the glomerular capillaries and visceral layer of the Bowman's capsule respectively. Each kidney contains approximately 1 million glomeruli which filter nearly one fifth of cardiac output. Glomerular capillaries (label 4) are surrounded by Bowman's capsule and contained within Bowman's space into which plasma is filtered. Endothelial cells in the glomerular capillaries are fenestrated, i.e., they have gaps which allow passage of water and molecules. These fenestrations not only provide a porous membrane but help protein filtration since they are covered with anionic proteoglycans and glycoproteins which absorb proteins and repel anions and large macromolecules. Structure labelled 6 corresponds to the cuboidal epithelium of the proximal convoluted tubule. They contain a brush border of microvilli which help increase the surface area. Lacis cells are extraglomerular mesangial cells of the juxtaglomerular apparatus. They are in close contact with macula densa cells and are located in a region with no capillaries, lymph or nerve fibres.

6.5.49 *B – Efferent arteriole*

Label 3 corresponds to the efferent arteriole; hence B is the correct response. Blood enters the glomerulus through the afferent arteriole at the vascular pole, undergoes capillary glomerular filtration and exits through the efferent arteriole at the vascular pole.

6.5.50 *C – Form a glomerular filtration barrier which help restrict passage of the anionic molecules and macromolecules*

Label 5 corresponds to the visceral epithelium of the Bowman's capsule which lines the glomerular capillaries. The fenestrated endothelium carries negative charges that restrict movement of anionic (not cationic) particles into Bowman's space; hence C is the correct response. This layer is composed of podocytes with finger-like projections called foot processes or pedicels. These are an added filtering mechanism. Mesangial cells are contractile cells that contribute to the central stalk of the glomerulus. They are irregularly shaped cells which have processes that extend towards the basement membrane that provide support to tufts via bundles of microfilaments.

6.6   Lower limb

6.6.1 *C – Adductor magnus*

There are six muscles in the medial compartment of the thigh: gracilis, adductor longus, adductor brevis, adductor magnus, obturator externus and pectineus. The tibial division of the sciatic nerve (L2, L3) innervates the hamstring part of the adductor magnus; hence C is the correct response. The obturator nerve innervates gracilis (L2), adductor longus (anterior division; L2, L3), the adductor part of adductor magnus (L2, L3) and obturator externus (posterior division; L4). The femoral nerve innervates pectineus (L2).

6.6.2 *D – Superior gemellus*

The superior gemellus originates at the ischial spine, while the inferior gemellus originates from the upper aspect of the ischial tuberosity. Together with the obturator internus tendon, the two gemelli insert onto the medial surface of the greater trochanter of the femur; hence D is the correct response. The obturator internus originates from the posterior surface of the obturator membrane and the anterolateral wall of the pelvis and inserts onto the medial side of the greater trochanter of the femur. The quadratus femoris originates on the lateral aspect of the ischium just anterior to the ischial tuberosity and inserts onto the quadrate tubercle on the intertrochanteric crest of the proximal femur. The tensor fasciae latae originates on the lateral aspect of the ischial crest between the anterior superior iliac spine and tubercle of the crest and inserts onto the iliotibial tract of the fasciae latae.

6.6.3 *D – The superior border is bound by the inguinal ligament*

The femoral triangle is a wedge-shaped depression in the anterior superior thigh. The borders of the femoral triangle (as shown below) are the inguinal ligament superiorly, the adductor longus medially, and sartorius laterally; hence D is the correct response. The floor is formed by pectineus and adductor longus medially and iliopsoas laterally. The roof, from superficial to deep, is composed of skin, subcutaneous tissue, superficial fascia, and fasciae latae. The apex of the triangle is formed distally by the intersection of sartorius and adductor longus. From lateral to medial, the contents include the femoral nerve, artery, vein, and empty space with lymphatics (NAVEL). These vessels (except the femoral nerve) are encased within the femoral (fascial) sheath which is a continuation of transversalis fascia of the abdomen and the inguinal ligament.

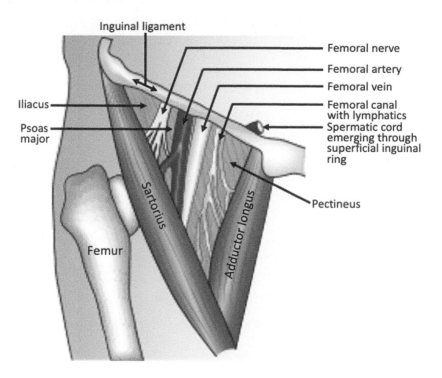

Inguinal ligament

Femoral nerve

Femoral artery

Femoral vein

Femoral canal
with lymphatics

Spermatic cord
emerging through
superficial inguinal
ring

Iliacus

Psoas
major

Sartorius

Adductor longus

Femur

Pectineus

6.6.4 *C – Medial circumflex*

The main arteries that supply the femoral head and neck are the medial and lateral femoral circumflex arteries which branch from the deep femoral artery (profunda femoris). The deep branch and the terminal nutrient arteries of the medial femoral circumflex artery are the primary blood supplies to the femoral head and neck; hence C is the correct response. The obturator artery supplies the medial compartment of the thigh. The descending genicular artery is the most distal branch of the femoral artery which anastomoses with the medial superior genicular artery to supply vastus medialis, adductor magnus and skin of the medial thigh. Perforating arteries (of which there are usually three) are branches of profunda femoris that perforate the tendon of adductor magnus to reach the posterior thigh.

6.6.5 *C – Femoral nerve*

Hunter's canal or adductor canal is a conical musculoaponeurotic passage through the distal middle third of the thigh that transmits neurovascular structures from the femoral triangle to the adductor hiatus. These include the femoral artery and vein, saphenous nerve, medial femoral cutaneous nerve, and nerve to vastus medialis. The femoral nerve is not contained with Hunter's canal; hence C is the correct response. The canal has three borders: vastus medialis anterolaterally, adductor longus and adductor magnus posterolaterally, and the aponeurosis of the vastoadductor membrane medially.

6.6.6 *B – Vastus intermedius*

Vastus intermedius originates from the superior two-thirds of anterior and lateral femur and inserts onto the lateral margin of the patella by forming the quadriceps femoris tendon; hence B is the correct response. Vastus medialis originates from the medial portion of the intertrochanteric line, pectineal line, medial lip of the linea aspera and the medial supracondylar line of the femur and inserts onto the medial border of the patella by forming the medial aspect of the quadriceps femoris tendon. Vastus lateralis originates from the lateral portion of the intertrochanteric line, anteroinferior border of the greater trochanter, lateral margin of the gluteal tuberosity and lateral lip of linea aspera and inserts onto the lateral base of the patella by forming the lateral aspect of the quadriceps femoris tendon. Adductor longus originates from the anterior surface of the body of the pubis and inserts onto the middle third of the linea aspera of the femur. Rectus femoris originates from the anterior inferior iliac spine (straight head) and the ilium (reflected head) and inserts onto the base of the patella forming the central part of the quadriceps femoris tendon. Sartorius originates from the anterior superior iliac spine and inserts onto the medial surface of the tibial shaft inferomedial to the tibial tuberosity.

6.6.7 *A – Semimembranosus*

Semimembranosus originates from the superior lateral quadrant of the ischial tuberosity and inserts onto the posterior surface of the medial tibial condyle; hence A is the correct response. Semitendinosus originates from the common tendon with the long head of biceps femoris from the inferomedial part of the upper part of the ischial tuberosity and inserts onto the medial surface of the tibial shaft. The long head of biceps femoris originates with semitendinosus, and the short head originates from the lateral lip of the linea aspera. Both heads insert onto the head of the fibula. The hamstring part of adductor magnus originates from the ischial tuberosity and inserts onto the adductor tubercle and supracondylar line.

Answers 6.6.8 to 6.6.12 relate to the following annotated axial MRI figure of the lower limb.

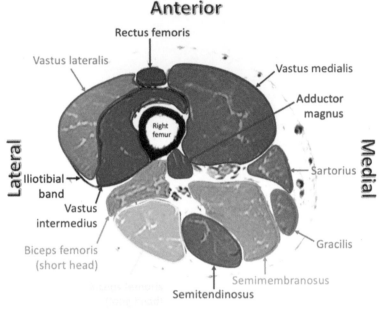

Muscles of the thigh are arranged in three compartments separated by intermuscular septa. The anterior compartment contains four large quadriceps femoris muscles – rectus femoris, vastus lateralis, vastus intermedius, and vastus medialis, sartorius, and the terminal ends of psoas major and iliacus. The medial compartment contains gracilis, pectineus, obturator externus and the adductor muscles – adductor longus, brevis and magnus. The posterior compartment contains biceps femoris, semitendinosus and semimembranosus.

6.6.8 *A – Quadriceps femoris tendon*

Muscle labelled 1 corresponds to the rectus femoris muscle, which inserts onto the quadriceps femoris tendon (with the vastus muscles); hence A is the correct response. Psoas major and iliacus insert onto the lesser trochanter of the femur. Pectineus and the adductor muscles (except the hamstring part of adductor magnus) insert onto linea aspera. Obturator externus inserts onto the trochanteric fossa. Biceps femoris inserts onto the head of the fibula.

6.6.9 *D – Medially rotates and adducts the thigh at the hip joint*

Muscle labelled 2 corresponds to adductor magnus, which medially rotates and adducts the thigh at the hip joint; hence D is the correct response.

6.6.10 *B – It laterally rotates the thigh at the hip joint*

Muscle labelled 3 corresponds to the long and short head of biceps femoris which flexes the leg at the knee joint, extends and laterally rotates the thigh at the hip joint, and laterally rotates the leg at the knee joint; hence B is the correct response. It is innervated by the sciatic nerve (S1). It distally attaches to the head of the fibula. The long head originates from the inferomedial part of the upper area of the ischial tuberosity (not spine).

6.6.11 *E – Sciatic*

Muscle labelled 4 corresponds to semitendinosus which is innervated by the sciatic nerve; hence E is the correct response.

6.6.12 *B – Gracilis*

Muscle labelled 5 corresponds to gracilis; hence B is the correct response.

Answers 6.6.13 to 6.6.17 relate to the following coronal MRI figure of the lower limb.

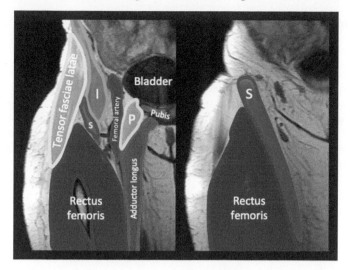

I: Iliopsoas; P: Pectineus; **S: Sartorius**

6.6.13 *C – Tensor fasciae latae*

6.6.14 *A – 1 and 5*

Muscles labelled 1 and 5 correspond to tensor fasciae latae and adductor longus, respectively. The tensor fasciae latae is innervated by the superior gluteal nerve and adductor longus is innervated by the obturator nerve; hence A is the correct response.

6.6.15 *D – 4*

Muscle labelled 4 corresponds to pectineus which adducts and flexes the thigh at the hip joint; hence C is the correct response. Tensor fasciae latae (label 1) stabilises the knee in extension. Sartorius (label 2) is not involved in adduction; it is a hip and knee flexor. Rectus femoris (label 3) flexes the thigh at the hip joint and extends the leg at the knee joint. Adductor longus (label 5) medially rotates and adducts the thigh at the hip joint; it is not involved in flexion.

6.6.16 *E – 4 and 5*

The external iliac artery becomes the femoral artery when it passes under the inguinal ligaments and enters the femoral triangle. The largest branch of the femoral artery in the thigh is the profunda femoris which arises from the posterolateral side of the femoral artery in the femoral triangle. It travels posteriorly between pectineus (label 4) and adductor longus (label 5); hence E is the correct response. It continues inferiorly between adductor longus and adductor magnus, eventually connecting with branches of the popliteal artery behind the knee. Profunda femoris has lateral and medial circumflex femoral branches and three perforating branches.

6.6.17 *C – 3*

Muscle labelled 3 corresponds to the rectus femoris which, along with vastus medialis, vastus intermedius and vastus lateralis, distally attaches to the quadriceps femoris tendon; hence C is the correct response. Tensor fasciae latae (label 1) distally attaches onto the iliotibial tract of the fasciae latae. Sartorius (label 2) distally attaches onto the medial surface of the tibia close to the tibial tuberosity. Pectineus (label 4) distally attaches onto the pectineal line of the femur – an oblique line extending from the base of the lesser trochanter to linea aspera on the posterior surface of the femur. Adductor longus (label 5) distally attaches onto linea aspera on the middle one-third of the shaft of the femur.

6.6.18 *E – Posterior tibial artery*

The popliteal fossa is a diamond-shaped fat-filled space in the posterior knee. It contains the popliteal artery and vein, short saphenous vein, tibial nerve, common fibular (peroneal) nerve, posterior femoral cutaneous nerve and the auricular branch of the obturator nerve. The posterior tibial artery is a branch of the popliteal artery, but it is not contained within the popliteal fossa; hence E is the correct response. Boundaries of the popliteal fossa are as follows:

- Superolateral – medial border of biceps femoris
- Superomedial – lateral border of semimembranosus and semitendinosus
- Inferolateral – medial border of the lateral head of gastrocnemius and plantaris

- Inferomedial – lateral border of the medial head of gastrocnemius
- Floor – knee joint capsule, popliteal surface of the femur and popliteal muscle
- Roof – superficial fascia and skin

6.6.19 *C – Sural*

The sural nerve is formed by terminal branches of the tibial and common peroneal nerves. It provides only sensation to the posterolateral aspect of the distal third of the leg and lateral aspect of the foot and ankle; hence C is the correct response. The tibial nerve terminates in the medial sural cutaneous nerve and the common fibular nerve terminates in the lateral sural cutaneous nerve. These two nerves unite in the distal third of the posterior leg as the sural nerve. The saphenous nerve provides sensory innervation to the medial, anteromedial, and posteromedial aspects of the distal thigh to the medial malleolus of the ankle. The tibial nerve, one of the two terminal branches of the sciatic nerve, provides a motor supply to the posterior compartment of the thigh and leg, and muscles of the sole of the foot. It provides a sensory supply to the posterior calf and sole of the foot, knee, ankle and foot joints. The common fibular (peroneal) nerve, the other terminal branch of the sciatic nerve, supplies muscles of the anterior and lateral compartments of the lower limb. It divides close to the fibular head into the superficial and deep fibular nerves. Most of the anterior and lateral sensation of the leg is carried by the superficial fibular nerve.

6.6.20 *D – Navicular and medial cuneiform*

Tibialis posterior is the deepest muscle of the deep posterior compartment of the lower leg. It is a primary inverter and secondary plantar flexor of the foot. As it travels distal to the medial malleolus, it courses along the plantar aspect of the foot, where it splits into three parts: the primary part inserts onto the navicular bone tubercle, the plantar part inserts onto the medial cuneiform, intermediate cuneiform, lateral cuneiform, the base of the second to fourth metatarsals, and cuboid, and the recurrent part which has a small insertion at the sustentaculum tali of the calcaneus; hence D is the correct response.

6.6.21 *B – Popliteus*

Alongside flexor hallucis longus, flexor digitorum longus, and tibialis posterior, popliteus is a deep muscle in the posterior compartment of the leg. It proximally attaches to the lateral femoral condyle and inserts onto the posterior surface of the proximal tibia; hence B is the correct response. The superficial muscles in the posterior compartment of the leg are plantaris, gastrocnemius and soleus. These muscles all insert onto the posterior surface of the calcaneus via the calcaneal tendon. Plantaris originates from the inferior aspect of the lateral supracondylar line of the femur and oblique popliteal ligament of the knee. The medial head of gastrocnemius originates from the posterior surface of the distal femur above the medial condyle, and the lateral head originates from the posterolateral surface of the lateral femoral condyle. Soleus is a large flat muscle which has multiple origins – the posterior aspect of the fibular head and adjacent surface of the fibular neck and upper shaft, the soleal line and medial border of the tibia, and the tendinous arch between the tibial and fibular attachments. Fibularis longus is a muscle of the lateral compartment of the leg which originates from the upper lateral surface of the fibula, fibular head, and the lateral tibial condyle (occasionally), and inserts onto the under and lateral surface of the medial cuneiform and base of the first metatarsal.

6.6.22 *B – Posterior tibial*

The popliteal artery is the major blood supply to the leg and foot. It descends in the posterior compartment of the leg and bifurcates in the deep region into the anterior tibial artery and posterior tibial artery. The posterior tibial artery passes posterior to popliteus and pierces soleus, and then descends between tibialis posterior and flexor digitorum longus. It divides into the medial and lateral plantar arteries at the level of the talus; hence B is the correct response. The popliteal artery also branches into two sural arteries which supply plantaris, gastrocnemius and soleus. It also gives rise to branches that contribute to an extensive anastomotic network around the knee joint via the superior medial and superior lateral genicular arteries above the knee joint, the middle genicular and sural arteries at the level of the knee joint, and the inferior medial and inferior lateral genicular arteries below the knee joint.

6.6.23 *A – Tibialis posterior*

Tibialis posterior inverts and plantarflexes the foot; hence A is the correct response. Fibularis longus everts and plantarflexes the foot. Flexor digitorum longus and flexor hallucis longus are flexes of the lateral four toes and great toe, respectively. Plantaris plantarflexes the foot.

6.6.24 *D – Calcaneus*

The sustentaculum tali is a triangular projection found on the plantaromedial aspect of the calcaneus; hence D is the correct response. This has a superior concave shelf which articulates with the middle calcaneal surface of the head of the talus. The inferior surface has a groove along which flexor hallucis longus runs into the sole of the foot. Several ligaments attach to the sustentaculum tali which helps to stabilise the ankle joint – medial (deltoid) ligament, plantar calcaneonavicular ligament and the medial talocalcaneal ligament.

6.6.25 *B – Superior fibular*

The retinacula of the ankle are localised thickenings of superficial aponeurosis covering deeper structures which maintain approximation of tendons to the underlying bone. There are three retinacula of the ankle:

- the fibular (peroneal) retinacula bind the tendons of fibularis longus and brevis to the lateral aspect of the foot. The superior fibular retinaculum extends between the lateral malleolus and calcaneus; hence B is the correct response. The inferior fibular retinaculum attaches to the lateral surface of calcaneus around the fibular trochlea.
- the extensor retinacula enclose the extensor tendons of the ankle. The superior extensor retinaculum attaches to the anterior borders of the fibula and tibia. The inferior extensor retinaculum is Y-shaped, where its base is attached to the lateral side of the upper surface of the calcaneus; it then crosses medially where one arm attaches to the medial malleolus and the other attaches to the medial side of the plantar aponeurosis.
- the flexor retinaculum is a band of connective tissue which attaches to the medial malleolus of the tibia, the medial and posterior surface of talus, the medial process of calcaneus, and the inferior surface of the sustentaculum tali. It forms the roof of the tarsal tunnel.

6.6.26 *D – Small saphenous*

Within the foot there are interconnected networks of deep and superficial veins. The deep veins follow a similar course to the arteries, while the superficial veins drain into a dorsal venous arch over the metatarsals. The small saphenous vein originates from the lateral side of the arch and passes posterior to the lateral malleolus; hence D is the correct response. The great saphenous vein originates from the medial side of the arch and passes anterior to the medial malleolus.

6.6.27 *E – Flexor digitorum brevis*

The tarsal tunnel acts as a passageway for vessels, nerves and tendons to travel from the posterior leg to the foot. Its contents from anterior to posterior are tibialis posterior tendon, flexor digitorum longus tendon, posterior tibial artery and vein, tibial nerve, and flexor hallucis longus tendon. Flexor digitorum brevis is not contained within the tarsal tunnel; hence E is the correct response.

6.6.28 *C – Subtalar*

The subtalar joint is a synovial articulation between the talus and calcaneus. The major ligaments of the subtalar joint include the lateral, medial, posterior and interosseous talocalcaneal ligaments which help stabilise the joint; hence C is the correct response. The talonavicular, bifurcate (which has arms that are attached to cuboid via the calcaneocuboid ligament, and to navicular via the calcaneonavicular ligament), and plantar calcaneonavicular ligaments stabilise the talocalcaneonavicular joint. The plantar calcaneocuboid and long plantar ligaments support the calcaneocuboid joint. Medial and lateral collateral ligaments, and plantar ligaments reinforce the interphalangeal and metatarsophalangeal joints.

6.6.29 *E – Flexor digiti minimi brevis*

The lateral plantar nerve is a smaller terminal division of the tibial nerve. It innervates abductor digit minimi, adductor hallucis, quadratus plantae, 2nd–4th lumbricals, dorsal and plantar interossei, and flexor digiti minimi brevis; hence E is the correct response. Abductor hallucis, flexor digitorum brevis, 1st lumbrical and flexor hallucis brevis are innervated by the medial plantar nerve, also a branch of the tibial nerve.

6.6.30 *D – They adduct toes three to five*

There are four dorsal interossei which abduct the 2nd–4th toes. The plantar interossei adduct the 3rd–5th toes; hence D is the correct response.

6.6.31 *A – Calcaneofibular*

The deltoid (medial) ligament of the ankle is composed of four parts: anterior tibiotalar, posterior tibiotalar, tibionavicular and tibiocalcaneal. The calcaneofibular, together with anterior and posterior talofibular ligaments, are components of the lateral ligament of the ankle; hence A is the correct response.

6.6.32 *A – Dorsiflexion of the ankle, eversion of the foot*

Fibularis tertius, with tibialis posterior, extensor hallucis longus, and extensor digitorum longus, is a muscle of the anterior compartment of the leg. Its action is to dorsiflex and evert the foot; hence A is the correct response. Tibialis anterior dorsiflexes the foot at the ankle joint and inverts the foot. All anterior compartment muscles are dorsiflexes of the foot. The posterior compartment muscles – gastrocnemius, plantaris and soleus are plantarflexes of the foot.

6.6.33 *E – Extensor digitorum longus*

The deep fibular (peroneal) nerve is composed of dorsal branches of L4 to S1. It innervates muscles of the anterior compartment of the leg. S2 does not contribute to the motor supply of extensor digitorum longus; hence E is the correct response. The superficial and deep muscles of the posterior compartment are innervated by the tibial nerve (predominantly S2).

Answers 6.6.34 to 6.6.36 relate to the following annotated MRI figure of the knee.

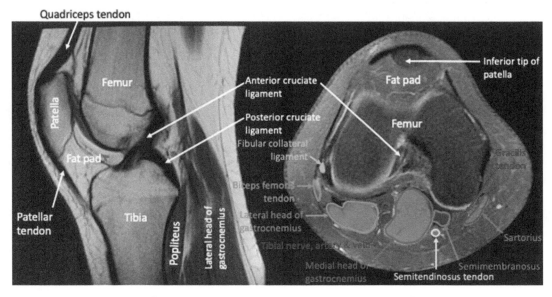

6.6.34 *D – Anterior cruciate*

6.6.35 *A – It serves to resist excessive posterior translation of the tibia*

Structure labelled 2 corresponds to the posterior cruciate ligament. It is one of the main stabilisers of the knee joint and serves to resist excessive posterior translation of the tibia relative to the femur; hence A is the correct response. It originates from the anterolateral surface of the medial femoral condyle and inserts onto the tibial plateau. It comprises two bundles: a larger anterolateral bundle, which tightens when the knee is flexed, and a smaller posteromedial bundle, which tightens when the knee is extended. It is accompanied by the anterior menisco-femoral ligament anteriorly (Humphrey's ligament) and the posterior menisco-femoral ligament posteriorly (Wrisberg's ligament). The primary function of the medial meniscus is to decrease the amount of stress on the knee joint.

6.6.36 *B – Tendon of semitendinosus*

6.6.37 *D – 1 everts the foot and 2 corresponds to abductor digiti minimi*

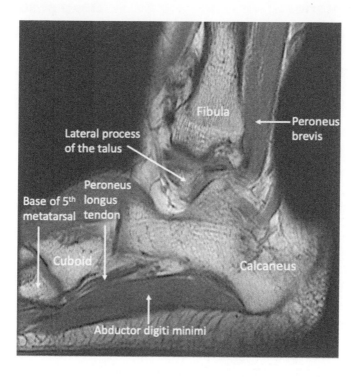

This is a sagittal MRI of the ankle and foot. It displays components of the lateral aspect of the foot, ankle and lower leg. The medial surface of the lateral malleolus articulates with the lateral surface of the talus. The lower part of the lateral surface of the body of the talus forms a bony projection – the lateral process. The calcaneus sits beneath talus and supports it. The cuboid articulates posteriorly with the calcaneus, and anteriorly with the bases of the 4th and 5th metatarsals. There are two muscles in the lateral compartment of the leg – peroneus (fibularis) longus and brevis. Therefore, muscle labelled 1 must correspond to one of these. Peroneus longus originates from the upper lateral surface of the fibula and head of the fibula. It then descends passing posterior to the lateral malleolus and curves forward under the fibular trochlea of the calcaneus, entering a deep groove on the inferior surface of the cuboid before attaching to the lateral aspect of medial cuneiform and base of the 1st metatarsal. Peroneus brevis lies deep to peroneus longus and originates from the lower two-thirds of the lateral surface of the shaft of the fibula. The tendon passes behind the lateral malleolus with peroneus longus but instead curves forwards across the lateral surface of calcaneus and attaches to the base of the 5th metatarsal. Hence muscle labelled 1 corresponds to peroneus brevis. Muscles of the lateral compartment are involved in eversion of the foot. Muscle labelled 2 corresponds to a muscle in the sole of the foot. There are four layers of muscles in the sole of the foot from superficial to deep. The first layer is composed of abductor hallucis, flexor digitorum brevis and abductor digiti minimi. As mentioned, this MRI slice is of the lateral aspect of the foot and the most lateral of these muscles is abductor digiti minimi. This muscle originates from the lateral and medial processes of the calcaneal tuberosity and inserts onto the lateral side of the base of the proximal phalanx of the little toe. Therefore, muscle labelled 2 corresponds to abductor digiti minimi; hence D is the correct response. This muscle abducts the little toe at the metatarsophalangeal joint. Abductor hallucis abducts and flexes the big toe at the metatarsophalangeal joint. Flexor digitorum brevis flexes the lateral four toes at the proximal interphalangeal joint.

Answers 6.6.38 to 6.6.40 relate to the following annotated axial MRI figure of the leg.

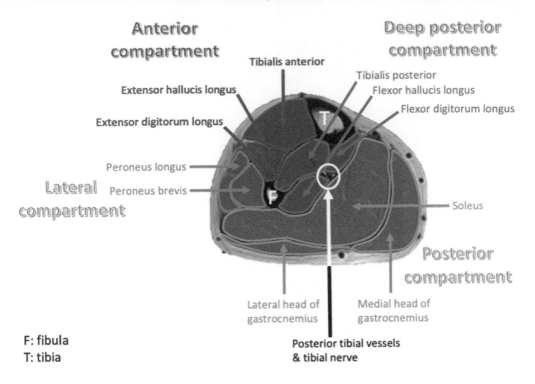

This may look daunting and somewhat complicated at first glance, therefore orientating the anatomy is the starting point. The tibia (T) is larger than the fibula (F) and the fibula lies on the lateral side of the leg. The leg is divided into anterior (extensor), posterior (flexor) and lateral (fibular or peroneus) compartments. There are four muscles in the deep posterior compartment – the popliteus, flexor hallucis longus, flexor digitorum longus and tibialis posterior. The popliteus is most superior and is not evident in this axial figure. Flexor digitorum longus originates from the medial side of the posterior surface of the tibia; hence C is the correct response. Flexor hallucis longus is more lateral and originates from the lower two-thirds of the posterior surface of the fibula. Tibialis posterior lies between flexor digitorum longus and flexor hallucis longus and originates from the adjacent posterior surfaces of the tibia and fibula.

The posterior tibial artery supplies the posterior and lateral compartments of the leg. It descends through the posterior compartment on the superficial surfaces of tibialis posterior and flexor digitorum longus. Following suit is the tibial nerve; hence A is the correct response.

Muscle labelled 3 corresponds to soleus. It lies under the gastrocnemius muscle. It is attached to the proximal ends of the fibula and tibia, and a tendinous ligament. More specifically, it originates from the soleal line and medial border of the tibia, the posterior aspect of the fibular head and adjacent surfaces of the neck and proximal shaft; hence D is the correct response. It is involved in plantarflexion of the foot. It is innervated by the tibial nerve (S1, S2). It is supplied by branches of the popliteal artery and posterior tibial artery. It inserts onto the posterior surface of calcaneus via the calcaneal tendon. Fibularis tertius inserts onto the dorsomedial surface of the base of the 5th metatarsal.

Answers 6.6.41 to 6.6.43 relate to the following annotated axial MRI figure of the lower limb.

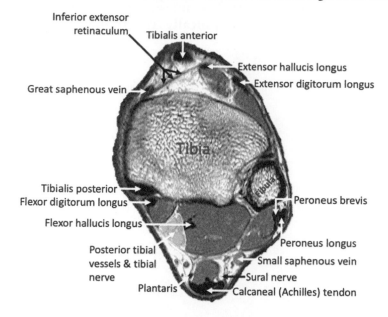

6.6.41 *C – Popliteus*

The tendons and associated muscles of the anterior, posterior and lateral compartments of the leg are evident in this MRI figure. It is an axial section of the distal tibia and fibula, and the popliteus muscle is far more proximal to the knee since it attaches to the lateral femoral condyle and inserts onto the posterior surface of the proximal tibia; hence C is the correct response.

6.6.42 *D – Inferior extensor retinaculum*

This fibrous band attaches to the medial malleolus of the tibia. It crosses over the foot anterior to the tendon of extensor hallucis longus and extensor digitorum longus and attaches to the upper surface of the calcaneus on the lateral side, and onto the medial side of the plantar aponeurosis. Therefore, structure labelled 1 corresponds to the inferior extensor retinaculum; hence D is the correct response. The superior extensor retinaculum is more superior, where it attaches to the anterior borders of the tibia and fibula.

6.6.43 *E – Great saphenous vein*

The great and small (lesser) saphenous veins originate from the medial and lateral sides of the foot as continuations of the medial and lateral marginal veins, respectively. The great saphenous vein ascends along the medial aspect of the tibia and thigh where it empties into the common femoral vein in the groin; hence E is the correct response. The small saphenous vein passes behind the lateral malleolus of the fibula and ascends in the posterior leg to join the popliteal vein in the knee. All other options are more posterior structures in the leg.

Answers 6.6.44 to 6.6.46 relate to the following annotated radiograph on a mortise AP view of the lower limb. The ankle mortise (or mortice) AP view allows the distal tibia, distal fibula, talus and proximal 5th metatarsal to be visualised radiographically. The 5th metatarsal is not shown in this figure.

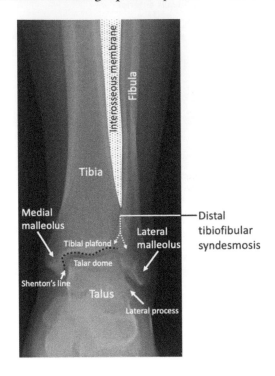

6.6.44 *B – Extensor hallucis longus*

Regions labelled 1 correspond to the interosseous membrane and the medial surface of the fibula to which extensor hallucis longus attaches; hence B is the correct response.

6.6.45 *E – Lateral plantar*

Structure labelled 2 corresponds to the talus bone. The blood supply to the talus is complex. The main blood supply is via the deltoid branches and artery of tarsal canal from the posterior tibial artery, dorsalis pedis from the anterior tibial artery, and lateral calcaneal branch and artery of the tarsal sinus from the peroneal artery. The lateral plantar artery is a branch of the posterior tibial artery which supplies the lateral side of the sole of the foot; hence E is the correct response.

6.6.46 *D – Syndesmosis*

Region labelled 3 corresponds to the distal tibiofibular syndesmosis; hence D is the correct response. A syndesmosis is a fibrous joint where two adjacent bones, in this case the tibia and fibula, are linked by strong ligaments and membranes. The ligament complex consists of the anterior inferior tibiofibular ligament, the posterior inferior tibiofibular ligament, the transverse tibiofibular ligament, and the interosseous membrane. Clinically, this complex can be damaged following injury through external rotation and ankle dorsiflexion. The syndesmosis can become distorted when the talar dome pushes the fibula and separates from the tibia. Shenton's line highlights that the two articular surfaces are parallel which is normal. Following trauma, this line can often be distorted which can be associated with syndesmosis damage.

Pseudoarthrosis describes what happens when bones do not fuse properly, often due to non-union, which leads to delayed healing of broken bones. It can also be called a false joint. Epiphysiodesis is a surgical technique that is performed on the growth plate (physis) of a longer bone and used to correct differences in bone length. It is also called growth plate fusion. Aponeurosis (pl: aponeuroses) is a connective tissue sheath found on the surface of pennate muscles which is continuous with tendons and serves as insertion points for muscle fascicles. Articulation is the meeting point for two or more bones at a joint.

Answers 6.6.47 to 6.6.50 relate to the following annotated radiograph of the ankle and foot.

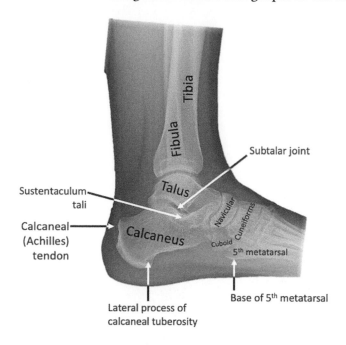

6.6.47 *D – S1–S2*

Structure labelled 1 corresponds to the calcaneal (Achilles) tendon. Gastrocnemius and soleus converge distally to form the Achilles tendon which inserts onto the middle part of the posterior surface of the calcaneus. Contraction of both muscles causes plantarflexion of the foot. Testing of the deep tendon reflex involves briskly striking the tendon which would normally cause plantarflexion of the foot. The sacral nerve roots S1 and S2 are being assessed; hence D is the correct response.

6.6.48 *A – Lateral plantar nerve Flexion of lateral four toes*

Region labelled 2 corresponds to the calcaneus, and more specifically the calcaneal tuberosity. There are several muscles of the foot which originate in this region. There are three muscles in the first layer in the sole of the foot: abductor hallucis, flexor digitorum brevis and abductor digiti minimi. Abductor hallucis and flexor digitorum brevis originate from the medial process of the calcaneal tuberosity, and abductor digiti minimi originates from the lateral and medial processes of the calcaneal tuberosity. The second layer of muscles in the sole of the foot include quadratus plantae and lumbricals. Quadratus plantae originates from the medial surface of calcaneus and the lateral process of the calcaneal tuberosity. It is innervated by lateral plantar nerve and assists flexor digitorum longus in flexion of the lateral four toes; hence A is the correct response. Abductor hallucis, flexor digitorum brevis, 1st lumbrical, and flexor hallucis brevis are all innervated by the medial plantar nerve. All remaining muscles of the sole of the foot are innervated by the lateral plantar nerve. The 1st and 2nd dorsal interossei are also innervated by the deep fibular nerve, which also innervates extensor digitorum brevis on the dorsal aspect of the foot. Extensor digitorum brevis originates on the superolateral surface of the calcaneus. None of the third (flexor hallucis brevis, adductor hallucis, and flexor digiti minimi brevis) or fourth (dorsal and plantar interossei) muscle layers in the sole of the foot originate from region labelled 2.

6.6.49 *E – Interosseous talocalcaneal*

Region labelled 3 corresponds to the subtalar joint. The interosseous talocalcaneal ligament is found within this region; hence E is the correct response. The talonavicular ligament is found more superior where it passes between the neck of the talus and adjacent regions of the navicular. The long plantar ligament lies inferior to the plantar calcaneocuboid ligament in the sole of the foot. The plantar calcaneocuboid ligament connects the calcaneal tubercle to the inferior surface of the cuboid. The calcaneofibular ligament connects the posteromedial surface of the lateral malleolus to the calcaneal tubercle.

6.6.50 *C – Flexor digiti minimi brevis*

Region labelled 4 corresponds to the base of the 5th metatarsal. Flexor digiti minimi brevis attaches to the base of the 5th metatarsal and inserts onto the lateral side of the base of the proximal phalanx of the little toe; hence C is the correct response. Abductor digiti minimi attaches to the band of connective tissue that connects the calcaneus with the base of the 5th metatarsal.

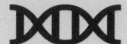

CHAPTER 7
Embryology

By 'life', we mean a thing that can nourish itself and grow and decay.

Aristotle

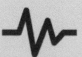

Single Best Answers for Medical Students: Basic Science, First Edition. Stuart Kyle.
© 2024 John Wiley & Sons Ltd. Published 2024 by John Wiley & Sons Ltd.

7.1 During spermatogenesis, which of the following cells undergo a second meiotic division?

  A Spermatogonia

  B Primary spermatocyte

  C Secondary spermatocytes

  D Spermatids

  E Spermatozoa

7.2 Which of the following comparisons between spermatogenesis and oogenesis is correct?

	Spermatogenesis	Oogenesis
A	Starts before birth	Starts from puberty
B	Two mitotic and two meiotic divisions occur	One mitotic and two meiotic divisions occur
C	No maturation phase	Maturation phase
D	After meiosis II, two haploid spermatids are produced	After meiosis II, one ovum and two polar bodies are produced
E	Equal cytokinesis	Unequal cytokinesis

7.3 After ovulation and no fertilization, which of the following is the correct sequence of events?

  A Corpus haemorrhagicum → Corpus albicans → Corpus luteum

  B Corpus haemorrhagicum → Corpus luteum → Corpus albicans

  C Corpus luteum → Corpus haemorrhagicum → Corpus albicans

  D Corpus albicans → Corpus haemorrhagicum → Corpus luteum

  E Corpus albicans → Corpus luteum → Corpus haemorrhagicum

7.4 Which of the following regarding hormonal changes during pregnancy is **not** correct?

  A Relaxin produced by the placenta helps relax the pelvic ligaments

  B Human placental lactogen stimulates breast development

  C Placental progesterone inhibits uterine contractions

  D Aldosterone from the adrenal cortex promotes sodium loss

  E Human chorionic gonadotrophin maintains the corpus luteum

7.5 Which of the following (A–E) correctly match hormones (1–3) in the graph?

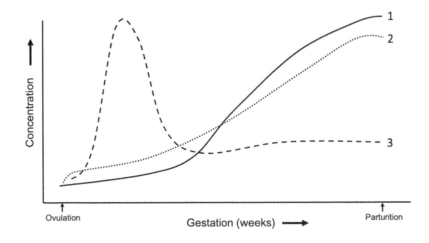

	(1)	(2)	(3)
A	HCG	Progesterone	Oestrogen
B	Oestrogen	HCG	Progesterone
C	Oestrogen	Progesterone	HCG
D	Progesterone	Oestrogen	HCG
E	Progesterone	HCG	Oestrogen

7.6 Which of the following hormones influences change of granulosa to lutein cells after ovulation?
A Progesterone
B LH
C FSH
D Oestrogen
E Testosterone

7.7 Columnar cells adjacent to the amniotic cavity refers to which layer of the human blastocyst?
A Hypoblast
B Epiblast
C Cytotrophoblast
D Syncytiotrophoblast
E Exocoelomic membrane

7.8 Which of the following predominantly produces human chorionic gonadotrophin?
A Cytotrophoblast
B Syncytiotrophoblast
C Epiblast
D Hypoblast
E Blastocoel

7.9 During embryonic development, which day does the syncytiotrophoblast begin to show large numbers of lacunae?
A Day 4
B Day 7
C Day 9
D Day 11
E Day 15

7.10 During which period of development do type II alveolar cells start producing lung surfactant, sufficient for alveolar stability?
A 12–14 weeks
B 16–18 weeks
C 20–22 weeks
D 24–26 weeks
E 30–32 weeks

7.11 On which of the following days does the primitive streak form?
A 9
B 11
C 13
D 15
E 17

7.12 Which of the following statements regarding the third week of development is **not** correct?
A Gastrulation begins with the formation of the primitive streak
B Epiblast is the source of all the germ layers
C Cells that remain in the epiblast form mesoderm
D Allantois appears around the 16th day of development
E The connecting stalk later develops into the umbilical cord

7.13 Which of the following regarding the notochord is **not** correct?
A It gives rise to the nucleus pulposus
B It forms during blastulation
C It is an early forming structure in the mesoderm layer
D It forms during week 3 of human development
E It secretes sonic hedgehog protein which helps regulate organogenesis

7.14 Following primary neurulation, neural crest cells form which of the following structures?
A Epidermis
B Hair
C Adrenal medulla
D Spinal cord
E Retina

7.15 Which of the following correctly matches the missing words (1–3) of the following sentence?
Embryologically around the 19ᵗʰ day, ...(1)...... tissue thickens and flattens to become the ......(2)...... which then elevates to become the ......(3)......

	(1)	(2)	(3)
A	endodermal	neural groove	neural tube
B	mesodermal	neural groove	neural tube
C	mesodermal	neural plate	neural folds
D	ectodermal	neural plate	neural folds
E	ectodermal	neural groove	neural folds

7.16 Which of the following regarding the embryonic period is **not** correct?
A The notochord secretes sonic hedgehog which induces the sclerotome
B The ectodermal germ layer gives rise to skin, including hair and nails
C The spleen is a mesodermal derivative
D Homeobox genes control craniocaudal patterning of the embryonic axis
E Lateral plate mesoderm forms somitomeres

7.17 Which of the following is the major growth-promoting factor during development before and after birth?
A Transforming growth factor beta (TGFβ)
B Insulin-like growth factor-1 (IGF-1)
C Vascular endothelial growth factor (VEGF)
D Epidermal growth factor (EGF)
E Fibroblast growth factor (FGF)

7.18 Which of the following regarding the structure of the placenta is correct?
A The foetal portion is formed by the decidua basalis
B Intervillous spaces are derived from lacunae in the cytotrophoblast
C There is no syncytium within the placenta
D It is considered to be haemochorial
E The maternal portion is covered by the chorionic plate

7.19 Which of the following does **not** cross the placental membrane?
A Arachidonic acid
B Vitamin B_{12}
C Cholesterol
D Uric acid
E Heparin

7.20 Which of the following conditions results from multiple CGG repeats within a chromosome?
A Turner syndrome
B Fragile X syndrome
C Trisomy 13
D Trisomy 18
E Trisomy 21

7.21 Which of the following teratogen associated with congenital malformations is **not** correct?
A Toxoplasmosis   Cerebral calcifications
B Isotretinoin   Cleft palate
C Valproic acid   Neural tube defects
D Cytomegalovirus   Hearing loss
E Hyperthermia   Glaucoma

7.22 Which of the following graphs most likely represents the risk of congenital malformations during pregnancy until parturition?

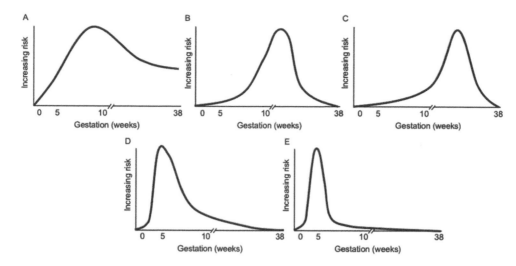

7.23 Which of the following changes occur at birth?
A The allantois (urachus) becomes the median umbilical ligament
B The umbilical artery becomes the ligamentum arteriosum
C The vitelline artery gives rise to the ascending aorta
D The left umbilical vein becomes the ligamentum venosum
E The ductus arteriosus becomes the ligamentum teres hepatis

7.24 Which of the following regarding development of the diaphragm is correct?
A It is formed by three separate components
B The septum transversum develops within the thoracic region
C The pleuroperitoneal folds project into the cephalic end of the pericardioperitoneal canals
D Ventral mesentery is derived from the septum transversum
E The right common cardinal vein develops into the inferior vena cava

7.25 Which of the following regarding limb development is correct?
A The development of each limb proceeds distoproximally
B Fingers and toes are formed when programmed cell death occurs
C Retinoic acid initiates differentiation of the zeugopod (radius/ulna and tibia/fibula) in the cascade of limb development
D Osteoclasts help deposit bone matrices
E Secondary ossification centres are found within the diaphysis

7.26 Which of the following heart defects results in an expanded right atrium and small right ventricle?
A Ostium primum
B Hypoplastic right heart syndrome
C Holt-Oram syndrome
D Tetralogy of Fallot
E Ebstein anomaly

7.27 Which of the following regarding development of the kidney is correct?
A There are four phases of kidney development
B The Wolffian duct penetrates the metanephric blastema
C The ureteric bud gives rise to the proximal convoluted tubules
D Growth of the embryo causes the kidneys to descend to their final position
E The mesenchyme expresses a transcription factor, WT1 that makes the tissue competent

7.28 Which of the following regarding the pharyngeal arches is correct?
A The muscles of mastication are derivatives of the second arch
B The superior laryngeal branch of the vagus nerve innervates muscles of the sixth arch
C The third arch gives rise to the stylohyoid ligament
D The parathyroid glands develop from the same pharyngeal pouch
E Meckel's cartilage forms the incus in the first arch

7.29   Which of the following pharyngeal arches forms Reichert's cartilage?
   A   1
   B   2
   C   3
   D   4
   E   6

7.30   Which of the following arteries does the fourth pharyngeal arch become?
   A   Stapedial
   B   Common carotid
   C   Pulmonary trunk
   D   Aortic arch
   E   External carotid

7.31   Which of the following regarding embryology of the muscular system is **not** correct?
   A   Cardiac muscle is derived from paraxial mesoderm
   B   The abaxial domain consists of lateral plate mesoderm
   C   Intercostal muscles and latissimus dorsi are derivatives of the primaxial domain
   D   Sphincter muscles of the pupil are derived from ectoderm
   E   Head musculature is derived from seven somitomeres

7.32   Which of the following regarding embryology of the cardiovascular system is **not** correct?
   A   Progenitor cells in the primary heart field are involved in formation of the atria and left ventricle
   B   Conus cordis and truncus arteriosus are derived from cells in the secondary heart field
   C   The inferior mesenteric arteries are derived from the umbilical arteries
   D   The medial umbilical ligaments are formed from the distal portions of the umbilical arteries
   E   The umbilical vein is obliterated to form the ligamentum venosum

7.33   Which of the following vessels is formed by anastomosis between the sacrocardinal veins?
   A   Inferior vena cava
   B   Left common iliac vein
   C   Azygos vein
   D   Hemiazygos vein
   E   Left renal vein

7.34   Which of the following regarding embryology of the respiratory system is **not** correct?
   A   Location of the lung bud is dependent on retinoic acid levels
   B   The lung bud appears as an outgrowth from the foregut at ~4 weeks
   C   Somatic mesoderm becomes the parietal pleura
   D   Alveoli mature from approximately 20 weeks
   E   Branches of the 6th pharyngeal arch is innervated by the recurrent laryngeal nerve

7.35   Which of the following regarding embryology of the digestive system is correct?
   A   Endocrine cells of the pancreas are derived from visceral mesoderm
   B   The lienorenal ligament connects the right kidney and the liver
   C   At ca. 3–4 weeks, the liver bud contains rapidly proliferating cells which penetrate the hepatoduodenal ligament
   D   The anorectal canal develops from the posterior region of the cloaca
   E   Development of the foregut results in formation of the primary intestinal loop

7.36   Which of the following regarding embryology of the urinary system is correct?
   A   Collecting ducts of the metanephros develop from the ureteric bud
   B   Nephrogenesis continues until ca. 8 weeks postnatally
   C   Urethral epithelium is mesodermal in origin
   D   The urachus is formed from the urogenital sinus
   E   Ureters are formed by an outgrowth of the vitelline duct

7.37 Which of the following regarding embryology of the genitals is correct?
A Primordial germ cells originate in the cytotrophoblast
B In the ovary, medullary cords degenerate, and the tunica albuginea thickens
C By week 5–6, only Müllerian and Wolffian ducts are present in the male and female, respectively
D Müllerian inhibiting substance (anti-Müllerian hormone) is produced by Leydig cells
E SRY and WNT4 are important genes for testes and ovary development, respectively

7.38 Gartner's duct cysts can develop on the lateral wall of the vagina. These are remnants of which embryological structure?
A Urogenital sinus
B Urachus
C Mesonephric duct
D Paramesonephric duct
E Urethral folds

7.39 Which of the following regarding embryology of external genitalia is correct?
A In the female, the genital tubercle elongates to form the labia majora
B In the male, the processus vaginalis forms the inguinal canal
C Internal oblique muscle does not contribute a layer covering the testes
D The gubernaculum only forms in males
E The urethral groove is derived from intermediate mesoderm

7.40 Which of the following male structures is homologous to the female clitoris?
A Prostate
B Seminal vesicles
C Scrotum
D Penis
E Epididymis

7.41 Which of the following facial prominences is a single, unpaired structure?
A Medial nasal
B Lateral nasal
C Frontonasal
D Maxillary
E Mandibular

7.42 Which of the following facial prominences forms the philtrum of the upper lip?
A Medial nasal
B Lateral nasal
C Frontonasal
D Maxillary
E Mandibular

7.43 Which of the following brain vesicles is correctly matched to its brain derivative?
A Telencephalon – Hypothalamus
B Diencephalon – Cerebral hemispheres
C Metencephalon – Pons
D Mesencephalon – Cerebellum
E Myelencephalon – Posterior colliculi

7.44 How many rhombomeres are found in the hindbrain?
A 5
B 6
C 7
D 8
E 9

7.45 Which of the following cranial nerves does **not** arise from a rhombomere?
A Trochlear
B Abducens
C Facial
D Optic
E Vagus

7.46 Which of the following cranial nerves sensory ganglia have the least contribution from placodes?
A Oculomotor
B Trigeminal
C Facial
D Accessory
E Vagus

7.47 On which of the following days does the developing eye appear?
A 20
B 22
C 24
D 26
E 28

7.48 Which of the following structures of the eye is derived from neuroectoderm?
A Lens
B Sclera
C Conjunctiva
D Cornea
E Retina

7.49 Which of the following regarding embryology of skin and nails is **not** correct?
A Periderm formation occurs at weeks 4–5
B In the limbs, the dermis is derived from lateral plate mesoderm
C Dermal papillae are formed from the corium
D Development of fingernails proceeds toenails by ca. 4 weeks
E Melanocytes develop from melanoblast neural crest cells

7.50 Which of the following regarding twin-twin transfusion syndrome is correct?

A The recipient twin is oligohydramniotic
B The donor twin is polyuric
C Dichorionic diamniotic twins are at a higher risk than monochorionic diamniotic twins
D The presence of bidirectional vascular anastomoses between twins causes a haemodynamic imbalance
E Fetoscopic laser ablation can be used to treat the most severe cases

Answers

Spermatogenesis, which begins at puberty, but is continuous during adult life takes place within seminiferous tubules. The process is divided into two phases:

1) spermatocytogenesis, where immature spermatogonia, derived from epithelial germ cells in the basement membrane, undergo mitosis and develop into primary spermatocytes. Several mitotic divisions maintain a large stem cell population of spermatogonia which undergo clonal expansion (stem cell renewal and proliferation). Primary spermatocytes which undergo meiosis I give rise to daughter cells (secondary spermatocytes), which then undergo meiosis II forming spermatids – a maturation stage; hence C is the correct response.
2) spermiogenesis, where metamorphosis of circular spermatids into oval-shaped, mature spermatozoa are released into the lumen of the seminiferous tubules. This is a non-division but cell differentiation stage where most of the cell cytoplasm is lost in order for flagella to develop.

Spermatogenesis takes ca. 65–75 days at different times and regions of the testis. Over 200 million spermatozoa are produced each day! The process is illustrated in the figure below.

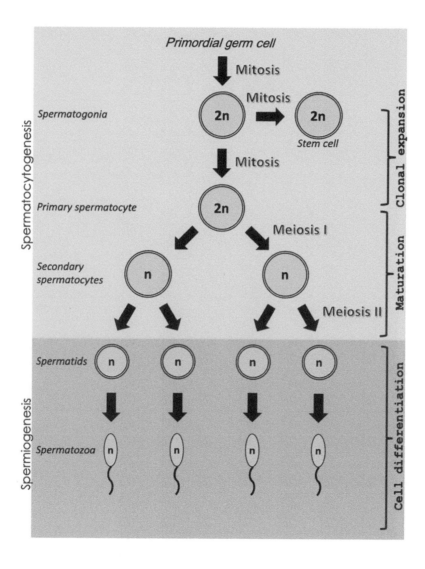

7.2 │ E │ *Equal cytokinesis* │ *Unequal cytokinesis* │

Oogenesis is differentiation of the ovum. During meiosis, cytokinesis occurs in both spermatogenesis and oogenesis. However, it is unequal in oogenesis. This is because only one of the four daughter cells produced during meiosis II develops into a mature gamete which retains most of the cytoplasm. The other three form polar bodies which receive little cytoplasm and ultimately degenerate. Hence one mature oocyte forms. Similarly, in meiosis I, a larger secondary oocyte and smaller first polar body form. In contrast, all four spermatids develop into mature gametes in spermatogenesis (equal cytokinesis); hence E is the correct response.

All other options are incorrect. In oogenesis, the initial stages of meiosis begin in the embryo after the seventh month of gestation and maintained until puberty. In contrast, spermatogenesis is initiated during puberty. Oogonia continue to divide by mitosis until a few weeks before birth, at which point mitosis ceases and no new oocytes are produced. Oogonia enter meiosis I early in gestation, progressing through the leptotene, zygotene and pachytene stages, terminating at the diplotene stage of prophase I. The oocyte then becomes surrounded by follicular cells (primordial follicle). Meiosis II follows meiosis I but arrests in metaphase, which remains until fertilisation. Only after ovulation and when a secondary oocyte is fertilised, is meiosis II completed. Similarly, in spermatogenesis, diploid spermatogonia undergo several mitotic divisions to generate primary spermatocytes, and then two meiotic divisions to form spermatids. However, in spermatogenesis meiosis is uninterrupted. Maturation is involved in both oogenesis and spermatogenesis. After meiosis II, four haploid spermatids are produced (not two) in spermatogenesis, and one ovum and two polar bodies are produced in oogenesis. The process is illustrated in the figure below.

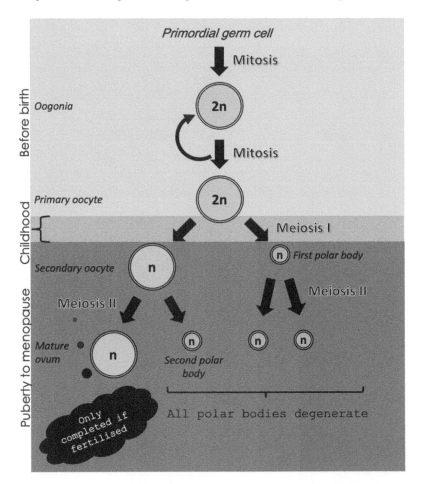

7.3 │ B – *Corpus haemorrhagicum* → *Corpus luteum* → *Corpus albicans*

Post ovulation and with no fertilisation, the lumen or cavity of a ruptured follicle fills with blood and a clot forms. This is known as the corpus haemorrhagicum. Clot dissipation and removal by phagocytes, cell infiltration and reorganisation of the collapsed follicular wall results in the corpus luteum. This develops from the remains of a Graafian follicle after ovulation. It produces progesterone and oestrogens. Granulosa cells secrete progesterone. They also produce oestradiol, the synthesis of which requires theca interna cells, which produce androgens (i.e. androstenedione, androstenediol and testosterone) in response to luteinising hormone. Granulosa cells convert androgens into oestrogens in response to follicle stimulating hormone. It is yellow in colour (from the Latin *luteus* meaning yellow) as a result of accumulation of steroid hormones. It is the hypertrophic granulosa and theca interna cells that develop a yellowish pigment and become lutein cells. If fertilisation does not occur, the corpus luteum begins to degenerate (luteolysis) after 10–14 days after ovulation and it stops secreting progesterone. Fibroblasts invade the regressing corpus luteum which is replaced by fibrotic connective tissue (collagen-rich white scar/body) known as the corpus albicans (from the Latin *albicans* meaning whitish). It is white due to the absence of steroid hormones; hence B is the correct response.

If pregnancy ensues following successful fertilisation of the oocyte, degeneration of the corpus luteum is prevented by human chorionic gonadotrophin (a product of the syncytiotrophoblast). It then forms the corpus luteum graviditatis which continues to produce hormones until the placenta takes over at ca. 3–4 months.

7.4 *D – Aldosterone from the adrenal cortex promotes sodium loss*

In pregnancy, there is increased activity of the renin-angiotensin system mediated by increased production of renin by the kidneys, ovaries and placenta. In addition, the production of oestrogens by the placenta causes an increased secretion of angiotensinogen by the liver which increases aldosterone levels. Therefore, increased plasma levels of renin and aldosterone leads to salt and water retention (not loss) in the distal convoluted tubules and collecting duct; hence D is the correct response.

Relaxin, structurally related to insulin, is produced by the ovaries, placenta and corpus luteum. It stimulates prostaglandin release, and collagen degradation by increasing the level of collagenase (inhibiting fibrosis). It may also have roles in cervical ripening, relaxing the pubic symphysis and pelvic ligaments, and inhibiting contractions of the uterus. Human placental lactogen (more recently known as human chorionic somatomammotropin), produced and secreted by the syncytiotrophoblast of the placenta, exerts both growth hormone-like and lactogenic effects. Although largely due to prolactin in tandem with oestrogen and progesterone, human placental lactogen promotes breast development during the third trimester (where levels peak at ca. 34 weeks). Progesterone has utero-relaxing properties and so inhibits the uterus from contracting. The opposite effect is seen with oxytocin, which stimulates uterine contractions. HCG, secreted from the syncytiotrophoblast, maintains the corpus luteum, in addition to supporting the uterine endothelium and maintaining quiescence of the myometrium.

7.5 | C | Oestrogen | Progesterone | HCG |

The figure below highlights that C is the correct response. Other key pregnancy hormones are also shown.

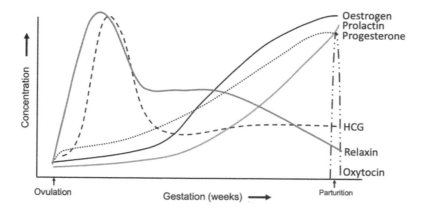

7.6 *B – LH*

After ovulation, granulosa cells (and theca interna cells) develop into luteal cells, which form the corpus luteum. Within ca. 35 hours of the LH surge, these cells begin secreting progesterone (and some oestrogen). The uterine endothelium now enters the secretory phase ready for embryo implantation; hence B is the correct response. Lutein cells, although no longer differentiate or divide, continue to secrete progesterone for ca. 10 days. Various reproductive hormones secreted in males and females, together with their origin and target organs are shown in the table below.

Hormone secreted	♂ or ♀	Origin	Target
LH	♀	Anterior pituitary	Thecal and luteal cells of ovaries
	♂		Leydig cells of testes
FSH	♀	Anterior pituitary	Granulosa cells of ovaries
	♂		Sertoli cells of testes
Progesterone	♀	Granulosa and luteal cells of ovaries Corpus luteum	Endometrium and myometrium
	♀+♂	Zona fasciculata of adrenal cortex Purkinje neurons of cerebellar cortex of brain Pineal gland	Mammary glands Hypothalamus

Hormone secreted	♂ or ♀	Origin	Target
Oestrogen (oestradiol)	♀	Granulosa cells of ovaries	Reproductive tract
	♂	Sertoli cells of testes	Hypothalamus Anterior pituitary
Testosterone	♀	Theca interna cells of ovaries	Granulosa cells of ovaries
	♂	Leydig cells of testicular interstitium	Sertoli cells of testes
	♂+♀	Zona reticularis of adrenal cortex	Skeletal muscle Anterior pituitary Skin
Oxytocin	♀	Synthesised in hypothalamus	Endometrium, myometrium and mammary glands
	♂	Stored in posterior pituitary	Smooth muscle (tail of epididymis, vas deferens)
Prolactin	♂	Anterior pituitary	Testes
	♀+♂		Hypothalamus Mammary glands
Inhibin	♀	Granulosa cells of ovaries	Anterior pituitary
	♂	Sertoli cells of testes	

7.7 B – Epiblast

Between the 3rd and 4th day of embryonic development, a 16-cell morula is formed which enters the uterine cavity. Fluid intersperses between the inner cell mass of the morula, and forms a confluent, single cavity known as the blastocele. The embryo is now a blastocyst consisting of a hollow ball of cells surrounding a smaller aggregation of cells. Between the 7th and 8th day of development, the blastocyst apposes the uterine epithelium and then penetrates it. The blastocyst consists of an embryoblast layer (inner cell mass) and trophoblast layer (outer cell mass).

The embryoblast differentiates into (1) a hypoblast layer (composed of cuboidal cells adjacent to the cavity), and (2) the epiblast layer (composed of columnar cells adjacent to the amniotic cavity); hence B is the correct response. The trophoblast also differentiates into (1) the syncytiotrophoblast, an outer zone of multinucleated cells with no cell boundaries, and (2) the cytotrophoblast, an inner zone of single layer, mononucleated cells. Fusion of cytotrophoblast cells form a syncytiotrophoblast syncytium, which develop finger-like projections which invade the endometrium. A blastocyst penetrating the endometrial stroma at ca. the 7th day of development is shown in the figure below. On the 8th day, a cavity forms between the epiblast layer which becomes the amniotic cavity, and the epiblast cells adjacent to the cytotrophoblast are known as amnioblasts, destined to form the amniotic epithelium.

The exocoelomic membrane (or Heuser's membrane) is a layer of flattened hypoblast cells that line the inner surface of the cytotrophoblast. This membrane and the hypoblast form the lining of the exocoelomic cavity or primitive yolk sac at ca. week 2 of development.

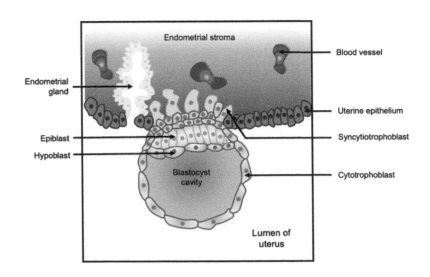

7.8 B – Syncytiotrophoblast

HCG is a glycosylated heterodimeric protein composed of α and β subunits, comprised of 92 and 145 amino acids, respectively. HCG maintains progesterone production by the corpus luteum until the maturing placenta assumes this role at ca. 10 weeks of gestation. There are five isoforms of hCG. HCG produced in pregnancy (hCG-1) is predominantly produced by syncytiotrophoblast cells; hence B is the correct response. It is this isoform that promotes fusion of cytotrophoblasts to form syncytiotrophoblasts, in addition to promoting angiogenesis of the uterine vasculature, and growth and development of the umbilical cord. Interestingly, hyperglycosylated hCG (hCG-2) promotes the growth of cytotrophoblast cells and invasion into the uterine epithelium (hence blastocyst and placental implantation). Hence in ca. weeks 1–5 of gestation, it is the hyperglycosylated hCG that is found in larger quantities (which then declines), thereafter hCG-1 levels rapidly rise. The levels peak ca. 8–10 weeks of pregnancy, and then decline, remaining low for the remainder of pregnancy.

7.9 C – Day 9

As the blastocyst continues to invade deep into the endometrium, the trophoblast progressively develops, distinctly at the embryonic pole. Within this region of the syncytium of syncytiotrophoblast, sporadic vacuoles form and fuse, creating large numbers of trophoblastic lacunae. This is known as the lacunar stage, occurring on day 9; hence C is the correct response. At the abembryonic pole, the exocoelomic membrane (which covers the inner part of the cytotrophoblast) forms, and in addition to the hypoblast, forms the primitive yolk sac.

Days 4 and 7 are too early for such development. On the 4th day, the morula formed on day 3 enters the uterine cavity and forms a blastocyst. The blastocyst has not yet penetrated the mucosa. On the 7th day, the uterine epithelium is in the secretory phase which prepares it for implantation of the blastocyst. The endometrium augments the process of implantation by providing an extensive glandular network with a rich blood supply. On day 11, the blastocyst has completely invaded the endometrial stroma. The syncytiotrophoblast continues to invade the stroma and the maternal endothelium (sinusoids). This continues as the maternal circulation advances into the trophoblast, hence establishing the uteroplacental circulation. On day 15, gastrulation occurs where the three defined germ layers are established (endoderm, ectoderm and mesoderm).

7.10 D – 24–26 weeks

During development and maturation of the lungs, bronchioles continually divide into smaller canal-like structures. This is known as the canalicular period, occurring between 16 and 26 weeks. Primitive alveoli or terminal sacs, arising from division of bronchioles and alveolar ducts, are lined with flat type I alveolar cells (pneumocytes). These cells form over 90% of the surface area lining the alveolar sacs. Type II alveolar cells are more cuboidal in shape, measuring ca. 6–9 μm in diameter, with a distinct foamy cytoplasm and are far more numerous than type I cells. They contain many microvilli on their surface. These cells produce phospholipids, proteins and glycosaminoglycans which are stored as lamellar or inclusion bodies (comprising ca. 25% of the cytoplasm), and form the basis of pulmonary surfactant.

Surfactant is a complex mixture of lecithins, the most important of which is dipalmitoylphosphatidylcholine. Sufficient quantities of surfactant are produced by 24–26 weeks, permitting expansion of the terminal sacs and providing the alveolar stability required for gas exchange. It is essential to reduce surface tension in the alveolar walls thus reducing lung recoil and increasing compliance; hence D is the correct answer. In fact, surfactant production by alveolar cells begins earlier, ca. weeks 20–22, but overall is insufficient to prevent atelectasis of the airways. In most foetuses, surfactant production gradually increases with advancing gestational age and mature levels are not achieved until ca. 35 weeks.

7.11 D – 15

The process which establishes all three germ layers (endoderm, mesoderm and ectoderm) is known as gastrulation which occurs in the third week of development. It begins with the formation of the primitive streak in the caudal region of the epiblast at ca. day 15–16; hence D is the correct response. An elevated and slightly thickened region at the cranial end of the primitive streak is known as the primitive node. Surrounding the node is a small primitive pit into which epiblast cells invade and migrate. They displace the hypoblast, replacing it with embryonic endoderm. Invaginating epiblast cells infiltrate the space between the epiblast and hypoblast and form the intraembryonic mesoderm. Cells remaining in the epiblast form the ectoderm. It is important to mention that the primitive node secretes morphogens (e.g. fibroblast growth factor, sonic hedgehog and retinoic acid) which play important roles in neurulation and establishment of the body axes. Remnants of the primitive streak or failure of the primitive node to regress can lead to formation of sacrococcygeal teratomas.

7.12 C – Cells that remain in the epiblast form mesoderm

Cells that remain in the epiblast form ectoderm (not mesoderm); hence C is the correct response. Gastrulation begins with the formation of the primitive streak (see Q7.11). Epiblast is the source of all the germ layers. The allantois, a small diverticulum that extends from the posterior wall of the yolk sac into the connecting stalk, appears on ca. day 16 of development. The blood vessels of the allantois become the umbilical arteries and vein. It gives rise to the urachus which contributes to the anterosuperior surface of the urinary bladder. The distal part becomes fibrotic and persists after birth as the median umbilical ligament. Foeto-placental circulation is established ca. 6–7 weeks through the connecting stalk, which later becomes the umbilical cord.

7.13   B – It forms during blastulation

The notochord begins to form ca. day 17. It is a midline structure that develops in the region lying between (1) the cranial end of the primitive streak (between the ectoderm and endoderm) to form the notochordal process, and (2) the caudal end of the pre-chordal plate, a component of the oropharyngeal membrane. The notochord is formed during gastrulation (not blastulation, which is the formation of the blastocyst from a morula); hence B is the correct response.

7.14   C – Adrenal medulla

Neural crest cells arise at the border between the neural and non-neural ectoderm at the dorsal region of the neural tube. Neural and non-neural ectoderm give rise to the central nervous system and epidermis, respectively. Cells migrate extensively to many different locations and generate a prodigious number of differentiated cell types within the embryo. These include cells of the peripheral nervous system, connective tissue and bone, epidermal pigment cells, and endocrine and paraendocrine derivatives. Neural crest cells undergo an epithelial-to-mesenchymal transition or delamination in which migration is initiated by displacement from the neuroectoderm. The adrenal medulla, a component of the sympathetic nervous system, arises from neural crest cells during embryonic development; hence C is the correct response. All other options are derivatives of ectoderm. The table below shows derivatives of various embryonic tissues. The figure below summarises the formation of primary germ layers that give rise to all tissues in the body.

Contributions of cells to tissues in the embryo

Neural crest cell derivatives

Cranial sensory ganglia	Enteric neurons	Carotid body type I cells
Sympathetic ganglia	Adipocytes	Connective tissue
Parasympathetic ganglia	Melanocytes	Tendons
Sensory dorsal root ganglia	Epidermal pigment cells	Extraocular muscles
Schwann cells	Pericytes	Corneal stroma and endothelium
Olfactory cells	Contruncal septum of heart	Tooth papillae
Meninges	Smooth muscle cells	Osteocytes
Neuroglial cells	C cells of the thyroid gland	Osteoblasts
Parasympathetic ganglia	Adrenal medulla cells	Chondrocytes

Neuroectoderm

Brain	Retina
Spinal cord	Neural pituitary
Motor neurons	Pineal gland

Surface ectoderm

Epidermis of skin	Olfactory epithelium	Anterior pituitary
Epidermal derivatives: hair, sebaceous glands and nails	Mouth epithelium	Tooth enamel
Anal canal	Lens, cornea	Cheek epithelium

Mesoderm

Nucleus pulposus of IV discs	Reproductive organs	Blood vessels
Axial and limb skeleton	Urogenital system (except bladder)	Wall of gastrointestinal and respiratory tracts (except epithelial lining)
Skeletal muscle	Connective tissue of body wall and limbs	
Connective tissue of skin	Heart	Adrenal cortex
Visceral serosa	Spleen	Notochord
Lymphatics		

Endoderm

Liver	Urinary bladder and urethral epithelium	Tonsils
Gallbladder	Respiratory tract epithelium	Gastrointestinal epithelium
Pancreas	Parathyroid	Reproductive ducts and gland epithelium
Thymus	Follicular cells of thyroid	

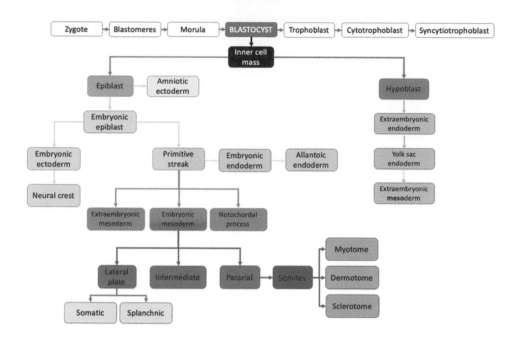

7.15 | *D* | *ectodermal* | *neural plate* | *neural folds* |

Molecular signals emitted from the notochordal process induce transformation of ectodermal cuboidal cells into elongated colum-nar cells. The overlying ectodermal epiblast cells undergo apicobasal thickening to form the neural plate. Neuroepithelial cells of the neural plate undergo structural changes that lead to the formation of the neural groove. Lengthening of the neural plate and folding of the lateral margins results in the neural folds. The neural groove, a depressed mid-region of the neural plate deepens, and the neural folds elevate, fusing along the posterior midline to form the neural tube. This process proceeds cranially and cau-dally. Failure of the neural tube to close most dorsally results in neural tube defects. This is commonly seen in spina bifida caudally, and anencephaly rostrally.

7.16 *E – Lateral plate mesoderm forms somitomeres*

Paraxial mesoderm (not lateral plate) organises into segments composed of whorls of cells known as somitomeres; hence E is the correct response. Somitomeres eventually become compacted and separate from the presomitic paraxial mesoderm to form somites. Somites give rise to sclerotome (cartilage of the vertebrae and ribs), myotome (muscle tissue of the rib cage, limbs and back), and dermatome (dermis of the dorsal skin). Cells in the medial and ventral walls of the somite lose their round epithelial characteristics and become mesenchymal cells which form the sclerotome. Paracrine factors such as sonic hedgehog secreted from the notochord and neural tube floor plate induce the sclerotome.

The ectodermal germ layer gives rise to structures that maintain contact with the external environment, such as the central and peripheral nervous system, sensory epithelium of eye, ear and nose, skin including hair and nails, teeth enamel and glands (pitui-tary, mammary and sweat). Mesoderm gives rise to the cardiovascular system (heart and blood vessels), urogenital system (kid-neys, gonads, and their ducts, but not the bladder), cortex of the suprarenal glands and the spleen (see also Q7.14). Homeobox genes are a family of transcription factors that are highly conserved between species and are temporospatially expressed during early embryological development. Hence, they control and regulate craniocaudal patterning of the embryonic axis.

7.17 *B – Insulin-like growth factor-1 (IGF-1)*

Embryogenesis relies on regulatory molecules, such as growth factors, that reach cells by an extracellular pathway and subse-quently influence intracellular signalling. Growth factors are ligands that bind to transmembrane receptors and are multifunc-tional in developmental biology. For example, they can regulate (1) cell proliferation, (2) cell differentiation (positively and negatively), (3) cell migration and (4) cell survival and apoptosis. Foetal growth and development are highly dependent on insulin-like growth factors and deficiency can result in marked growth restriction. IGFs are mitogenic and anabolic, they can stimulate foetal metabolism and co-ordinate foeto-placental metabolism. Studies have also shown that IGFs are important in limb morphogenesis, and infants with intrauterine growth restriction have low circulating levels of IGFs; hence B is the correct response. All other growth factors also play an important role in embryogenesis, but not as significant as IGFs on prenatal and postnatal growth. On an interesting note, growth hormone in the foetus has no effect on prenatal growth which explains why infants with congenital hypopituitarism have no growth deficiencies.

7.18 *D – It is considered to be haemochorial*

In primates, tissues of the chorionic villi separate maternal and foetal blood. The foeto-maternal interface is formed by direct contact of the placental trophoblast layer and maternal blood. The syncytiotrophoblast of the chorionic villi is now bathed in maternal blood in the intervillous space (similar to a mop in a bucket of water). This placental barrier is described as haemochorial; hence D is the correct response.

The placenta has two components: the foetal portion (chorionic plate) derived from the chorion frondosum (trophoblastic ectoderm and extraembryonic mesoderm), and the maternal portion (basal plate) derived from the uterine endometrium (decidua basalis, uterine vessels and glands). Intervillous spaces are derived from lacunae found within syncytiotrophoblast (not cytotrophoblast). Early in gestation, placental barriers include cytotrophoblast, embryonic connective tissue, endothelium and a syncytium. From ca. 4 months until term, most cytotrophoblast and connective tissue disappear leaving only the syncytium and endothelial walls of blood vessels to separate maternal and foetal circulations.

7.19 *E – Heparin*

The placenta is the interface between mother and foetus. The main functions of the placenta include (1) exchange of gases, such as oxygen and carbon dioxide, (2) exchange of nutrients and electrolytes, such as glucose, amino acids, fatty acids, vitamins and water, (3) production of hormones, such as hCG, somatomammotropin (HPL), oestrogens and progesterone, and (4) transmission of maternal IgG to foetus. Most drugs and their metabolites traverse the placenta with ease, as do many viruses (such as measles, varicella, rubella, cytomegalovirus, and coxsackie). Generally, drugs smaller than 500 Da in weight cross the placenta, whereas those over 1000 Da do not. Low-molecular-weight heparins (ca. 2000–5000 Da) and unfractionated heparin (ca. 12,000–15,000 Da) are too large to cross the placental membrane; hence E is the correct response. All other options can traverse the placental membrane. Arachidonic acid, a polyunsaturated essential fatty acid; vitamin B_{12}, a water-soluble vitamin; and uric acid, a product of purine metabolism are all transferred by active transport. Cholesterol is taken up by receptor-mediated endocytosis.

7.20 *B – Fragile X syndrome*

Fragile X syndrome is an X-linked recessive disease which causes intellectual disability and autistic spectrum disorders, in addition to prominent ears, facial coarsening, enlarged testes and joint hyperextensibility. It affects 1 in 4000 males and females. It is associated with expansion of trinucleotide repeats of CGG (>200) within the *FMR1* gene (fragile X mental retardation 1). This leads to aberrant hypermethylation which induces gene silencing; hence B is the correct response. Turner syndrome is a monosomy disorder that only occurs in females and affects 1 in 2000–5000 live female births. It results from either partial or complete loss of the second X chromosome hence has the karyotype 45,X (or 45,XO). Presenting features include short stature, neck webbing, gonadal dysgenesis, and congenital renal and cardiac anomalies. Trisomy 13, or Patau syndrome, results from an extra copy of chromosome 13 secondary to translocation or non-disjunction. It affects 1 in 5000–20,000 live births. Main abnormalities include neurological impairment, congenital heart defects (ventricular septal defects, patent ductus arteriosus, dextrocardia), holoprosencephaly, omphalocoele, cleft lip/palate, eye defects (microphthalmia, anophthalmia, coloboma, retinal dysplasia) and postaxial polydactyly. Most infants will not survive the new-born period. Trisomy 18, or Edwards syndrome, results from an extra copy of chromosome 18 secondary to non-disjunction. It affects 1 in 6000–8000 live births. Infants are born with dysmorphic features, low-set ears, micrognathia, microcephaly, and congenital anomalies (cardiac and renal). Prognosis is extremely poor and less than 5% survive at 1 year. Trisomy 21, or Down syndrome, results from an extra copy of chromosome 21 secondary to non-disjunction (ca. 95%), translocation (ca. 3%) and mosaicism (ca. 2%). Risk is associated with maternal age. It affects 1 in 600–1000 live births. Clinical presentation includes developmental disability, growth retardation, hypotonia, craniofacial abnormalities (up-slanting palpebral fissures, epicanthal folds, flat facies, small ears and mouth), Brushfield spots, short and broad hands and feet, and clinodactyly of the fifth finger. Multiple medical complications can co-exist including congenital heart anomalies (atrioventricular septal defect), eye disorders (congenital cataracts, strabismus, nystagmus), hearing loss, gastrointestinal malformations (atresias, imperforate anus, Hirschsprung's disease), thyroid dysfunction, gonadal deficiency, leukaemia and infections.

7.21 *E – Hyperthermia Glaucoma*

Hyperthermia is associated with an increased risk of miscarriage, seizures, hypotonia, gastroschisis, anencephaly, intellectual disability, impairment of distal limb development and spina bifida (not glaucoma); hence E is the correct response. Rubella can lead to glaucoma, cataracts, deafness and mental retardation. Toxoplasmosis is caused by an intracellular protozoan parasite, and neonatal congenital toxoplasmosis can lead to cerebral calcifications, hydrocephalus, microcephaly, microphthalmia, retinochoroiditis, epilepsy, thrombocytopenia and anaemia. Isotretinoin (Accutane) is a vitamin A metabolite used to treat severe acne. In higher doses it can cause mental retardation, ear and eye defects, cleft lips/palate, heart defects and microcephaly. Valproic acid (sodium valproate) is used to treat both epilepsy and bipolar disorder. Congenital malformations include neural tube defects (spina bifida), atrial septal defects, cleft palate, hypospadias and polydactyly. Congenital cytomegalovirus causes mental retardation, cerebral palsy, microcephaly, visual impairment and sensorineural hearing loss.

7.22 *D*

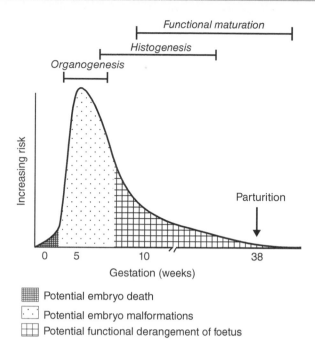

Potential embryo death
Potential embryo malformations
Potential functional derangement of foetus

The period of teratogenesis most susceptible to the induction of birth defects is the embryonic period during the third to eight weeks post-fertilisation. Recent studies involving axes formation (especially in heterotaxy) during embryogenesis have shown the most sensitive period should also include the second week post-fertilisation. The foetal period begins ca. eight week and progresses until parturition. The risk of structural anomalies being induced during this period reduces gradually with time; hence D is the correct response. The embryonic period is too broad, with peak risk shifted too far to the right in graphs A–C. E shows an appropriate peak risk ca. 5 weeks gestation but the risk decreases too rapidly.

7.23 *A – The allantois (urachus) becomes the median umbilical ligament*

The allantois appears ca. the 16th day of embryological development as a diverticulum from the posterior wall of the yolk sac, which extends into the connecting stalk. Involution of the allantois results in the formation of a thick tubular canal (urachus). Embryologically, the urachus connects the cloaca to the umbilicus. In early foetal development, the urachus facilitates drainage and removal of waste through the placenta via the umbilical cord. Normally, the urachus closes rapidly at parturition. As gestation proceeds, the bladder descends into the pelvis, lengthening and narrowing the urachus, and obliterating its lumen. This leads to the formation of a permanent fibrous cord (median umbilical ligament); hence A is the correct response. The ligamentum arteriosum is a fibrous remnant of the foetal ductus arteriosus, which connects the aortic arch and pulmonary trunk. Vitelline arteries supply the yolk sac and primitive gut. These fuse and form arteries that supply the dorsal gut mesentery. In adults, they remain as the coeliac trunk (which supplies the foregut), the superior mesenteric artery (which supplies the midgut), and the inferior mesenteric artery (which supplies the hindgut). At birth, the left umbilical vein regresses into the ligamentum teres hepatis which forms the free border of the falciform ligament. The right umbilical vein is obliterated during the embryonic period. The ligamentum venosum is a remnant of the ductus venosus of the foetal circulation.

7.24 *D – Ventral mesentery is derived from the septum transversum*

Ventral mesentery results from a thin sheet of mesoderm of the septum transversum that appears on ca. day 22 rostral to the developing heart; hence D is the correct response. This septum separates the heart from the developing liver. The liver grows into the ventral mesentery as it outgrows the developing diaphragm. There is no ventral mesentery of the midgut or hindgut as it exists only from the caudal foregut to the upper portion of the duodenum. All ligaments associated with the liver and lesser curvature of the stomach are derived from the ventral mesentery (falciform, hepatogastric, hepatoduodenal, coronary, peritoneal and triangular ligaments, lesser omentum). The septum transversum becomes the central tendon of the adult diaphragm. It develops within the cervical region (not the thoracic).

The diaphragm develops from four separate components (not three): (1) septum transversum, (2) two pleuroperitoneal membranes, (3) dorsal mesentery of the oesophagus (within which the crura of diaphragm develops) and (4) muscular ingrowth from the dorsolateral thoracic wall (from cervical somites 3–5). As the name suggests, pleuroperitoneal membranes separate the pleural and peritoneal cavities. They are attached dorsolaterally to the body wall, and their free edges extend into the caudal end (not cephalic) of the pericardioperitoneal canals (openings on both sides of the foregut). The pleuroperitoneal membranes fuse with the septum transversum and seal off the pericardioperitoneal canals, which is complete ca. week 7. The left canal is larger than the right and closes later (probably due to growth of the liver and muscle tissue which extend into the membranes).

Pleuropericardial folds separate the pleural and pericardial cavities that develop from the lateral body walls. These folds and their associated serous membrane form the pericardial sac. Pleuropericardial membranes, extensions of the pleuropericardial folds, transmit the common cardinal veins and phrenic nerves. Eventually these membranes fuse with each other and with lung roots to form the definitive pericardial cavity and two pleural cavities. In adults, the fibrous pericardium is derived from pleuropericardial folds.

The cardinal veins carry the venous return from the embryo. The paired anterior and posterior cardinal veins drain into short common cardinal veins, which drain directly into the sinus venosus. The right common cardinal vein forms the superior vena cava which empties into the right atrium. The left common cardinal vein persists as the coronary sinus into which coronary veins drain. At the level of the vitelline vein connecting to the right atrium, the inferior vena cava is formed by connections of the posterior cardinal, supracardinal and subcardinal veins. The azygos and hemiazygos veins originate from the supracardinal vein.

7.25 *B – Fingers and toes are formed when programmed cell death occurs*

Initial limb growth and patterning occurs during weeks 4–8. Lateral plate mesoderm migrates into limb buds at ca. 4 weeks. These are outpouches from the ventrolateral body wall which are covered by ectoderm. During the 5th–6th week, hand and footplates appear at ends of limb buds and ridges form digital rays. The distal ends of the limb buds flatten into paddle-shaped hand or foot plates, and respective digits form at the margins of these plates. Interdigital ray cells and tissue regress by programmed cell death (apoptosis) to produce separate digits; hence B is the correct response.

Limb outgrowth occurs as the distal border of the ectodermal layer starts to thicken and form the apical ectodermal ridge (AER). Limb development proceeds proximodistally into three segments: the most proximal stylopod (humerus and femur), followed by zeugopod (radius/ulna and tibia/fibula) and the most distal autopod (hand/foot). Morphogenesis is similar in the upper and lower limb, but lower limb development is behind the upper limb by 1–2 days. The process is heavily reliant on growth factors, especially FGF signalling from the AER, and HOX genes, which direct proximodistal limb patterning. Limb malformations due to complete or partial loss of signalling from the AER include amelia, meromelia and adactyly. Conversely, if the AER is duplicated, additional limbs can form as seen in diplopodia. The AER influences a population of cells to remain undifferentiated by expressing FGFs, meaning cells furthest away from the AER begin to differentiate into cartilage and muscle. However, mesenchymal cells at the proximal end are no longer influenced by FGFs, and instead differentiate under the control of other signalling molecules. One such molecule is retinoic acid, which has morphogenic properties and can initiate differentiation of the stylopod (not zeugopod). Hence retinoic acid abundance in the proximal limb but lack of it most distally suggests a crucial role in limb proximodistal patterning.

For completeness, it is important to mention that ca. 7th–8th week, the limbs rotate in opposite directions. The upper limb rotates laterally through 90°, and as a result, the extensor muscles lie on the posterolateral surface with the thumbs lying laterally. On the other hand, the lower limb rotates medially through 90°, and as a result, the extensor muscles lie on the anterior surface with the great toe lying medially.

Osteoclasts are bone resorbing cells and degrade bone during remodelling. Osteoblasts are responsible for bone formation and depositing bone osteoid matrices, composed predominantly of collagen type I. Osteoblasts mature into osteocytes, which are embedded in lacunae within the bone matrix and maintain mineral concentration of the matrix.

Bone formation or ossification begins at ca. 6th–7th week of embryonic development and continues until the mid-twenties. There are two types of ossification: intramembranous and endochondral. In intramembranous ossification, mesenchymal progenitor cells differentiate into osteoblasts and group into ossification centres. This mechanism generates the flat bones of the skull, clavicle and most of the cranial bones. Endochondral ossification involves the formation of a hyaline cartilage template (model) which is later replaced with mature lamellar bone. Peripheral chondrocytes organise into a perichondrium and undergo hypertrophy and then degenerate (by apoptosis). The extracellular matrix surrounding these cells undergoes calcification which is initiated in the middle of the diaphysis. Perichondrium is transformed into periosteum, and osteoblasts create a thickened region of compact bone (periosteal collar) – *primary ossification centres*. Ossification expands toward the metaphyseal regions. Chondrocytes and cartilage continue to proliferate at the ends of bone, which increases bone length at the same time as bone is replacing cartilage in the diaphysis. *Secondary ossification centres* form at the ends of long bones but remain separated from primary ossification centres by epiphyseal plates (growth plates). After birth, the process repeats itself in the epiphyseal region, thus mediating longitudinal bone growth until adulthood, when the epiphyseal plate disappears and the epiphyses fuse with the shaft of the bone.

7.26 *E – Ebstein anomaly*

Ebstein anomaly is a rare congenital heart malformation in which the tricuspid valve becomes apically displaced as a result of abnormal positioning of the tricuspid leaflets. The anterior leaflet is usually enlarged, dysplastic and hypomobile which leads to tricuspid regurgitation. Valvular displacement means parts of the right ventricle are incorporated into the right atrium (atrialisation). As a result, the right atrium expands, and the right ventricle gets smaller; hence E is the correct response. Ostium primum is an atrial septal defect which results from partial fusion of the primary septum and the endocardial cushions in the atrio-ventricular canal, which can lead to anomalies in the atrioventricular valves. As defect size increases, the associated left-to-right shunt will also increase which may lead to right atrial and right ventricular enlargement, and pulmonary overload. Hypoplastic right heart syndrome is a rare cyanotic congenital heart defect in which the right atrium and right ventricle are underdeveloped (hypoplasia). There may be pulmonary and/or tricuspid valve atresia, pulmonary artery stenosis and/or tricuspid regurgitation. It is associated with atrial septal defects leading to right-to-left shunting. Holt-Oram syndrome (the most common heart-hand syndromes) is an autosomal dominant disorder caused by mutations in the gene encoding the T-box transcription factor *TBX5*. Subsequently, various cardiac and limb malformations can occur such as atrial and ventricular septal defects, absence or hypoplasia of the radius, absent or triphalangeal thumb, and underdevelopment of the shoulder, clavicle, humerus and/or scaphoid. Tetralogy of Fallot is the most common of the cyanotic congenital heart defects. It is characterised by four major features: (1) ventricular septal defect, (2) overriding aorta, (3) right ventricular hypertrophy and (4) right ventricular outflow tract obstruction (pulmonary artery stenosis, or in extreme cases, pulmonary atresia).

7.27 E – The mesenchyme expresses a transcription factor, WT1, that makes the tissue competent

Molecular regulation of kidney development is complex. The tumour suppressor gene, human Wilms' tumour-1 (*WT1*), has been shown to be critical during kidney development and embryogenesis. It is a transcription factor which encodes a zinc finger protein. WT1 is essential for mesenchymal survival, conversion and competence, such that a mutation in WT1 leads to Wilms' tumours and a deletion leads to renal agenesis; hence E is the correct response.

In mammals, there are three phases of kidney development (not four) that develop from the intermediate mesoderm. (1) The pronephric kidney forms first from mesenchyme at the beginning of the 4th week. Groups of cells in the cervical region of the embryo form vestigial excretory units (nephrotomes). These degenerate by the end of the 4th week and never form complete nephrons (interestingly, the pronephros remains functional in frogs!). (2) During regression of the pronephric system, the mesonephric duct forms, which extends caudally within the body of the intermediate mesoderm. The first excretory tubules start to appear on either side of the midline which progressively lengthen in a longitudinal course, forming the mesonephric kidney. Tubules form which contain a glomerulus, a Bowman's capsule and laterally, a collecting duct known as the mesonephric duct (or Wolffian duct). This duct continues to elongate and eventually fuses with the cloaca, which gives rise to the bladder. By the end of the second month, all pronephros and mesonephros have disappeared in females (apart from a small portion found in the epoophoron). In males, portions of mesonephros and mesonephric duct persist as vas deferens, epididymis, rete testis, seminal vesicles and prostate. However, in both males and females, an outgrowth of the Wolffian duct close to its entrance to the cloaca leads to formation of the ureteric bud. (3) At ca. week 5, the permanent kidney, known as the metanephros, appears which is composed of the ureteric bud and metanephric mesenchyme. The ureteric bud gives rise to the collecting system, which includes the ureters, renal pelvis, renal calyces and collecting tubules. Epithelial cells of the ureteric bud (not the Wolffian duct) penetrates and invades the intermediate mesenchyme and branches within the body, known as the metanephric blastema. The metanephric mesenchyme proliferates, condenses and ultimately differentiates into epithelium which comprises the mature nephron, which includes the proximal and distal convoluted tubules, ascending and descending limbs of loop of Henlé, and podocytes of the glomerulus. This process of mesenchymal-epithelial transitions and interactions is regulated by *WT1* and other factors.

Finally, the kidneys develop in the pelvis and ascend (not descend) to the lumbar region in the abdomen as the body changes shape (less curvature) and growth occurs in the lumbar and sacral regions.

7.28 E – Meckel's cartilage forms the incus in the first arch

The pharyngeal arches are bilateral swellings that surround the foregut of the embryo. They give rise to the structures of the head and neck. They appear in the 4th–5th week and develop in a rostrocaudal direction. There are initially six arches, separated by pharyngeal clefts, but the fifth arch regresses before development is complete. Each arch contains an artery, nerve and musculoskeletal component, as shown in the table below.

Meckel's cartilage forms the incus and malleus in the first arch; hence E is the correct response. The muscles of mastication are derivatives of the first arch (not second). The superior laryngeal branch of the vagus nerve innervates muscles of the fourth arch (not sixth). The recurrent laryngeal nerve innervates the sixth arch. The second (not third) arch gives rise to the stylohyoid ligament. Progressive development of the arches and clefts leads to outpouches between each arch known as the pharyngeal pouches, which develop from endoderm. There are four pairs of pouches in the human embryo which give rise to different structures, as shown in the table below. The parathyroid glands do not develop from the same pharyngeal pouch. The inferior parathyroid (and thymus) develops from the third pouch, and the superior parathyroid develops from the fourth pouch.

Pharyngeal arches are also important in embryological development of the face and nose. The centre of the face and mouth develop from a large primitive stomodeum. Neural crest cells proliferate and form the facial primordia which appear as prominences around the stomodeum. There are five prominences: paired mandibular and maxillary prominences, and a single median frontonasal prominence.

Derivatives of the pharyngeal arches.

Pharyngeal arch	Artery	Nerve	Muscles	Bones, cartilage and ligaments
I (Mandibular)	Maxillary External carotid	V2 V3	Tensor tympani Muscles of mastication Mylohyoid Anterior belly of digastric Tensor veli palatini	Incus, malleus, mandible, maxilla, zygomatic, part of temporal Anterior ligament of malleus Sphenomandibular ligament Meckel's cartilage
II (Hyoid)	Stapedial Hyoid	VII	Stapedius Stylohyoid Facial expression (buccinator, frontalis, orbicularis oris, orbicularis oculi, auricularis) Posterior belly of digastric	Stapes, styloid process, hyoid (lesser cornu, upper body) Stylohyoid ligament Reichart's cartilage
III	Common carotid Internal carotid	IX	Stylopharyngeus	Hyoid (greater cornu, inferior body)
IV	Right: aortic arch, subclavian Left: aortic arch	Superior laryngeal branch of X	Pharyngeal and extrinsic laryngeal muscles Levator veli palatini	Thyroid cartilage Corniculate cartilage Cuneiform cartilage
VI	Right: pulmonary Left: pulmonary, ductus arteriosus	Recurrent laryngeal branch of X	Intrinsic laryngeal muscles	Arytenoid cartilage

Derivatives of the pharyngeal pouches

Pharyngeal pouch	Derivatives
1	Middle ear cavity Auditory (eustachian) tube
2	Palatine tonsils Tonsillar crypts
3	Inferior parathyroid gland (dorsal region) Thymus (ventral region)
4	Superior parathyroid gland (dorsal region) Ultimobranchial body which incorporates into the thyroid giving rise to parafollicular cells (C cells) (ventral region)

7.29 B – 2

As shown in the first table in Q7.28, Reichert's cartilage is formed by the 2nd pharyngeal arch; hence B is the correct response. Most of this cartilage disappears but parts of this cartilaginous continuation of the 2nd arch leads to the formation of the stapes, parts of the temporal and hyoid bones, and the stylohyoid ligament. Specifically, the styloid process of the temporal bone is formed by ossification of Reichert's cartilage.

7.30 D – Aortic arch

As shown in the first table in Q7.28, the 4th pharyngeal arch becomes the aortic arch (on the left side) and the right subclavian (on the right side); hence D is the correct response. The 1st and 2nd arches give rise to parts of the maxillary and stapedial arteries, respectively (branches of the external carotid artery). The 3rd arch joins with the dorsal aorta to form the common carotid and internal carotid arteries. The 6th arch gives rise to the pulmonary artery and ductus arteriosus (connecting the pulmonary trunk and aortic arch in the foetus; upon closure at birth, this becomes the ligamentum arteriosum).

7.31 A – Cardiac muscle is derived from paraxial mesoderm

Cardiac muscle is derived from prechordal splanchnic mesoderm (not paraxial mesoderm); hence A is the correct response. Skeletal muscle is derived from paraxial mesoderm, which forms somites on either side of the neural tube and notochord. Smooth muscle derives from splanchnic mesoderm around the primitive gut and its derivatives, and from ectoderm in muscles of the iris (sphincter and pupillary muscles), myoepithelial cells of the mammary gland and sweat glands.

During embryonic development, cells that form critical elements of the musculoskeletal system arise from two populations of mesoderm: the somites and lateral plate. There is a well-defined boundary between the somites and parietal layer of lateral plate mesoderm which is known as the lateral somitic frontier. This frontier led to the identity of two distinct mesodermal domains in the developing embryo: (1) the primaxial domain which is populated exclusively by cells from the somites, and (2) the abaxial domain which is populated by both cells from the somites and lateral plate mesoderm. Muscle cells that cross this frontier and enter lateral plate mesoderm comprise abaxial muscle cell precursors, whereas those that remain in the paraxial mesoderm and do not cross, comprise primaxial muscle cell precursors. Primaxial muscle cell precursors form muscles of the back (epaxial muscles innervated by the dorsal primary rami), shoulder girdle and intercostal muscles. Abaxial muscle cell precursors form limb muscles (hypaxial muscles innervated by the ventral primary rami), infrahyoid and muscles of the abdominal wall.

The body of vertebrates initially segment during gastrulation into somitomeres which are whorls of mesenchymal cells in the paraxial mesoderm that form in a craniocaudal sequence. Head musculature is derived from seven somitomeres. These do not form somites but contribute to mesoderm of the head and neck. The remaining somitomeres condense and form somites in the trunk.

7.32 E – The umbilical vein is obliterated to form the ligamentum venosum

At the time of birth, the umbilical vein is obliterated and forms the ligamentum teres hepatis in the falciform ligament of the liver. The ductus venosus collapses at birth and obliterates into the ligamentum venosus; hence E is the correct response.

7.33 B – Left common iliac vein

Symmetrical cardinal veins form ca. 4th week. During the 5th–7th weeks, additional veins form which include (1) subcardinal veins which drain the kidneys, (2) sacrocardinal veins which drain the lower extremities and (3) supracardinal veins which drain the body wall by intercostal veins. Several venous anastomoses are also formed between:

- sacrocardinal veins which form the left common iliac vein; hence B is the correct response
- subcardinal veins which form the left renal vein
- anterior cardinal veins which form the left brachiocephalic vein

The vena cava is formed from anastomoses of the left and right cardinal veins. The superior vena cava is formed from the proximal portion of the right anterior cardinal vein and the right common cardinal vein. The inferior vena cava is formed from a hepatic portion of the vitelline vein, a renal portion of the right subcardinal vein and a portion from the sacrocardinal vein. Bilateral anterior cardinal veins form the internal jugular veins. The right and left supracardinal veins become the azygos and hemiazygos veins, respectively.

7.34 D – Alveoli mature from approximately 20 weeks

At term there are ca. 20 million primitive alveoli (terminal sacs). These mature postnatally and connect mature alveoli to one another through pores of Kohn. Mature alveoli have a well-developed epithelium and capillary network. During the alveolar period of lung development (ca. 36 weeks–10 years), alveoli expand and increase in size until a baby is ca. 3 years old. New alveoli continue to be formed until aged ca. 8–10 years with the formation of ca. 300 million mature alveoli. The process of alveolarization continues until ca. 21 years of age; hence D is the correct response (20 weeks is too early for alveoli maturation).

7.35 D – The anorectal canal develops from the posterior region of the cloaca

At ca. 33 days, the terminal portion of the hindgut enters the posterior subdivision of the cloaca which later becomes the anorectal canal; hence D is the correct response. The allantois enters the anterior subdivision and later expands as the urogenital sinus. Endocrine cells of the pancreas (islets) develop from the pancreatic parenchyma at ca. 3 months of foetal life. At ca. 5–6 months, alpha and beta cells begin to secrete glucagon and insulin, respectively. The connective tissue surrounding the parenchyma is formed from visceral mesoderm. The lienorenal (or splenorenal) ligament is derived from peritoneum and connects the spleen to the body, close to the left kidney. It contains the tail of the pancreas and splenic vessels. At between 3 and 4 weeks, the liver bud (hepatic diverticulum) contains rapidly proliferating cells which penetrate the septum transversum (not the hepatoduodenal ligament, which connects the liver with the duodenum and encloses the hepatic artery, portal vein and bile duct). At ca. 6–8 weeks, the primary intestinal loop is formed from the midgut (not foregut) and eventually projects into the umbilical cord (herniation). The proximal loop limb forms the distal duodenum, jejunum and ileum, and the distal loop limb forms the lower part of the ileum, caecum, appendix, ascending colon and proximal two-thirds of the transverse colon.

7.36 A – Collecting ducts of the metanephros develop from the ureteric bud

The metanephric kidney develops ca. 5th week and forms the definitive kidney. During ca. 6th week of development, the ureteric bud (an outpouch of the Wolffian duct), begins to branch which subsequently creates the collecting tubules; hence A is the correct response. Nephrogenesis, the formation of nephrons commences early in development and is complete by birth when a baby is born at term. The majority of nephrons are formed in the second half of gestation. There are ca. 1 million nephrons in each kidney at birth. Urethral epithelium is endodermal in origin (not mesodermal). However, the surrounding connective tissue and smooth muscle is derived from visceral mesoderm. The urachus is a fibrous remnant of the allantois (not the urogenital sinus). The urogenital sinus is formed from the cloaca. Ureters, alongside the renal pelvis, calyces and collecting tubules are formed from the ureteric bud, an outgrowth of the mesonephric or Wolffian duct (not vitelline duct). The vitelline duct provides communication between the yolk sac and the midgut during development. It is normally obliterated ca. 7th week.

7.37 E – SRY and WNT4 are important genes for testes and ovary development, respectively

The *SRY* gene (sex-determining region of the Y chromosome) determines sex in humans. Males develop when the SRY gene is present, and females develop when it is absent. *WNT4* gene (wingless-related MMTV integration site 4!) regulates ovarian development and prevents testis formation; hence E is the correct response. Primordial germ cells originate in the epiblast (not cytotrophoblast). They infiltrate the primitive streak and integrate within endodermal cells in the yolk sac wall ca. 3rd–4th week. Ovary formation is reliant on a plethora of regulatory genes which cause cortical (ovarian) cords to develop, medullary cords to degenerate and disappear, and there is no development of the tunica albuginea (it does not thicken). During the indifferent stage ca. the 5th–6th week, both males and females have two pairs of genital ducts: mesonephric or Wolffian ducts, and paramesonephric or Müllerian ducts. Müllerian inhibiting substance or anti-Müllerian hormone is produced by Sertoli cells (not Leydig cells). Testosterone is produced by Leydig cells.

7.38 C – Mesonephric duct

In females, the mesonephric duct degenerates and remains as a vestigial system which can become a Gartner's duct cyst when remnants secrete fluid. They are benign, solitary and unilateral cysts and located in the anterolateral wall of the superior vagina; hence C is the correct response. The urogenital sinus is a subdivision of the cloaca. The urachus is formed from the allantois. In females, oestrogens and absence of testosterone regulate development of paramesonephric ducts which form the upper third of the vagina, cervix, uterus and both fallopian tubes.

At ca. weeks 3–4, mesenchymal cells migrate around the cloacal membrane to form cloacal folds. These folds unite cranially to form the genital tubercle which becomes the penis, and caudally to form urethral folds (anteriorly) and anal folds (posteriorly). Lateral to urethral folds are another pair of genital swellings which give rise to parts of the scrotum in males, and labia majora in females. Remember, it is still impossible to distinguish between sexes in the 6th week of development. Between weeks 7 and 12, male and female differentiation begins.

7.39 B – In the male, the processus vaginalis forms the inguinal canal

The processus vaginalis forms in both males and females ca. the 8th week. It is an outpouch of parietal peritoneum which attaches to the ventral surface of the developing gubernaculum (a fibrous strand). Together with guidance by the gubernaculum, the processus vaginalis creates a trajectory for gonad descent through the inguinal canal and into the scrotum (in males); hence B is the correct response. In females, the processus vaginalis (also called the canal of Nuck) also accompanies the gubernaculum giving rise to the round ligament of the uterus. The processus vaginalis pushes through the three layers of abdominal wall and forms the inguinal canal. Its entry point of herniation becomes the deep inguinal ring and the exit point is through the aponeurosis of external oblique at the superficial inguinal ring. Indirect inguinal hernias are due to congenital patent processus vaginalis. If the processus vaginalis fails to close off in foetal life, peritoneal fluid can travel into the scrotum forming a hydrocele.

In the female, the genital tubercle elongates slightly to form the clitoris (not the labia majora which is formed from enlargement of genital swellings). In males, the genital tubercle elongates to form the phallus (corpus cavernosum of the penis). The testes are covered by two layers of peritoneum (derived from the processus vaginalis) – the visceral and parietal layers of the tunica vaginalis, in addition to muscles of the anterior abdominal wall such that the internal spermatic fascia is formed from the transversalis fascia, the cremasteric fascia and muscle is formed from internal oblique, and the external spermatic fascia is formed from external oblique. Transversus abdominis does not contribute a layer covering the testes. The gubernaculum aids in descent of gonads in males and females, albeit in females this descent is much shorter than in males. In males, the gubernaculum persists as the scrotal ligament. In females, it persists as the ovarian ligament (superior portion) and round ligament of the uterus (inferior portion). The suspensory ligament of the ovary is not a remnant of the gubernaculum nor is it a true ligament, more a peritoneal reflection or fold that serves to supply the ovaries with blood vessels, nerves and lymph.

In males, at the caudal end of the cloacal folds, urethral folds form anteriorly. As the genital tubercle elongates to form a phallus, the urethral folds are pulled forwards and form the lateral walls of the urethral groove. This groove extends caudally to form the urethral plate, and as the urethral folds close over the plate, a penile urethra is formed. The lining of the groove is derived from endoderm (not intermediate mesoderm) and the outer edges of the urethral folds are derived from ectoderm. A failure in proper closure and fusion of the urethral folds results in hypospadias.

7.40 *D – Penis*

The glans penis and corpora cavernosa in the male are homologous to the clitoris in the female; hence D is the correct response. The male prostate is homologous to Skene glands (paraurethral glands) which are located around the urethral opening in the female. The seminal vesicles and epididymis in the male degenerates in females, leaving only remnants. The scrotum in the male is homologous to the labia majora in the female. For completeness, the spongy urethra in the male is homologous to the labia minora in the female. The corpus spongiosum and bulb of the penis is homologous to the bulbs of the vestibule in the female. The bulbourethral glands in males are homologous to greater vestibular glands in females.

7.41 *C – Frontonasal*

Facial prominences are formed mainly from neural crest-derived mesenchyme by the end of the 4th week of development. Three swellings surround the stomodeum and form the:

- central, unpaired frontonasal prominence which constitutes the upper border of the stomodeum and gives rise to the forehead and bridge of the nose; hence C is the correct response. On either side of the frontonasal prominence are ectodermal thickenings called nasal placodes which form two nasal pits on the ventrolateral aspect of the frontonasal prominence. The prominence on the outer aspect of the pits are lateral nasal prominences (which form the alae of the nose), and those on the inner aspect are medial nasal prominences (which form the philtrum of the upper lip and the tip of the nose).
- paired maxillary prominences which are lateral to the stomodeum and derived from the first pharyngeal arch. They give rise to the lateral portions of the upper lip and upper portions of the cheeks.
- paired mandibular prominences which are caudal to the stomodeum and are also derived from the first pharyngeal arch. They give rise to the lower part of the face, lower lip and jaw.

7.42 *A – Medial nasal*

The philtrum of the upper lip is formed from the medial nasal prominence; hence A is the correct response. See response to Q7.41.

7.43 *C – Metencephalon – Pons*

The three primary brain vesicles differentiate into five secondary vesicles by ca. the 5th week of development. As shown in the table below, the hindbrain or rhombencephalon differentiates into the metencephalon, from which the pons and cerebellum are derived; hence C is the correct response.

Primary vesicle	Secondary vesicle	Adult derivatives	
		CNS	**Ventricles**
Prosencephalon (forebrain)	Telencephalon	Cerebral hemispheres	Lateral ventricles
	Diencephalon	Thalamus Hypothalamus Pituitary Optic vesicle	Third ventricle
Mesencephalon (midbrain)	Mesencephalon	Anterior and posterior colliculi	Cerebral aqueduct
Rhombencephalon (hindbrain)	Metencephalon	Pons Cerebellum	Fourth ventricle
	Myelencephalon	Medulla oblongata	

7.44 *D – 8*

Rhombomeres are transverse subdivisions of the brain stem along the antero-posterior (AP) axis. The hindbrain is divided into eight rhombomeres ([rostral] r1–r8 [caudal]) which give rise to cranial motor nerves; hence D is the correct response. Neural crest cells associated with r1 and r2 form the first pharyngeal arch, those of r4 form the second arch and those of r6 and r7 form the third arch. Neural crest cells form in r3 and r5 but most of these cells undergo apoptosis due to the presence of BMP-4. Interestingly, recent research has found that there are repulsive agents (semaphorins) within these rhombomeres that prevent neural crest cells from entering. Cranial nerves V, VII and IX innervate the first, second and third pharyngeal arches, respectively. Cell bodies of cranial nerves V, VII and IX are found exclusively in rhombomeres 2, 4 and 6, respectively. *HOX* gene expression occurs in a sequentially overlapping pattern which is unique to specific rhombomeres. Under tight regulation by retinoic acid (and other transcription factors), these genes are expressed in a temporospatial manner at specific rhombomere boundaries which determines the identity of the rhombomeres and their derivatives. For example, *HOXB1* is expressed in higher quantities in rhombomere 4, whereas *HOXA4, B4* and *D4* are expressed in higher quantities in rhombomeres 6–8. So, although these are all involved in the development of head and neck structures, specific structural derivatives of the head and neck are different. Hence correct rhombomere patterning is critical. It has also been postulated that the first and last rhombomeres may represent transitional neuromeres (segments of neural tube beyond the hindbrain) at the junctions between the mesencephalon and hindbrain, and spinal cord and hindbrain.

7.45 *D – Optic*

Segmentation of rhombomeres and their derived structures in the mature central nervous system are highlighted in the table below. The optic nerve does not attach to rhombomeres; hence D is the correct response. All cranial nerves arise from the brain stem, except the olfactory and optic nerves. The only cranial nerve found in the diencephalon of the forebrain is the optic nerve. In a similar manner to the hindbrain segmenting into rhombomeres, the diencephalon is segmented into prosomeres 1–3 ([caudal] p1–p3[rostral]).

Rhombomere	Derived structures
1	Entire cerebral cortex, lateral hemispheres, vermis and rostral pons
2	Cerebellar nuclei, caudal pons, cranial nerves IV and V
3	Caudal pons, cranial nerve V
4	Medulla oblongata, cranial nerves VI and VII, neural crest
5	Medulla oblongata, cranial nerves VI and VII, no neural crest
6	Medullar oblongata, cranial nerves VIII and IX
7	Medulla oblongata, cranial nerves IX and X, neural crest
8	Entire spinal cord, caudal medulla oblongata, cranial nerves XI and XII

7.46 *A – Oculomotor*

Placodes are specialised regions of ectodermal thickenings which give rise to a range of sensory ganglia. Ectodermal placodes include four epipharyngeal placodes, which contribute to ganglia for nerves of the pharyngeal arches (V, VII, IX and X), otic, trigeminal, olfactory and adenohypophyseal placodes; hence A is the correct response. The parasympathetic nerve supply of the oculomotor nerve develops from parts of the midbrain and hindbrain neural crest cells. Research has shown that a limited number of cells may originate from ectodermal placodes which migrate towards the optic vesicle.

7.47 *B – 22*

The developing eye appears on day 22; hence B is the correct response. Two small optic grooves develop on each side of the developing forebrain in the neural folds. Closure of the neural tube allows these grooves to form outpocketings which are now called the optic vesicles. The optic vesicles extend from the forebrain toward the surface ectoderm and the connection between the two forms the optic stalk, which transforms into the optic nerve. Cells of the surface ectoderm interact with the optic vesicle which leads to cell elongation and development of thickenings called the lens placode. Ultimately this induces lens formation.

Invagination of the optic vesicle leads to the formation of a double-layered optic cup. The anterior rim (1/5) forms the iris and ciliary body, and the remaining posterior (4/5) forms the retina. The outer layer of the posterior 4/5 becomes the pigmented layer of the retina, and the inner layer becomes the neural retina; and both are separated by the intraretinal space. Cells of the posterior aspect of the inner layer that border the intraretinal space differentiate into photoreceptors (rods and cones). Adjacent to this is a layer of supporting cells and bipolar neurons, and the more superficial, innermost layer gives rise to ganglion cells which later becomes the optic nerve.

At ca. the 6th week, the loose mesenchymal tissue that surrounds the optic cup differentiates into an inner, highly vascularised and pigmented layer known as the choroid, and an outer fibrous layer known as the sclera. Mesenchymal tissue overlying the eye anteriorly also differentiates into two layers that surround the anterior chamber of the eye. The inner layer which is continuous with the choroid is called the iridopupillary membrane, and the outer layer which is continuous with the sclera is the substantia propria of the cornea. The iridopupillary membrane eventually disappears completely allowing communication between the anterior and posterior chambers (and filled with fluid called aqueous humor produced by ciliary bodies).

Finally, molecular regulation of eye development is heavily reliant on a key transcription factor, *PAX6*. Up- and downregulation of this gene in response to the expression of other genes such as sonic hedgehog, *PAX2*, *BMP4*, and *FGF* is critical for cell proliferation and differentiation of various structures of the eye.

7.48 *E – Retina*

Structures of the eye derived from neuroectoderm include the retina (pigmented and non-pigmented epithelium), sphincter and dilator muscles of the iris, pigmented iris epithelium, pigmented and non-pigmented epithelium of the ciliary body and optic nerve; hence E is the correct response. Structures derived from surface ectoderm include the lens, conjunctiva, cornea (surface epithelium), skin of the eyelids, caruncle and lacrimal apparatus. Structures derived from neural crest cells include corneal stroma and endothelium, stroma of the iris and choroid, ciliary muscles, connective tissue of extraocular muscles and trabecular meshwork. Structures derived from mesoderm include fibres of extraocular muscles, endothelium of orbital and ocular blood vessels, temporal sclera and vitreous.

7.49 *D – Development of fingernails proceeds toenails by ca. 4 weeks*

Nails begin to develop ca. 9th–10th week, where epidermal thickenings at the tips of the digits begin to form (nail fields). These migrate dorsally and eventually keratinise as they grow towards the distal end of the nail plate. This process is completed by ca. the 32nd week in the fingers and ca. the 36th week in the toes; hence D is the correct response, as the fingernails precede (not proceed) toenail development by ca. 4 weeks.

7.50 *E – Fetoscopic laser ablation can be used to treat the most severe cases*

Twin-to-twin transfusion syndrome (TTTS) is a disease of the placenta that affects identical twin pregnancies (or other multiples), where a monochorionic placenta is shared. Minimally invasive endoscopic surgery known as fetoscopic laser ablation can be performed *in utero* to correct this blood sharing imbalance; hence E is the correct response. The progressive stages of blood volume imbalance can be assessed by using the Quintero staging system which gives an indication of the severity of cases and prognosis of TTTS.

The recipient twin is hypervolaemic which results in polyuria and polyhydramnios (not oligohydramnios). The donor twin has progressive hypovolaemia which results in oliguria and oligohydramnios. TTTS can occur in monochorionic diamniotic and monochorionic monoamniotic twin pregnancies. Monochorionic diamniotic twin pregnancies are at a much higher risk of TTTS than their dichorionic counterparts as a result of the vascular anastomoses that connect the two foetal circulations. In fact, MCDA twins are at a higher rate of complications than DCDA twins, even without TTTS. Bidirectional vascular anastomoses are in fact a protective factor in TTTS as a balanced blood flow is maintained.

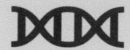

CHAPTER 8

Medical Statistics and Ethics, Epidemiology and Drug Calculations

Statistics is the grammar of science.
Karl Pearson

8.1 A respiratory physician gathered data on two antibiotics (clarithromycin and doxycycline) used to treat community-acquired pneumonia. The physician looked at improvement or no improvement in symptoms at 7 days on the same patients. A statistical test was performed and found no statistical difference in treatments.

Which of the following was the most appropriate statistical test to be used in this study?
A Unpaired t – test
B Chi-square (χ^2)
C Paired t – test
D Wilcoxon signed-rank test
E Pearson's correlation

8.2 A clinical trial compared four different treatments for knee pain in male and female patients with osteoarthritis. The trial underwent stratified randomisation. Patients were advised to use the assigned medication at the onset of pain and record the time when it subsided.

Which of the following was the most appropriate statistical test to be used in this study?
A ANCOVA
B Student's t-test
C Chi-square (χ^2)
D One-way ANOVA
E Two-way ANOVA

8.3 A neurologist investigated the effect of onabotulinum toxin A injections for the treatment of chronic migraines. Patients were asked to report their pain on a scale of 0–10 at 4 and 12 weeks after receiving the injections.

Which of the following was the most appropriate statistical test to be used in this study?
A Mann-Whitney test
B Paired t-test
C Wilcoxon signed-rank test
D McNemar test
E Kruskal-Wallis test

8.4 Which of the following would be the most suitable method of presenting frequency distribution data on diastolic blood pressure in pre-eclamptic, multiparous women?
A Histogram
B Pie chart
C Box plot
D Regression line
E Scatter plot

8.5 Which of the following is equal to the square root of the sample variance?
A Standard error
B Standard deviation
C Sample mean
D Population mean
E Quadratic mean

8.6 Which of the following is required to calculate a p-value?
A Power
B Standard error of mean
C Variance
D Covariance
E Degrees of freedom

8.7 Which of the following regarding the Delphi method is correct?
A Findings of each round are shared openly with the whole group
B They are smaller versions of focus groups
C Drop-out rates are usually low
D Participants can see results of previous rounds
E Expert consensus is highly reliable and valid

8.8 A haematologist hypothesises that men and women diagnosed with chronic myeloid leukaemia also live a sedentary lifestyle. Which of the following study designs would be most appropriate in investigating this possible association?
A Randomised controlled trial
B Prospective cohort
C Prospective observational
D Randomised crossover trial
E Retrospective case-control

8.9 What level of evidence does a systematic review of cohort studies offer?
A 1a
B 1b
C 2a
D 2b
E 3

8.10 Which of the following types of bias would result from systematically recruiting subjects into different groups for a study?
A Sampling
B Allocation
C Loss-to-follow-up
D Interviewer
E Recall

8.11 Which of the following data distributions does the following graph represent?

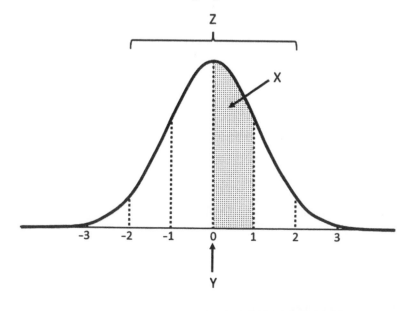

A Binomial
B Normal
C Positively skewed
D Negatively skewed
E Bimodal

Questions 8.12 to 8.14 relate to the following figure.

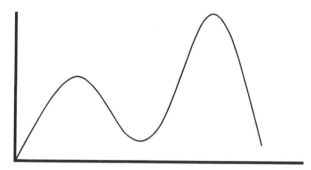

8.12 Which of the following does shaded region X represent?
  A 0.1%
  B 2.1%
  C 13.6%
  D 34.1%
  E 68.3%

8.13 Which of the following regarding Y is correct?
  A Mean > Mode > Median
  B Mean ≥ Median ≥ Mode
  C Median > Mode > Mean
  D Mode ≥ Mean ≥ Median
  E Mean = Median = Mode

8.14 Which of the following regarding Z is correct?
  A 95.4% of data falls within two standard deviations from the mean
  B 99.7% of data falls within two standard deviations from the mean
  C 68.3% of data falls within one standard deviation from the mean
  D 95.4% of data falls within four standard deviations from the mean
  E 99.7% of data falls within four standard deviations from the mean

8.15 A biomedical scientist investigated the accuracy and precision of four assays used to measure haemoglobin concentration in a single patient. Five replicates were used on each assay. The patient's 'true' haemoglobin level was known to be 135.2 g/dl. The results obtained are highlighted below:

Assay	Hb concentration (g/dl)					Mean (g/dl)
A	135.3	135.1	135.2	135.1	134.9	135.1
B	130.7	138.4	136.8	137.4	139.8	136.6
C	135.5	134.7	135.8	135.6	134.6	135.2
D	134.7	137.4	138.2	140.2	145.1	139.1
E	132.2	132.6	132.9	131.9	132.1	132.3

Which of the assays are accurate but not precise?
  A Assay A
  B Assay B
  C Assay C
  D Assay D
  E Assay E

8.16 A 1-month-old baby presents with signs of encephalitis. To prevent treatment delay, the paediatricians commence intravenous aciclovir. The recommended dose of aciclovir for a 1-month-old is 20 mg/kg every 8 hours for 14 days. It is available in concentrations of 25 mg/mL. The baby weighs 4.5 kg. What volume of aciclovir should be administered every 8 hours?

[ ] mL

8.17a A 92-year-old male has been prescribed 30 mg slow-release morphine twice daily. This appeared to be controlling his pain, but he has now started to experience more pain during the day. What is the maximum hourly immediate-release morphine that should be prescribed for his breakthrough pain?

[ ] mg

8.17b One week later, the palliative care team decide to change oral morphine to subcutaneous morphine. The patient was requiring 60 mg slow-release oral morphine twice daily and 40 mg immediate-release oral morphine in 24 hours. What is the total subcutaneous morphine dose required in 24 hours?

[ ] mg

8.18 A 6-year-old girl is prescribed trimethoprim for a urinary tract infection. The recommended dose is 4 mg/kg twice daily for 3 days. Trimethoprim is available in concentrations of 50 mg/5 mL. The child weighs 20 kg. What is the total volume that should be dispensed?

□ mL

8.19 A 10-year-old child has acute anaphylaxis to peanuts. Which of the following adrenaline/epinephrine regimens should be implemented immediately?
A 150 micrograms (1:1000) IM
B 300 micrograms (1:1000) IM
C 500 micrograms (1:1000) IM
D 500 micrograms (1:10,000) IV
E 1000 micrograms (1:10,000) IV

Questions 8.20 – 8.26 relate to the following scenario.

A new diabetic retinopathy screening test was developed. An investigation was carried out to find out how effective this screening test was in a population of 50,000 patients, aged over 50 with diabetes. The data is shown in the table below:

		Diabetic retinopathy		
		Present	**Absent**	**Total**
Screening test result	**Positive**	7856	2097	9953
	Negative	241	39,806	40,047
	Total	8097	41,903	50,000

8.20 What is the sensitivity?
A 2.98%
B 78.93%
C 83.52%
D 95.00%
E 97.02%

8.21 What is the specificity?
A 5.00%
B 89.69%
C 95.00%
D 97.02%
E 99.40%

8.22 What is the positive predictive value?
A 0.60%
B 10.31%
C 78.93%
D 97.02%
E 99.40%

8.23 What is the negative predictive value?
A 21.07%
B 78.93%
C 83.52%
D 95.00%
E 99.40%

8.24   What is the disease point prevalence?
   A   4.68%
   B   16.19%
   C   19.91%
   D   83.81%
   E   95.32%

8.25   What is the positive likelihood ratio (LR+)?
   A   0.05
   B   0.21
   C   0.59
   D   19.39
   E   35.01

8.26   What is the negative likelihood ratio (LR-)?
   A   0.03
   B   0.79
   C   1.02
   D   31.92
   E   131.16

Questions 8.27 – 8.29 relate to the following scenario.

800 patients with depression were randomly assigned to receive either sertraline (n = 425) or placebo (n = 375) for 20 weeks. During the randomised controlled trial, sexual dysfunction was recorded in patients treated with sertraline and placebo. The results are shown in the table below:

		Developed sexual dysfunction		
		Yes	No	Total
Treated with	Sertraline	97	328	425
	Placebo	24	351	375
	Total	121	679	800

8.27   What is the odds ratio?
   A   0.02
   B   0.23
   C   0.26
   D   3.78
   E   4.33

8.28   What is the relative risk?
   A   0.60
   B   0.82
   C   2.44
   D   3.57
   E   12.06

8.29   What is the number needed to treat (harm)?
   A   1.14
   B   3.14
   C   3.51
   D   6.09
   E   6.74

Questions 8.30 and 8.31 relate to the following scenario.

In a randomised controlled trial, 160 asthmatic patients were given a new treatment for asthma and 160 were given standard therapy. A total of 8 patients receiving the new asthma treatment continued to have asthma attacks, compared to 24 in the control group.

8.30 What was the relative risk reduction?
  A 5%
  B 10%
  C 15%
  D 33%
  E 67%

8.31 What was the number needed to treat (NNT)?
  A 6
  B 10
  C 20
  D 26
  E 40

Questions 8.32 – 8.33 relate to the following scenario.

8.32 The Kaplan-Meier survival curve in patients with mantle cell lymphoma treated with a novel drug A compared to placebo is shown below. Patients were followed up for 5 years.

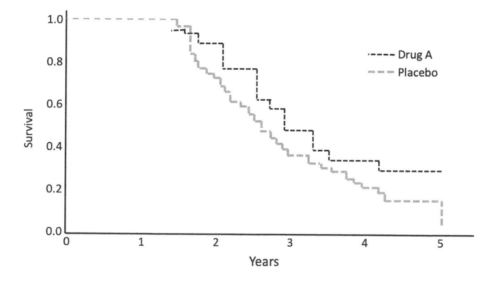

Which of the following can be concluded directly from this curve?
A Drug A is better in treating mantle cell lymphoma than placebo
B There is a statistically significant difference between the treatments
C There is a 50% survival probability beyond 2.5 years with drug A
D The median survival with placebo is approximately 3 years
E The 5-year survival rate with drug A is approximately 30%

8.33 A Cox regression was used to compare the hazard ratio of drug A to placebo. Which of the following hazard ratios would most likely be obtained from this model?
  A > 1
  B < 1
  C = 0
  D ≥ 1
  E ≤ 1

Questions 8.34 – 8.36 relate to the following hypothetical figure.

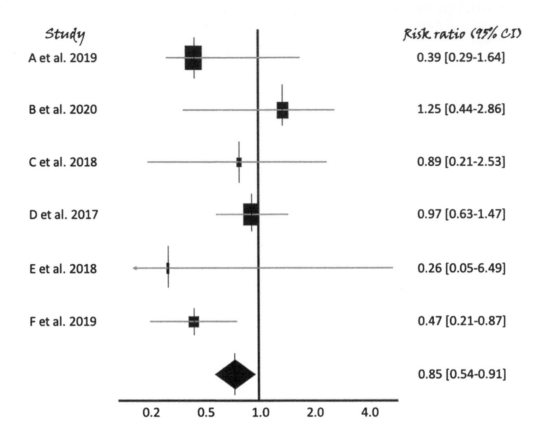

8.34   Which of the following has been used to display the data shown in the figure?
    A   Forest plot
    B   Funnel plot
    C   Stem and leaf plot
    D   L'Abbé plot
    E   Galbraith plot

8.35   Which of the following represents the 95% confidence interval (CI) in the figure?
    A   Rectangle/square width
    B   Rectangle/square vertical black line
    C   Central vertical black line at 1.0
    D   Diamond width
    E   Grey horizontal line width

8.36   Which of the following can be concluded from these studies shown in the figure?
    A   Study A shows a 39% risk increase
    B   Study B shows that the new treatment is the most effective
    C   Study D shows the most uncertainty about the result
    D   Study E shows data that is the most precise
    E   Study F shows data that is the most statistically significant

Questions 8.37 – 8.40 relate to the following figure.

Impact of dietary advice on cardiovascular events over 10 years

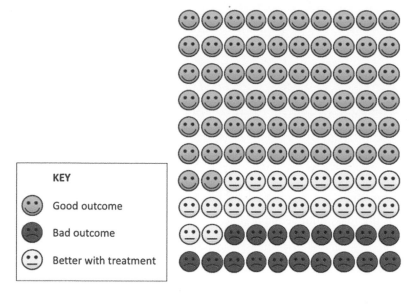

8.37 Which of the following has been used to display the data shown in the figure?
A Lineweaver-Burk plot
B de Finetti diagram
C Carpet plot
D Cates plot
E Q–Q plot

8.38 What is the numbers needed to treat (NNT)?
A 2
B 5
C 7
D 18
E 20

8.39 What is the relative risk of having a cardiovascular event in patients given dietary advice compared to those who are not?
A 18%
B 38%
C 47%
D 62%
E 82%

8.40 Which of the following can be concluded from this study shown in the figure?
A Relative risk reduction equates to the yellow faces
B 20 patients will die, even though they used dietary advice
C The Numbers Needed to Harm (NNH) is 6
D 18 patients will be saved from having a cardiovascular event because they have improved their diet
E Approximately $\frac{3}{5}$ of patients will not have a cardiovascular event, whether they use dietary advice or not

8.41   Daunorubicin can be used to treat neuroblastoma. A paediatrician had a difficult conversation with the parents of a 7-year-old child with neuroblastoma and was open, honest and transparent about the drugs side effects. Which of the following ethical principles is the paediatrician abiding by?
   A   Beneficence
   B   Non-maleficence
   C   Justice
   D   Respect for persons
   E   Double effect

8.42   Which of the following is the maximum period of time allowed for a patient to be detained in hospital by a nurse under Section 5(4) of the Mental Health Act 1983?
   A   3 hours
   B   6 hours
   C   12 hours
   D   18 hours
   E   24 hours

8.43   Which of the following is the maximum period of time allowed for a patient to be detained in hospital by a doctor under Section 5(2) of the Mental Health Act 1983?
   A   24 hours
   B   36 hours
   C   48 hours
   D   60 hours
   E   72 hours

8.44   Which section of the Mental Health Act 1983 allows police officers without a warrant to take a member of the public to a place of safety if it appears that they are suffering from a mental disorder?
   A   Section 17
   B   Section 116
   C   Section 135
   D   Section 136
   E   Section 138

8.45   Which of the following time periods must **not** be exceeded if a patient is detained under Section 2 of the Mental Health Act 1983?
   A   72 hours
   B   5 days
   C   7 days
   D   14 days
   E   28 days

8.46   Which of the following regarding the Mental Health Act 1983 is correct?
   A   Two Section 12 approved responsible clinicians are required to undertake a Section 2 assessment
   B   Under Section 3, there is no right to a tribunal
   C   Patients are eligible for Section 117 aftercare following detention under Section 2
   D   Under Section 3, a nearest relative, who is usually the next of kin, can make an application for admission for treatment
   E   Section 17A deals with community treatment orders

8.47   Which of the following is **not** outlined in the Mental Capacity Act 2005?
   A   Prohibition of discrimination
   B   Independent mental capacity advocates
   C   Lasting powers of attorney
   D   Deprivation of liberty
   E   Best interests

8.48   Which of the following is **not** correct regarding the Mental Capacity Act 2005?
   A   Lack of capacity cannot be established merely by reference to age
   B   Lack of capacity nullifies voting rights
   C   It does not matter whether the impairment is permanent or temporary
   D   An unwise decision is not the same as being unable to make a decision
   E   The Act does not apply to under 16s

8.49 In 2020, according to the World Health Organisation, which of the following estimated worldwide cancer deaths for men and women of all ages is correct?

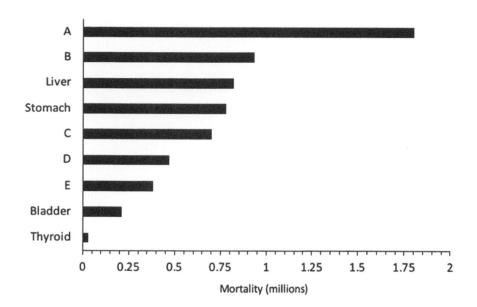

A Colorectal
B Lung
C Breast
D Prostate
E Oesophagus

8.50 Which of the following can be concluded from the following population pyramid?

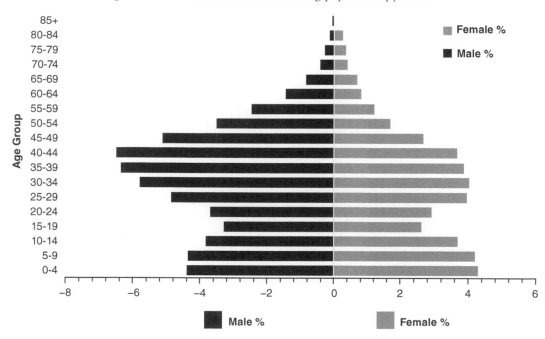

A There are more females aged 25–29 than males
B The country has high birth rates and low death rates
C More younger men are emigrating than women
D Women live longer than men
E There is rapid growth in the population

A quick note on hypotheses. Any scientific process must start with the generation of a hypothesis which can then be critically tested. A good hypothesis should be simple, specific and not retrospective or post-hoc. The null hypothesis states that there is no association or statistical relationship between the predictor and outcome variables in the population. Hypothesis testing leads to a dichotomous decision – the null hypothesis is either accepted or rejected. On the other hand, the alternative hypothesis states that there is a relationship between the two variables being studied. In statistics, there is still a degree of uncertainty whereby the wrong decision can be made. In hypothesis testing, there are two types of 'wrong decisions' that can occur (by chance). If the null hypothesis is true, but it is rejected, this is known as a type I error (false-positive errors). For example, stating that there is an effect/difference when none exists. The probability of making a type I error is called alpha (α) or p, the level of statistical significance. However, if the null hypothesis is false, but it is not rejected, this is known as a type II error (false negative errors). The probability of making a type II error is called beta (β). For example, stating that there is not an effect/difference when one exists. The statistical power of a hypothesis test is $(1 - \beta)$ which is the probability that the null hypothesis is correctly rejected. It is useful in medicine as it helps us decide on how many patients to enrol in clinical trials, i.e., when the sample size is large, power will be much less of an issue. As a rule of thumb, type I errors can be reduced by using a lower significance level and type II errors can be reduced by increasing the sample size.

A quick note on numerical data. It is important to remember that the data distribution that is being examined determines what method of analysis pursues (see figure below). Parametric tests involve making assumptions about the parameters of the distribution, i.e., the population data is normally distributed. Non-parametric tests make no assumptions about the distribution, i.e., the distribution is skewed (non-Normal distribution). Hence non-parametric tests are valid for both normal and non-normal distributions, so why are these tests not used every time? There are a number of reasons for this. Parametric tests have greater statistical power, i.e., if an actual effect exists, then a parametric test is more likely to detect it. It can also be challenging to perform complex modelling with non-parametric tests, especially when confounding factors are involved. Parametric analyses also allow unequal variances to be analysed. This can cause problems with non-parametric analysis where the distribution must have the same variability or dispersion. However, non-parametric tests can also be very useful in certain situations, such as when assessing the median of a study rather than the mean (parametric tests assess group means), and when analysing ranked and ordinal data, and outliers (parametric tests only analyse continuous data). Non-parametric testing is also valid when there is a small sample size; however, extreme caution must be taken here, as a reduced statistical power will only be exacerbated with a smaller sample size.

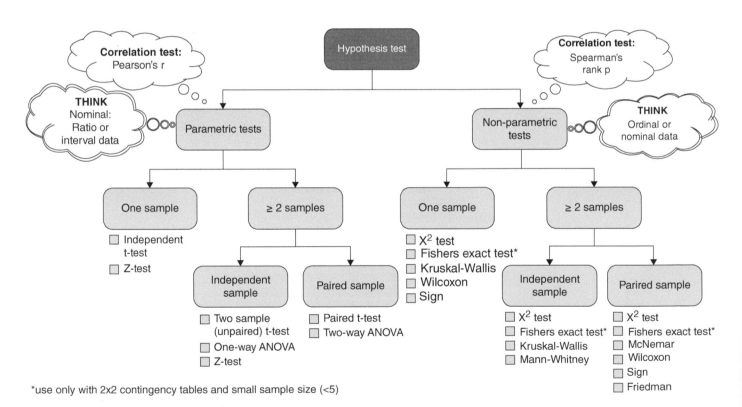

*use only with 2x2 contingency tables and small sample size (<5)

As a general rule of thumb, if the data distribution is <u>parametric</u>, and the groups are

1) independent, a two-sample t-test can be carried out.
2) paired, a paired t-test can be carried out.

If the data distribution is <u>non-parametric</u>, and the groups are

1) independent, a Mann-Whitney test can be carried out.
2) paired, a Wilcoxon Rank test can be carried out.

So, under what circumstances should these tests be used?

z-tests are a method of testing a hypothesis when (a) population variance is known, or (b) population variance is unknown but the sample size (n) $\geq$ 30. When the population variance is unknown AND n < 30 AND the data is normally distributed, a t-test must be used. When the population variance is unknown AND n < 30 AND the data is skewed (non-normal), a sign test must be used.

A one-sample z-test can be used when the sample mean is compared with the population mean, expressed mathematically as

$$z\,\text{score} = \frac{\bar{x} - \mu}{\sigma / \sqrt{n}}$$

where $\bar{x}$ is the sample mean, μ is the population mean, σ is the standard deviation of the population and n is the sample size.

A two-sample z-test can be used when the mean of two samples is compared, expressed mathematically as

$$z\,\text{score} = \frac{(\bar{x}_1 - \bar{x}_2) - (\mu_1 - \mu_2)}{\sqrt{\dfrac{\sigma_1^2}{n_1} + \dfrac{\sigma_2^2}{n_2}}}$$

where $(\bar{x}_1 - \bar{x}_2)$ is the difference between the sample means, $(\mu_1 - \mu_2)$ is the difference between the population means, σ is the standard deviation of the populations and n is the sample sizes.

A one-sample t-test can be used when the sample mean is compared with the population mean, but since there is no information on population variance, the sample standard deviation is used instead of the population standard deviation, expressed mathematically as

$$t = \frac{\bar{x} - \mu}{s / \sqrt{n}}$$

where $\bar{x}$ is the sample mean, μ is the population mean, s is the standard deviation of the sample and n is the sample size.

A two-sample t-test can be used when the mean of two samples is compared, expressed mathematically as

$$t = \frac{(\bar{x}_1 - \bar{x}_2) - (\mu_1 - \mu_2)}{\sqrt{\dfrac{s_1^2}{n_1} + \dfrac{s_2^2}{n_2}}}$$

where $(\bar{x}_1 - \bar{x}_2)$ is the difference between the sample means, $(\mu_1 - \mu_2)$ is the difference between the population means, s is the standard deviation of the samples and n is the sample sizes.

The sign test is a non-parametric test which compares the sizes of two groups. The two groups must also have the same sample size. It focusses on the median rather than the mean as a measure of central tendency. The main assumption in using this test is that the dependent variable arises from a continuous distribution or ordinal level, and the independent variable is categorical. It is useful in analysing binomial data where observed data values are either above or below the median, but it does not measure the magnitude of the pair difference. In a one-sample sign test, the median for a single sample is analysed. A paired sample sign test is essentially a one sample test but on the differences between the paired data entries. A positive (+) or negative (-) sign is assigned if the data entry is above or below the median, respectively.

Analysis of variance (ANOVA) is a parametric test used to analyse the difference between the means of more than two groups. The difference between a one-way and two-way ANOVA is that one-way uses one independent variable and two-way uses two. Remember, if you want to compare only two groups, use a t-test. ANOVA uses the F-test for statistical significance which compares the variance of multiple means between groups from the overall group variance. ANOVA tells us if there are differences between independent variables; however, it does not tell us which differences are significant. To compare group means, a post-hoc test is required. Examples of post-hoc tests include Tukey's HSD and Bonferroni tests.

The non-parametric equivalent to ANOVA is the Kruskal-Wallis test which is used when one nominal and ranked variable is used, and the measurement variable is not normally distributed. Similar to ANOVA, this test tells us if there is a significant statistical difference between two or more groups of an independent variable on a continuous/ordinal dependent variable. However, it does not tell you which groups are statistically significant and so a post-hoc test is again required.

The non-parametric equivalent to the independent (unpaired) t-test is the Mann-Whitney U test. It is used to compare differences that two samples come from the same population, i.e., have the same median when the dependent variable is continuous or ordinal. It is also used to compare whether observations in one sample are ranked higher than observations in another.

The non-parametric equivalent to the paired t-test is the Wilcoxon signed rank test for matched or paired data. It is similar to the sign test, but in addition to analysing the signs of the differences, it also takes into account the magnitude of the observed differences. This test is used when two interval or ratio level variables are measured, and we want to see if there is a difference in the distribution for the two variables, but the data is not normally distributed. This tests differences in the median rather than the mean (as used in the t-test).

Friedman's test is a non-parametric test equivalent to the one-way ANOVA when data distribution is unknown. It is identical to the sign test when only two treatments are involved. It is used to find statistically significant differences between the distributions of three or more paired groups across multiple attempts. It can also be used to compare ranked outcomes.

Chi-square is a non-parametric test which tests whether there is an association between two or more categorical variables (independent or related). This test does <u>not</u> compare continuous variables and it only tells us about associations between these variables. This test is not appropriate when categorical variables represent pre- and post-test observations as there is no independence in observations. Data cannot be paired and there must be no relationship between the subjects. McNemar's test (also known as paired/matched chi-square) would be more appropriate in this situation, as it assesses the dependence of categorical dichotomous data that are matched or paired. Mathematically, chi-square can be calculated using

$$\chi^2 = \sum \frac{(O - E)^2}{E}$$

where O is the observed frequencies and E is the expected frequencies.

Fisher's exact test is a non-parametric test that is used as an alternative to chi-square when testing significance in 2 by 2 tables, especially when the sample size is small. It is used to compare two sets of discontinuous, quantal data (categorical data such as response and no response). It has been commented upon widely throughout the literature that Fisher's exact test is preferred when the expected values in a cell of the contingency table is less than 5, otherwise chi-square can be used.

Pearson's correlation coefficient (r) (also called product moment correlation coefficient) is a measure of the linear association between two continuous, quantitative variables. Positive and negative values denote positive and negative linear correlations, respectively. A value of 0 denotes no linear correlation, but this does not imply that there is <u>no</u> relationship between the variables. For example, there may be a cubic or quadratic relationship. Pearson's correlation coefficient is sensitive to skewed distributions and outliers. The data must be linearly related and normally distributed; hence it is a parametric test. If these conditions are not met, then Spearman's rank correlation must be used. Mathematically,

$$r = \frac{\sum (x_i - \bar{x})(y_i - \bar{y})}{\sqrt{\sum (x_i - \bar{x})^2 (y_i - \bar{y})^2}}$$

where x_i and y_i are the values of the x and y variables in the sample, respectively, and $\bar{x}$ and $\bar{y}$ are the means of the values of the x and y variables, respectively.

Spearman's rank correlation coefficient (ρ) is the non-parametric version of the Pearson's correlation coefficient and measures the strength and direction of association between two ranked variables. The variables must either be ordinal or interval/ratio. Spearman's correlation determines the strength and direction of the monotonic relationship between two variables. A monotonic relationship is a relationship shown when either one variable increases, the other variable also increases, or when one variable increases, the other variable decreases. Mathematically,

$$\rho = 1 - \frac{6 \sum d^2}{n(n^2 - 1)}$$

where d is the difference between the two ranks of each observation and n is the number of observations.

Both correlation coefficients can range from $+1$ to -1. Correlation coefficients are never greater than $+1$ and never less than -1, and a correlation of 0 means that two variables don't have either any linear relationship in Pearson's correlation or monotonic relationship in Spearman's correlation.

Finally, regression analysis employs a variety of models that describe the relationship between dependent and independent variables in a simplified mathematical form. Regression analysis is useful in predicting the value of the dependent variable based on at least one independent variable; it can help forecast future trends and it can be useful in determining the strength of different predictors. Linear regression is used to study the linear relationship between a dependant variable (continuous) and one (univariable) or more (multivariable) independent variables (continuous, categorical or binary). The linear regression model describes the dependent variable with a straight line that is defined by the equation $y = mx + c$ where m is the gradient of the line and c is the y intersect. The regression line enables the value of the dependent variable (y-axis) to be predicted from that of the independent variable (x-axis). The gradient m of the regression line is called the regression coefficient. The coefficient of determination, r^2, is a measure of how close the data are to the fitted regression line. In univariable regression analysis, r^2 is simply the square of Pearson's correlation coefficient. Generally, the higher the r^2, the better the model fits the data.

Logistic regression analysis is used to examine the association of (categorical or continuous) independent variable(s) with one dichotomous dependent variable. For example, this would be the most appropriate type of analysis to use when there are only two possible scenarios or binary outcomes, such as the event happens or it does not, or 'yes' or 'no'.

Answers

8.1 *B – Chi-square* (χ^2)

Tabulating clarithromycin and doxycycline versus improvement and no improvement means a 2 × 2 table can be constructed. The research question could be 'Is there an association between using clarithromycin or doxycycline in improving symptoms in patients with community acquired pneumonia at 7 days?' In order to reject the null hypothesis that there is no association between using either antibiotic in improving symptoms at 7 days, a chi-square test can be performed, which compares the observed data with the expected data if the null hypothesis was true; hence B is the correct response. There is no indication in the question regarding the data being normally distributed and no reference has been made to the differences in means between the groups; therefore, an unpaired or paired t-test cannot be used. There is no reference to the data being scored or ranked; therefore, the Wilcoxon signed-rank test is not appropriate. There is no evidence that there is any linear relationship existing between two continuous variables; they are in fact categorical, and therefore Pearson's correlation is not appropriate.

8.2 *E – Two-way ANOVA*

In this example, the quantitative dependent variable is time, from the onset of pain to when it subsided. The independent variables include the four different treatments and gender, and these are categorical variables. Analysis of Variance (ANOVA) is a statistical test used to analyse the differences between the means of more than two groups. A two-way ANOVA uses two independent variables, whereas a one-way ANOVA uses one; hence E is the correct response. When using ANOVA, both variables should be categorical and if one is continuous, i.e., quantitative, then Analysis of Covariance (ANCOVA) should be used. It combines ANOVA with the principles of regression. For example, ANCOVA could be used in a study that tests the effects of two antihypertensives (categorical variables) on systolic blood pressure (a continuous variable) between the ages of 50 and 60 (a continuous variable). A t-test can only be used when the means of two independent groups are being compared, whereas ANOVA extends the t-test to more than two groups. The t-test compares means of a data set compared to the reference mean. For example, a two-tailed t-test could be used if elevated <u>and</u> reduced glucose values were to be compared to a reference value, whereas a one-tailed t-test could be used if elevated <u>or</u> reduced values were to be compared to a reference value. Chi-square would not be appropriate as this assesses associations between categorical variables. It does not make comparisons between continuous and/or categorical variables.

8.3 *C – Wilcoxon signed-rank test*

The question does not give an idea on the sample size, and potentially the data could be skewed, i.e., not normally distributed, so the most appropriate test to use would be a non-parametric test. These tests do not assume the data fits a specific distribution type and include the Mann-Whitney, Wilcoxon-signed rank, McNemar and Kruskal-Wallis tests. In this example, the dependent variable is pain scale, a continuous variable. The independent variable is the number of weeks after receiving the injections, 4 and 12. Therefore the Wilcoxon-signed rank test would be the most appropriate test to be used in this study; hence C is the correct response. It is equivalent to a one-sample and paired-sample t-test. This test assumes the dependent variable is ordinal or continuous, and the independent variables should be two categorical or matched pairs. Kruskal-Wallis is an extension of the Wilcoxon signed-rank test in the situation where there are several groups. It is equivalent to a one-way ANOVA. Kruskal-Wallis is also an extension of the Mann-Whitney test, which compares only two groups. The Mann-Whitney test compares whether there is a difference in the dependent variable (numerical, continuous or ordinal) for two independent groups (nominal). It is equivalent to an unpaired t-test. Do not get confused with the Mann-Whitney aka Wilcoxon rank-sum test, and the Wilcoxon signed-rank test. The McNemar test is used to determine if there are differences on a dichotomous dependent variable between two related groups. Dichotomous variables include two groups such as 'yes and no', 'high and low', 'pass and fail' etc. This test assumes that there is one categorical dependent variable with two categories and one categorical independent variable with two related groups. There should also be no overlap between groups. This test is equivalent to the paired t-test. The paired t-test is a parametric test so would not be appropriate in this example.

8.4 *A – Histogram*

Frequency distribution does exactly what the name suggests – it tells us how frequencies are distributed in a data set. Frequency distributions are useful for summarising categorical variables. Histograms would be the most appropriate method in displaying this data as it is easier to visualise frequencies for interval values rather than many distinct values; hence A is the correct response. The main difference between a histogram and bar chart is the x-axis of histograms show numerical intervals whereas a bar chart they are categorical. A bar chart can also compare two categorical data sets. A pie chart is used to represent the percentage/weight of components that belong to one category. They are used only with continuous data. A box plot and histogram are similar in that they both show the distribution of data and outliers can be identified. In addition, a box plot can show skewness, the median and the 25th and 75th percentiles. Box plots also allow multiple data sets to be compared. A histogram however shows the overall shape of the data better than a box plot and is far easier to create. A regression line is a line that best fits the data. It shows the relationship between the dependent and independent variable. Scatter plots use legends that represent values for two different numerical variables. They too show relationships between variables. They both would be inappropriate in this example.

8.5 B – Standard deviation

Sample variance, $s^2 = \dfrac{\sum (x_i - \bar{x})^2}{n-1}$ where x_i = the value of the ith term in the data set, $\bar{x}$ = the sample mean and n = the sample size. Therefore, standard deviation, $s = \sqrt{\dfrac{\sum (x_i - \bar{x})^2}{n-1}}$; hence B is the correct response. Standard error, $SE = \dfrac{s}{\sqrt{n}}$ where s = the standard deviation and n = the sample size. Sample mean, $\bar{x} = \dfrac{\sum x}{n}$. Population mean, $\mu = \dfrac{\sum x}{N}$ where N = the number of data items in the whole population. Sample mean is the arithmetic mean from only a subset of the population of interest, whereas the population mean represents the mean of the whole population. Quadratic mean (or root mean square) is a type of mean that is useful when trying to measure the average 'size' of numbers, regardless of whether they are positive or negative values. Quadratic mean, $x_{rms} = \sqrt{\dfrac{x_1^2 + x_2^2 + \ldots + x_n^2}{n}}$.

8.6 E – Degrees of freedom

A p value (probability value) is used to help accept or reject the null hypothesis. It is the evidence against the null hypothesis and smaller values support rejecting it. Hence smaller p values highlight a greater statistical significance. For example, a p value of 0.05 means there is a 5% probability that the results are due to chance. In order to conduct the hypothesis test for a population mean, a t-statistic is used which follows a t-distribution with n – 1 degrees of freedom. The p value can then be calculated; hence E is the correct response. It is important to set a significance level, α, which equates to a small probability of making a type I error (0.001, 0.01, 0.05 etc.). The p value is then compared to α and if p ≤ α, the null hypothesis is rejected and if p ≥ α, the null hypothesis is accepted. Power is an important aspect of statistics, but it is not an absolute requirement for calculating a p-value. Power tells us the likelihood that a significance test detects an effect in a study when there actually is an effect, i.e., sensitivity. Hence a study with a higher power indicates a higher probability that the test detects a true effect. Power is significantly influenced by sample size and often a power analysis is performed in order to determine a minimum sample size for the study. This also considers the significance level and the expected effect size (which can often be correlated with similar studies or pilots). Standard error of the mean, variance and covariance are not required to calculate a p-value.

8.7 D – Participants can see results of previous rounds

Delphi studies aim to gain reliable expert consensus through a series of rounds where opinions and views are sought. The questions for each round are based on previous findings which allows the study to continually evolve. Participants can see results from previous rounds which is an important part of the study as it allows reflective practice of individual and group opinions; hence D is the correct response. Findings of each round are shared but this is done anonymously in order to avoid bias. Delphi studies are not smaller versions of focus groups as the primary purpose is to allow participants to change their views in light of opinions from others, which tends to not happen in focus groups. A major limitation of Delphi studies is the high drop-out rate often as a direct consequence of the multiple rounds that are required. Unfortunately, these studies are not highly reliable and valid since experts can often disagree with each other and consensus may not always be reached. This is a further limitation, given the subjectivity of a consensus, which potentially leads to further bias.

8.8 E – Retrospective case-control

Prospective and retrospective refer to the timing of the study in relation to the development of the outcome. In retrospective studies, participants are sampled, and information is collected about their past, i.e., from their medical records or interviews in which they are asked to recall exposures. The key to these studies is that the outcome has already occurred (or not in control groups) by the time participants are enrolled in the study, but they are not followed-up. In prospective studies, the outcome has not occurred when the study commences, and participants are followed-up over time as circumstances/characteristics change. In this example, the haematologist is trying to find an association between men/women with chronic myeloid leukaemia and living a sedentary lifestyle. This would be an analytical study rather than descriptive, and it would be observational rather than experimental (as no exposure has been determined). The outcome is being set at the start of the study, so therefore a retrospective case-control study is most appropriate; hence E is the correct response. Most cohort studies are prospective, although some can be retrospective, whereas case-control studies are retrospective. In cohort studies, participants are selected based on exposure status whereas in case-control studies they are selected based on outcome status. In cross-sectional studies, the outcome and exposure are measured at the same time. Randomised controlled trials (RCT) are studies where participants are randomly assigned to 2 (or more) groups to test an intervention. Participants are followed up and outcomes are measured at specific times. Randomised crossover trials are specific types of RCTs where multiple interventions are being assessed. All participants receive all interventions but the order in which they receive the interventions are randomised.

Here are some basic questions to ask yourself when considering research study designs:

1) Is the study descriptive (characteristics are being described) or is it analytical (inferences are being made between variables)?
   a) Descriptive studies include case series, case reports, cross-sectional and ecological.
2) If it is analytical, has the exposure been determined?
   a) Yes – it is an experimental study which includes randomised and non-randomised controlled trials.
   b) No – it is an observational study.
3) If it is observational, when was the outcome determined?
   a) At the start – a case-control study
   b) At the end following follow-up – a cohort study
   b) At the same time as the exposure – a cross-sectional study

8.9 *C – 2a*

As shown in the table and figure below, cohort studies are classified into level 2, where level 2a is systematic review and 2b is individual; hence C is the correct response.

Level of evidence	Type of study
1a	Systematic review of randomised controlled trials
1b	Individual randomised controlled trials
2a	Systematic review of cohort studies
2b	Individual cohort study
3a	Systematic review of case-control studies
3b	Individual case-control studies
4	Case series or case reports
5	Expert opinions or editorials

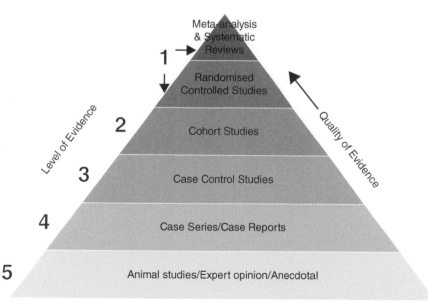

8.10 *B – Allocation*

Bias is unfortunately unavoidable since all experiments are designed by humans. Bias can have a huge impact on validity and reliability and therefore minimising this variable is critical. Allocation is a type of selection bias that relates to how participants are allocated to groups in a study. The aim to preventing allocation bias is to ensure that there is no influence on how participants are assigned to a given intervention group; hence B is the correct response. Sampling bias occurs when participants in a study are more likely to be selected over others. Loss-to-follow-up bias can occur when participants who leave a study are different to those who remain in the study with respect to exposure and outcome. This type of bias can be common in RCTs and cohort studies.

Interviewer bias relates to participants responses being distorted by the person questioning them. This often results in the interviewer influencing the responder in some form. Recall bias refers to responses made by participants about past exposures or outcomes which are more likely to be recalled than the controls. It is common in case-control and retrospective studies.

8.11   *E – Bimodal*

This graph is typical of a bimodal distribution where two peaks (bi) are evident; hence E is the correct response. In contrast, a normal distribution only has one peak and therefore is unimodal. Try not to confuse bimodal with binomial distributions. Binomial is a discrete probability distribution that takes only two possible outcomes: yes or no, success or failure etc. This describes the distribution of binary data from a finite sample which contrasts with normal distribution which describes continuous data which have a symmetric distribution. Skewness refers to asymmetry that deviates from the symmetrical bell curve seen in a normal distribution. If the curve is shifted to the left, it is positively skewed and to the right, negatively skewed. These graphs can also give us information on the mean, mode and median as shown in the figure below.

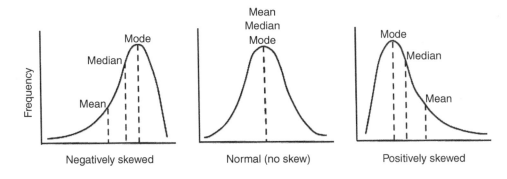

8.12   *D – 34.1%*

Normal distribution is a continuous probability distribution which is symmetrical. The area under the curve represents probability and the total area under it sums to one. Most of the data in a normal distribution cluster around the mean, and the further the data deviates from this, the less likely it is to occur. Using a normal distribution, it is possible to determine the proportion of values that fall within a certain distance from the mean. What this means is that 68.3% of data falls within the first standard deviation, i.e., there is a 68.3% probability of random selection between −1 and +1 standard deviations from the mean, as shown in the figure below. Half of this probability (+1 or −1 standard deviation from the mean) equals 34.1% (rounded); hence D is the correct response.

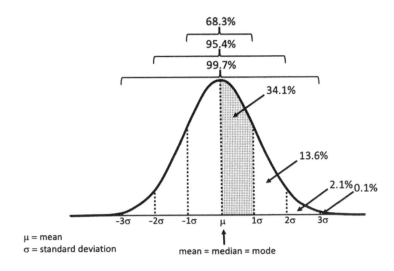

8.13   *E – Mean = Median = Mode*

As seen in the figure in Q8.12, mean equals the median which equals the mode in a normal distribution; hence E is the correct response. This is true for any symmetrical distribution. You could use both mean or median as a measure of central tendency, i.e., the value that attempts to describe a data set by identifying the central position within it. The mean would be the preferred measure of central tendency since it would include all values in the data set, and any change in data values would affect the mean. Yet this would not be the case for the median or mode. This is particularly the case in skewed data, as seen in Q8.11.

8.14 *A – 95.4% of data falls within two standard deviations from the mean*

As seen in the figure in Q8.12, 68.3%, 95.4% and 99.7% of data falls within one, two and three standard deviations from the mean, respectively; hence A is the correct response.

8.15 *C – Assay C*

Accuracy refers to the deviation of a measurement from its true value, i.e., a method is said to be accurate when it measures what it is supposed to measure. For example, if body temperature was set at 37 °C and it was measured using a thermometer and found to be 37 °C, then the thermometer is accurate. A method is said to be precise when repeats are performed which yield similar results, i.e., how close the measurements are to each other. For example, if body temperature was measured every day for a week and the thermometer consistently recorded a temperature of 37 °C, then the thermometer is precise. Now let's say the temperature recorded was 38 °C and this temperature was recorded every day for a week. The thermometer is now not accurate as it is consistently one degree above the true value, but it is precise as it has consistently recorded 38 °C.

In this question, C is the correct response. Assay A is both accurate and precise. Assays B and D are neither accurate nor precise. Assay E is precise but not accurate.

For completeness, let's look at two other terms – reliability and validity. Reliability refers to the consistency of a measure, i.e., a method is said to be reliable when the results can be reproduced consistently under the same conditions. For example, the thermometer records the same temperature every time under exactly the same conditions each time, then the results are reliable. Validity refers to the accuracy of a measure, i.e., the results represent what they are supposed to measure. For example, if the thermometer had not been calibrated for some time and the results were one degree higher as a result of this, then the measurement is not valid.

8.16 *3.6 mL*

Firstly, the dose required should be calculated: $20 \times 4.5 = 90$ mg aciclovir. Aciclovir is available as a stock concentration of 25 mg/mL; hence

$$\text{Dose} = \frac{\text{Stock required}}{\text{Stock strength}} \times \frac{\text{Volume}}{1} = \frac{90}{25} \times \frac{1}{1} = 3.6 \, \text{mL}$$

8.17a *10 mg*

Breakthrough pain is best managed with as required (prn) doses of oral immediate-release opioids. This is calculated as one-sixth of the 24-hour long-acting opioid dose. In this example, the total long-acting slow-release morphine prescribed is 60 mg. Therefore, one-sixth of this is 10 mg, which can be given hourly (max).

8.17b *80 mg*

To convert a patient from oral morphine to a 24-hour subcutaneous infusion of morphine, the total daily dose should be divided by two. Similarly, the prn dose of oral morphine should be divided by two to give a prn dose of subcutaneous morphine. In this example, the total oral morphine in 24 hours is 160 mg. Therefore, the total subcutaneous morphine dose in 24 hours is $160/2 = 80$ mg. Equivalent doses for opioid drugs in adults are important to practice as time progresses through medical school. Other common conversions include:

Oral	Subcutaneous	Conversion factor
Morphine	Diamorphine	Divide by 3
Morphine	Oxycodone	Divide by 4
Oxycodone	Diamorphine	Divide by 1.5
Oxycodone	Alfentanil	Divide by 15

8.18 *48 mL*

The total daily dose is $20 \times 4 \times 2 = 160$ mg, and for 3 days = $160 \times 3 = 480$ mg. Trimethoprim is available as a stock concentration of 50 mg/5 mL; therefore, $\frac{480}{50} \times 5 = 48$ mL.

8.19 *B – 300 micrograms (1:1000) IM*

Remembering emergency treatment for acute anaphylaxis and CPR is critical during medical training. This is an area commonly examined in undergraduate and postgraduate exams. Anaphylaxis is always treated with IM adrenaline/epinephrine (1:1000), which is age specific. Children up to 6 months are given 100–150 micrograms, children aged 6 months to 5 years are given 150 micrograms, children between 6 and 11 years are given 300 micrograms, and children aged over 12 (and adults) are given 500 micrograms. Doses are repeated after 5 minutes if there is no response, and further doses can be given every 5 minutes until critical care is available; hence B is the correct response. In CPR, adults are given 1 mg of adrenaline (1:10 000) at 100 micrograms/mL every 3–5 minutes by slow intravenous injection. Children are given 10 micrograms/kg every 3–5 minutes (max dose 1 mg) of adrenaline (1:10 000) at 100 micrograms/mL.

8.20 *E – 97.02%*

Sensitivity is the proportion of patients <u>with</u> the disease who have a positive test result i.e., the probability/percentage that the test will correctly identify a person who has the disease.

$$\text{Sensitivity} = \frac{\text{True positives}}{\text{True positives} + \text{False negatives}} = \frac{A}{A+C} \times 100$$

$$\text{Sensitivity} = \frac{7856}{7856+241} = \frac{7856}{8097} \times 100 = 97.02\%$$

8.21 *C – 95.00%*

Specificity is the proportion of patients <u>without</u> the disease who have a negative test result, i.e., the probability/percentage that the test will correctly identify a person who does not have the disease.

$$\text{Specificity} = \frac{\text{True negatives}}{\text{True negatives} + \text{False positives}} = \frac{D}{D+B} \times 100$$

$$\text{Specificity} = \frac{39,806}{39,806+2097} = \frac{39,806}{41,903} \times 100 = 95.00\%$$

8.22 *C – 78.93%*

Positive Predictive Value (PPV) is the proportion of patients who have a positive test result who have the disease.

$$\text{PPV} = \frac{\text{True positives}}{\text{True positives} + \text{False positives}} = \frac{A}{A+B} \times 100$$

$$\text{PPV} = \frac{7856}{7856+2097} = \frac{7856}{9953} \times 100 = 78.93\%$$

8.23 *E – 99.40%*

Negative Predictive Value (NPV) is the proportion of patients who have a negative test result who do not have the disease.

$$\text{NPV} = \frac{\text{True negatives}}{\text{True negatives} + \text{False negatives}} = \frac{D}{D+C} \times 100$$

$$\text{NPV} = \frac{39,806}{241+39,806} = \frac{39,806}{40,047} \times 100 = 99.40\%$$

8.24 *B – 16.19%*

Point prevalence is the proportion of people in a population who have the disease at a given time. This is different to the period prevalence which reports on the proportion of people having the disease over a period of time.

$$\text{Point prevalence} = \frac{\text{Number of people who have the disease}}{\text{Total number of people in the population}} = \frac{A+C}{A+B+C+D} \times 100$$

$$\text{Point prevalence} = \frac{7856 + 241}{7856 + 2097 + 241 + 39{,}806} = \frac{8097}{50{,}000} \times 100 = 16.19\%$$

It is important to remember that sensitivity and specificity are characteristics of a specific test. They <u>do not</u> indicate the likelihood of a patient having the disease when the test result is positive or negative. On the other hand, PPV and NPV rely on the prevalence of the disease in order to determine the likelihood of a specific test diagnosing the disease. Prevalence has no bearing on sensitivity or specificity. Hence, a higher prevalence increases the positive predictive value, i.e., it is more likely that those who test positive for a disease actually have the disease. Conversely, increased prevalence results in a lower negative predictive value.

8.25 *D – 19.39*

Likelihood Ratio (LR) is the proportion of patients <u>with</u> the disease having a positive or negative test result compared to the proportion of patients <u>without</u> the disease having a positive or negative test result. The higher the LR, the more likely the patient has the disease.

A positive LR refers to the likelihood of patients with the disease who tested positive compared to patients without the disease.

$$LR(+) = \frac{\text{Sensitivity}}{(1 - \text{Specificity})} \ or \ \frac{A/(A+C)}{B/(B+D)}$$

$$LR(+) = \frac{0.9702}{(1 - 0.9500)} \ or \ \frac{7856/8097}{2097/41{,}903} = 19.39$$

If LR+ > 1, a <u>positive</u> test is <u>more likely</u> to occur in people <u>with</u> the disease than in people without the disease, i.e. 'rule in' the disease.

If LR+ < 1, a <u>positive</u> test is <u>less likely</u> to occur in people <u>with</u> the disease than in people without the disease, i.e. 'rule out' the disease.

8.26 *A – 0.03*

A negative LR refers to the likelihood of patients with the disease who tested negative compared to patients without the disease.

$$LR(-) = \frac{(1 - \text{Sensitivity})}{\text{Specificity}} \ or \ \frac{C/(A+C)}{D/(B+D)}$$

$$LR(-) = \frac{(1 - 0.9702)}{0.9500} \ or \ \frac{241/8097}{39{,}806/41{,}903} = 0.03$$

If LR- > 1, a <u>negative</u> test is <u>more likely</u> to occur in people <u>with</u> the disease than in people without the disease, i.e., 'rule in' the disease.

If LR- < 1, a <u>negative</u> test is <u>less likely</u> to occur in people <u>with</u> the disease than in people without the disease, i.e., 'rule out' the disease.

LRs are a useful tool in the clinician's arsenal as they allow for the sensitivity and specificity of various tests to be adapted for individual patients. Following a focussed history and clinical examination, the clinician will usually have an idea of the probability of a patient having the disease. This is an estimate before the test result has been obtained and is based on clinical experience and published or prevalence data. It is known as the *pre-test probability*. This may be increased or decreased depending on a positive or negative test, respectively. The probability that the patient has the disease after the test results is known as the *post-test probability*. This is particularly helpful to clinicians as it allows decisions to be made with the patient regarding the confirmation or elimination of a diagnosis, or whether further testing is necessary. The more complex Bayes theorem allows the post-test probability to be estimated by combining the LR of the test and the pre-test probability. However, a simpler graphical tool (shown below) known as the *Fagan nomogram* allows the post-test probability of the disease to be estimated by revising a patient's pre-test probability and LR of a test.

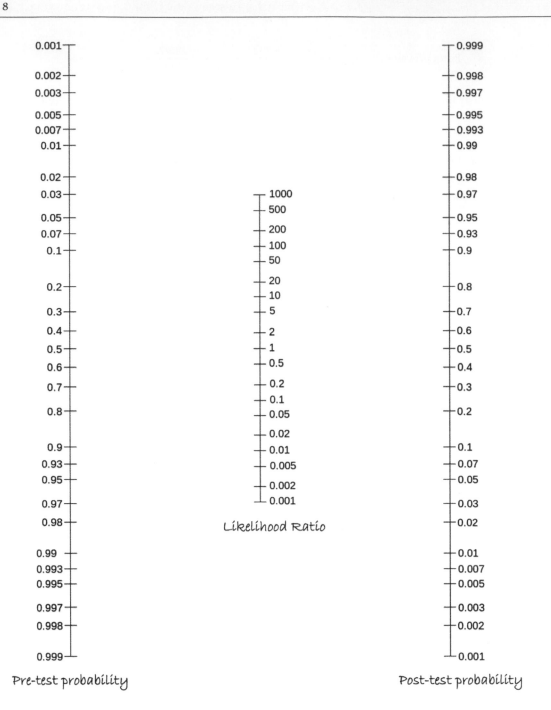

The Fagan Nomogram.

In the population described in this question, the prevalence of diabetic retinopathy in diabetic patients aged over 50 was 16.19% – the pre-test probability. The LR+ of the screening test was 19.39. By extrapolating a line from 16.19% which intersects at 19.39, the post-test probability is approximately 75%. This means that the probability of a diabetic patient aged over 50 with diabetic retinopathy in this population increases from 16.19% to 75% when they had a positive test result (A).

Similarly, the LR- of the screening test was 0.03. Applying the same principles, the post-test probability is approximately 0.7%. This means that after a negative test result, the chance of a diabetic patient having diabetic retinopathy reduces from 16.19% to 0.7% (B).

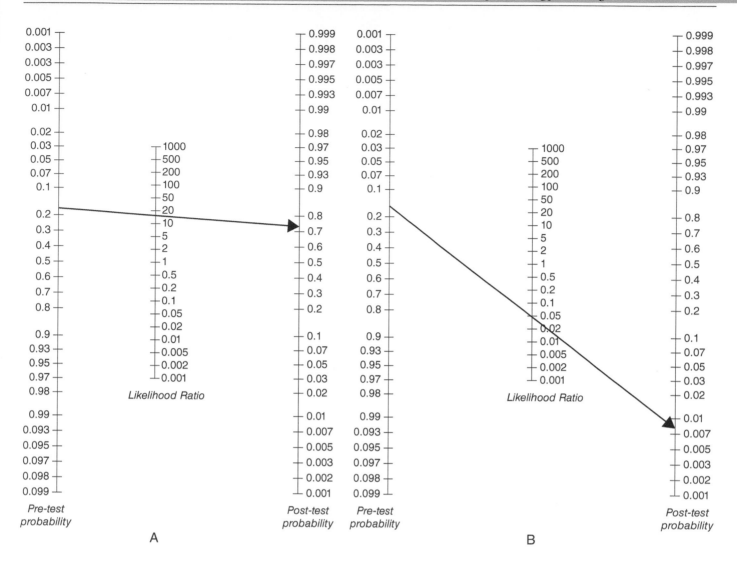

8.27 *E – 4.33*

Odds ratio (OR) is a measure of association between two binary variables, an exposure and an outcome. It represents the odds that an outcome will occur given a particular exposure, compared to the odds of the outcome occurring without that exposure. It is commonly used in case-control studies as it allows patients who have a disease (cases) to be compared with those who do not (controls).

$$OR = \frac{\text{Cases with exposure} / \text{Cases without exposure}}{\text{Controls with exposure} / \text{Controls without exposure}} = \frac{A/C}{B/D} = \frac{A \times D}{B \times C}$$

$$OR = \frac{97 \times 351}{328 \times 24} = \frac{34,047}{7872} = 4.33$$

If OR > 1, the odds of exposure among cases is higher than the odds of exposure among controls, i.e., the exposure may be a risk factor for the disease.

If OR < 1, the odds of exposure among cases is lower than the odds of exposure among controls, i.e., the exposure may be a protective factor against the disease.

If OR = 1, the odds of exposure among cases is the same as the odds of exposure among controls, i.e., the exposure is not associated with the disease.

8.28 *D − 3.57*

Relative Risk (RR) is the proportion of an event occurring in the exposed group (i.e. incidence in the risk factor group) compared to the proportion of an event occurring in the unexposed group (i.e. incidence in the no risk factor group). It is important in cohort studies which are prospective studies that follow a group (cohort) over a certain period of time which aims to investigate the effects of an intervention or risk factor.

$$RR = \frac{\text{Event rate in treated group (EER)}}{\text{Event rate in control group (CER)}} = \frac{A/(A+B)}{C/(C+D)}$$

$$RR = \frac{97/(97+328)}{24/(24+351)} = 3.57$$

If RR > 1, the risk in the exposed group is greater than the risk in the unexposed group (positive association).
If RR < 1, the risk in the exposed group is less than the risk in the unexposed group (negative association).
If RR = 1, the risk in the exposed group is equal to the risk in the unexposed group (no association).

Absolute Risk Reduction (ARR) is the risk difference between the outcome in the control group (CER) compared with the outcome in the experimental/intervention group (EER).

$$ARR = |CER - EER| = \left| \frac{C}{C+D} - \frac{A}{A+B} \right|$$

Relative Risk Reduction (RRR) is the proportion of risk reduction in the experimental/intervention group relative to the control group.

$$RRR = 1 - RR \text{ or } \frac{CER - EER}{CER}$$

8.29 *D − 6.09*

Numbers Needed to Treat/Harm (NNT/NNH) is the number of patients that need to be treated (NNT) in order to (a) prevent one bad outcome, or (b) for one of them to benefit. It measures the effectiveness of a particular intervention. Conversely, the number of patients that need to be harmed (NNH) would need to be exposed to a risk factor before one patient had an event. N.B. NNT is the reciprocal of ARR. NNH is the reciprocal of absolute risk increase.

$$NNT = \frac{1}{ARR}$$

$$NNT = \frac{1}{\left| \frac{C}{C+D} - \frac{A}{A+B} \right|} = \frac{1}{\left| \frac{24}{24+351} - \frac{97}{97+328} \right|} = 6.09$$

Therefore, approximately 6 people need to be treated with sertraline for 1 more person to experience sexual dysfunction.

8.30 *D − 67%*

$$RR = \frac{\text{Event rate in treated group (EER)}}{\text{Event rate in control group (CER)}} = \frac{A/(A+B)}{C/(C+D)} = \frac{8/160}{24/160} = \frac{1}{3}$$

$$RRR = 1 - RR = 1 - \frac{1}{3} = \frac{2}{3}$$

Hence D is the correct response.

8.31 *B – 10*

$$ARR = |CER - EER| = \left| \frac{24}{160} - \frac{8}{160} \right| = \frac{16}{160} = \frac{1}{10}$$

Hence B is the correct response.

8.32 *E – The 5-year survival rate with drug A is approximately 30%*

Kaplan-Meier is a method used to analyse 'time-to-event' data. This simply means the time from entry into a study until a subject has a particular outcome or event, such as death, disease onset, relapse etc. It is useful in survival analysis as it can highlight the patients who were lost to follow up or dropped out of the study, those who developed the disease or survived it and the method can be used to compare treatment and control groups in a particular study.

In understanding these survival curves further (see below), they have a monotonic (one direction) stair-step appearance. The horizontal x-axis shows the time variable in a linear manner, and the y-axis shows the proportion/probability of patients surviving. When a patient experiences an event, this is shown as a 'step-down' on the graph. Patients who have not experienced an event by the last follow-up, possibly being lost to follow-up, or a patient withdrawing from the study are shown as small vertical lines on the graph and are known as *censored observations*. The survival of these patients is still taken into account but only up until their maximum follow-up time. Survival curves with many small steps have larger sample sizes, and those with larger steps have a smaller sample size and are thus less accurate. In most studies, median survival is reported as survival times tend to be skewed. In addition, a mean cannot be calculated as there is no way of knowing if patients at the end of the study (alive or uncensored) will experience the particular event.

In analysing the data in this question, the 5-year survival rate with drug A is approximately 30%; hence E is the correct response. It 'appears' at first hand that drug A is better than placebo in treating mantle cell lymphoma. However, there are a number of issues with the displayed data that would go against this assumption. Firstly, there is no statistical analysis evident from this data. Secondly, there is no censored data displayed. Censored data can have a significant effect on the curve, and must be included when fitting the model, otherwise there would be bias in the results (N.B. having no censored data would be very unusual in a clinical trial!). If for whatever reason there was no censored observations, then it may be more appropriate to use a statistical rank test such as the Mann-Whitney test rather than analysing survival data. The added advantage over the latter is survival curves are a useful way of displaying survival data and they provide an estimate of risk. Finally, caution must be taken when survival curves cross each other. The data shown in this question identifies an intersection between drug A and placebo at ca. 1.75 years. In general, this means that there is an interaction between drug A and placebo which often will not yield significant *p* values. It is therefore essential that appropriate statistical tests are performed in studies like this; hence A and B are incorrect. There is ca. 65% survival probability beyond 2.5 years with drug A, not 50%; hence C is incorrect. The median survival with placebo is ca. 2.5 years (not 3 years); hence D is incorrect.

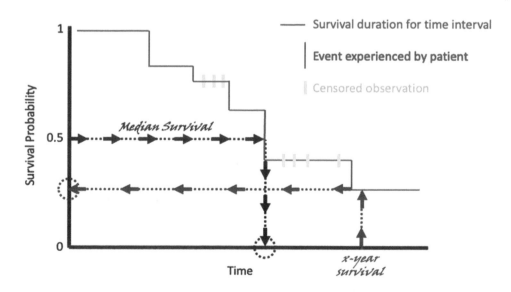

8.33 *B – < 1*

It is important to assess whether there are differences in survival among independent groups. Generally, there are two methods for this: [1] The log-rank test is used to test the null hypothesis which would state that there is no difference between the independent groups. This is a useful test as it compares the entire survival experience between the groups. This test sums the calculated chi-square (χ^2) for each event time and each arm. [2] Cox proportional hazards regression analysis is used to measure the effect of the hazard rate, i.e., the risk of failure or probability of suffering the event of interest, which is then used to calculate the hazard ratio (HR). HR is the ratio of the risk of hazard occurring at a given time in one group compared with another group at that exact time.

The log-rank helps to generate a *p* value which can tell us whether there is any significant difference between the two treatment arms, but it does not tell us what this difference is. The HR can do this as it incorporates data from across the whole Kaplan-Meier curve. Obviously, a crude and more simplistic way of gathering information from the direction for survival outcomes would be through median survival, which compares the survival time at a specific time point on the Kaplan-Meier curve.

Both log-rank and Cox regression analysis assume that the HR is constant over time. To calculate the HR, the Cox regression test must be used, which accounts for censoring times. If the HR is equal to 1, then there is equal efficacy of the experimental and control treatments. If the HR is less than 1, the experimental treatment is better than the control. If the HR > 1, the experimental treatment is worse than the control; hence the correct answer is B. Theoretically, it is possible for the HR to equal zero when the numerator is equal to zero. However, for this to happen, the numerator group would have to experience no achievement of outcome throughout the entire study period, which would be very unlikely. In the rare event of this happening, there would simply be no added benefit in calculating the HR under these circumstances.

8.34   A – Forest plot

Forest plots (or blobbograms) are a useful way of displaying data from meta-analyses (quantitative, epidemiological study designs used to systematically assess the results from multiple studies); hence A is the correct response.

Funnel plots are a useful way of checking if studies show publication bias in meta-analyses and systematic reviews. It is a scatter plot of the effect estimates from individual studies (often the standard error on a reversed scale with larger, more powerful studies are shown near the top) on the y-axis against a measure of individual studies size or precision (often odds ratio on a logarithmic scale) on the x-axis. In the absence of bias and between study heterogeneity, the plot will resemble a symmetrical inverted funnel. As a rule of thumb, if there are few or no dots scattered in the lower left of the funnel plot, consider publication bias! Other possible sources of asymmetry in funnel plots include aspects of the methodology employed such as inadequate analysis or poor design features, reporting bias, artefacts resulting from a lack of statistical scrupulousness and chance. A note on heterogeneity: this refers to the data differences between studies being due to something other than chance. Statistical tests have been developed to test for this, such as Egger's regression which is often used to test for funnel asymmetry, specifically publication bias. Tests should not be used when there are less than 10 studies in the meta-analysis as any statistical differences are far more likely to be due to chance.

Stem and leaf plots are used to organise data as they are collected. They are used to classify *discrete* (a variable with <u>finite</u> number of values, e.g., 1, 2, 3, 4 …, gender, yes/no etc.) or *continuous* variables (a variable with <u>infinite</u> number of values, e.g., age, temperature, time, speed, distance etc.). These plots are similar to histograms, but the data is often tabulated. Each data value is split into a 'stem' which equates to the first digit(s) and a 'leaf' which is usually the last digit. For example, times of 2.3, 2.5 and 2.7 seconds would be tabulated as 2 | 3 5 7 (2 being the 'stem' and 3, 5 and 7 being the 'leaf'). These plots allow the mean, mode, median and interquartile range from a set of data to be calculated.

L'Abbé plots are scatter plots of results from individual studies in a meta-analysis of clinical trials that compare the proportion of patients achieving the outcome with the intervention group on the y-axis against the event rate in the control group on the x-axis (as shown below). They are only applicable to studies with binary outcomes. Each circle on the plot equates to one trial in the review and the size of each circle is proportional to the sample size. Plots often contain a regression line and a diagonal line which represents equality, i.e., identical risks in each group.

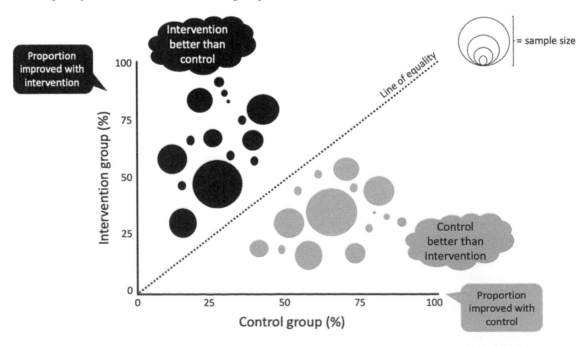

Galbraith (or radial) plots are a means of graphically presenting funnel plot asymmetry and are an alternative to confidence interval and forest plots. It is a plot of the standardised intervention effect (study effect estimate divided by the standard error (SE), the z score/statistic) on the y-axis against the reciprocal of the standard error on the x-axis (as shown below). Individual studies are represented by single dots and a regression line runs centrally through the plot. Two 95% confidence interval (CI) lines are created which run parallel to the regression line and are set at a 2-standard deviations distance. In the absence of heterogeneity, all plotted points would lie within the confidence bounds of these two lines. These plots are useful in examining heterogeneity between studies in a meta-analysis and can be used to detect outliers. The greater the vertical scatter, the greater the heterogeneity. More precise estimates and larger studies with smaller standard errors lie farthest from the origin.

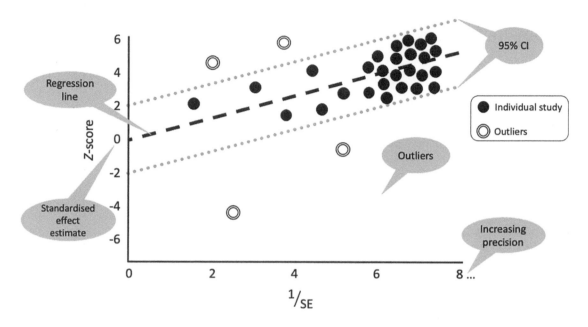

8.35 D – Diamond width

The diamond represents the overall aggregated effect which is obtained by combining all studies. If the diamond crosses the vertical line of no effect, there is no overall statistical difference. If the diamond lies to the left of this line, the intervention/treatment is favoured. If the diamond lies to the right of this line, the control/placebo is favoured. The width of the diamond represents the overall 95% confidence interval; hence D is the correct response.

Rectangle/square boxes or blobs represent the findings from each study. The position of these is a point estimate (i.e. the mean) of the odds ratio. The size/area of each box/blob is proportional to the precision/weight of the study (i.e., sample size and statistical power, so the bigger the box, the more participants in the study). The vertical black lines associated with each box/blob is the point estimate (mean) of that individual study. The overall measure of effect is represented as a black vertical line in the centre of the diamond. The central vertical line at 1.0 represents an odds ratio of 1, i.e., the line of no effect. The width of the horizontal grey line running through each box represents the 95% confidence interval. Longer lines mean more uncertainty and less precision.

N.B. Forest plots often report on another statistic called I^2 (i-squared) which gives us an understanding of heterogeneity. One way of looking at this is to ask the question *If all the studies reported are testing the same treatment/intervention, then why do they not get the same results?* It is less of a concern if the results are due to chance; however, if the results are not due to chance, tentative, questionable conclusions will be drawn. I^2 can help in these circumstances as it gives us an assessment of how consistent the analysis was between the studies. As a rule of thumb, the lower the I^2, the better the consistency, i.e., the studies are more similar and can be compared together.

8.36 E – Study F shows data that is the most statistically significant

If the horizontal grey line passes the vertical line of no effect, it means that the study is not statistically significant. Study F is the only study in which the horizontal line does not cross the vertical line, meaning the data from this study is the most statistically significant; hence E is the correct response.

Study A shows a 39% risk reduction (not increase). N.B. Any box/blob to the left or right side of the line of no effect implies a reduction or increase in the risk, respectively. Box/blobs towards the left side of line of no effect indicate that the new intervention is more effective, whereas those to the right indicate that the control/placebo is more effective; hence Study E (not B) shows that the new treatment/intervention is the most effective. Study D shows the least uncertainty (not most) about the result, as it has the narrowest horizontal grey line (or narrower CI). The wider the horizontal grey line, the more uncertainty about the result. Study E shows data that is least precise (not most) as it has the smallest box/blob. The area/size of the box/blob is proportional to the precision of the study, i.e., the size of the sample; hence Study A shows data that is the most precise.

8.37 *D – Cates plot*

Cates plots or 'smiley face' plots are an effective visual method in communicating risks and benefits of treatment to patients; hence D is the correct response. They can help explain how the effect of the treatment applies to high-risk and low-risk patients, and they also help communicate how the benefits and risks of treatments can be compared. The plots use four face categories: patients who are not affected by the treatment – green faces highlight a good outcome and red faces highlight a bad outcome, patients who had a bad outcome but because of the treatment now have a good outcome (yellow), and patients who have experienced an adverse event and change from a good outcome to a bad outcome (green face with a cross through it).

Lineweaver-Burk is a graphical representation of the Lineweaver-Burk equation of enzyme kinetics. A de Finetti diagram is used to display genotype frequencies of populations in genetics. A carpet plot is a means of displaying data that shows the interaction between multiple variables in a simplified manner. A Q–Q plot (or quantile–quantile) is a graphical technique for determining if two data sets come from populations with the same distribution.

8.38 *B – 5*

Let's recap: the green faces are the patients who will NOT have a cardiovascular event, whether they have dietary advice or not, i.e., 62 patients. The yellow faces are patients who will NOT have a cardiovascular event because they have taken dietary advice, i.e., 20 patients. The red faces are patients who will have a cardiovascular event whether they have taken dietary advice or not, i.e., 18 patients. The absolute risk of having a cardiovascular event in patients NOT taking dietary advice is 38% (yellow and red faces). The absolute risk of having a cardiovascular event in patients who take dietary advice is 18% (red faces). Therefore, the absolute risk reduction (ARR) is 20% and the NNT is 1/ARR = 5; hence B is the correct response.

8.39 *C – 47%*

The relative risk of having a cardiovascular event in patients who take dietary advice compared to those who do not is 47%, i.e., (the number of red faces) / (the number of red + yellow faces) = 18 / 38; hence C is the correct response.

8.40 *E – Approximately $\frac{3}{5}$ of patients will not have a cardiovascular event, whether they use dietary advice or not*

62% of patients will not have a cardiovascular event, whether they use dietary advice or not which is approximately $\frac{3}{5}$; hence E is the correct response. Relative risk reduction equates to 1 − (red faces / red + yellow faces). Absolute risk reduction equates to yellow faces. 20 patients will NOT have a cardiovascular event because they have taken dietary advice. There are no patients who experienced adverse effects as a result of dietary advice; therefore, there is no number needed to harm. 18 patients will have a cardiovascular event whether they take dietary advice or not. 20 patients will be saved from having a cardiovascular event because they took dietary advice.

8.41 *D – Respect for persons*

Respect for persons aims at acknowledging a person's right to make informed choices, to hold personal views and opinions, and it allows them to act based on their own values and beliefs. This principle is linked closely with autonomy which allows responsible people to make their own decisions and it also aims at protecting those who lack autonomy, such as with young children and patients who lack capacity. Furthermore, it allows for informed consent and confidentiality. One important aspect of the doctor–patient relationship is being open, honest and transparent about treatment options which includes side effects to drugs, an example of respect for persons; hence D is the correct response.

Beneficence is the principle of doing good. This is not just about avoiding harm but allowing people to take actions which then provide benefits and promotes the welfare of others. This principle is all about being positive – defending peoples' rights, preventing harm, removing conditions that could potentially cause harm, helping people with disabilities and rescuing those who are in danger. It is important to remember that this is situation specific, and what is good for one patient may not be good for another, or a doctor suggests one treatment and the patient chooses another. This is where ethical principles are closely interconnected and beneficence is balanced with patient autonomy, veracity (patients who are told true facts may inadvertently become more stress/worried) or justice (patients who live in one location may have access to better resources than others).

Non-maleficence is the principle of doing no harm. The guiding maxim 'First, do no harm' means if for whatever reason you cannot do good (beneficence), you must at least do no harm, i.e., actions must be intentionally avoided that cause harm. This principle is important when considering futile treatments for patients approaching end of life, where treatments may cause more harm by allowing them to endure a slow and painful death.

Justice is the principle of treating others equitably without prejudice and distributing benefits and burdens fairly. In healthcare, distributive justice refers to fair and appropriate distribution of healthcare resources in an equitable manner. Examples include scarce resources such as equipment, investigations, drug treatment and allocation of time. Prioritisation and rationing are important components of this principle.

Double effect is the principle by which a good outcome is followed by a less favourable outcome. In these circumstances, a balance exists between the intended benefits and the potential adverse effects. For example, a patient with metastatic disease may require morphine for pain control and respiratory distress as they near end of life. By giving higher doses or more frequent increments of morphine to help these symptoms, there is the possibility of respiratory arrest. Hastening death using morphine would obviously be morally impermissible.

8.42 *B – 6 hours*

Section 5(4) of the Mental Health Act 1983 permits nurses (of the prescribed class) to detain an informal in-patient who is already receiving treatment for a mental disorder for a period up to 6 hours; hence B is the correct response.

8.43 *E – 72 hours*

Section 5(2) of the Mental Health Act 1983 permits a doctor to detain an informal in-patient for a period up to 72 hours; hence E is the correct response.

8.44 *D – Section 136*

Section 136 of the Mental Health Act 1983 gives the police the power to remove a person from a public place, when they appear to be suffering from a mental disorder to a place of safety. A place of safety is usually a Mental Health Unit or the Emergency Department. A person can be detained on a Section 136 for up to 24 hours. This can be extendable by up to 12 hours if the person cannot be assessed for clinical reasons; hence D is the correct response. Section 17 allows detained patients to be granted leave of absence from hospital in which they are detained. Section 116 relates to in-patient welfare whilst under the MHA 1983. It allows social services to arrange in-patient visits whereby the local authority is the patient's guardian/nearest relative whilst they remain under section, or a child/young person who is in the care of a local authority. Section 135 is the power to remove a person from a dwelling if it is considered they have a mental disorder. It allows police via a warrant from the Court to gain entry so that a mental health assessment can be made, or the person is removed to a place of safety. Section 138 provides the police with a power to detain or recover an absconded patient from lawful custody if under Section 135 or 136, or following sectioning but before admission to hospital.

8.45 *E – 28 days*

Section 2 of the Mental Health Act 1983 allows compulsory admission for assessment, or for assessment followed by treatment for up to 28 days; hence E is the correct response.

8.46 *E – Section 17A deals with community treatment orders*

Section 17A of the Mental Health Act 1983 allows patients to be treated for a mental disorder but can be treated in the community rather than in hospital. These are known as community treatment orders. It lasts for 6 months and can be renewed for a further 6 months and then annually. A person must consent to the treatment; hence E is the correct response. This should not be confused with Section 17 which grants detained patients to a leave of absence from hospital. Section 2 is an admission for assessment which is undertaken by an Approved Mental Health Professional and two doctors, one of who is Section 12 approved, and one who is a registered practitioner. Section 3 is admission for treatment which can last up to six months. Patients can appeal via the Mental Health Tribunal to apply for discharge from detention. You can also appeal against Section 2. There are no rights to appeal against Sections 5(2), 5(4) or 136. Section 117 aftercare is a legal duty that provides services for patients who have been detained under Section 3, 37, 47, 48 and 45A. It comes into effect upon discharge from hospital. There is no Section 117 aftercare following detention under Section 2. Section 3 assessments are made by an Approved Mental Health Professional and two doctors (one who is Section 12 approved). Family members and nearest relatives cannot make an application for admission for treatment under Section 3.

8.47 *A – Prohibition of discrimination*

The Mental Capacity Act 2005 is designed to empower and protect those who lack mental capacity. The five main principles are as follows:

1) A person must be <u>assumed to have capacity</u> unless it is established that they lack capacity.
2) A person is not to be treated as unable to make a decision unless <u>all practical steps</u> to help them to do so have been taken without success.
3) A person is not to be treated as unable to make a decision merely because they makes an <u>unwise decision</u>.
4) An act done, or decision made, under this Act for or on behalf of a person who lacks capacity must be done, or made, in their <u>best interests</u>.
5) Before the act is done, or the decision is made, regard must be had to whether the purpose for which it is needed can be as effectively achieved in a way that is <u>less restrictive</u> of the person's rights and freedom of action.

Independent mental capacity advocates (IMCA), lasting powers of attorney, deprivation of liberty and best interests are all found within the Mental Capacity Act 2005. Prohibition of discrimination is found within Article 14 of The Human Rights Act 1998; hence A is the correct response.

Part I: The Convention Rights and Freedoms of The Human Rights Act 1998 include:

- Article 2 – Right to life
- Article 3 – Prohibition of torture
- Article 4 – Prohibition of slavery and forced labour
- Article 5 – Right to liberty and security
- Article 6 – Right to a fair trial
- Article 7 – No punishment without law
- Article 8 – Right to respect for private and family life
- Article 9 – Freedom of thought, conscience and religion
- Article 10 – Freedom of expression
- Article 11 – Freedom of assembly and association
- Article 12 – Right to marry
- Article 14 – Prohibition of discrimination
- Article 16 – Restrictions on political activity of aliens
- Article 17 – Prohibition of abuse of rights
- Article 18 – Limitation on use of restrictions on rights

8.48 *B – Lack of capacity nullifies voting rights*

A lack of mental capacity is not a legal incapacity to vote and Section 73 of the Electoral Administration Act 2006 abolished common law restrictions that a person was unable to register to vote due to a lack of capacity; hence B is the correct response.

8.49 *C – Breast*

Cancer is a leading cause of death worldwide. They can be prevented by avoiding risk factors and implementing preventative strategies. Cancer mortality can be reduced by early detection and treatment. As shown in the figure below, lung cancer is the most common cause of cancer deaths in 2020, followed by colorectal. Thyroid cancer is the least common. Breast cancer is the fifth most common; hence C is the correct response. These statistics are likely to change with better preventative strategies and treatment with modern technological advances; therefore, up-to-date figures should be referenced via the World Health Organisation, or other reputable cancer-related websites.

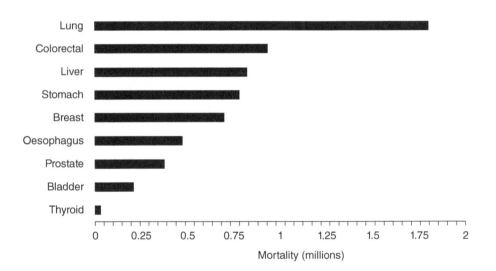

8.50 *D – Women live longer than men*

Epidemiology is the study of the distribution, causes, and possible prevention and control of diseases in populations. It is helpful for understanding and improving global health. A key feature of epidemiology is the measurement of disease outcomes in relation to a population at risk. Moreover, the health and healthcare needs of the population cannot be measured or met without knowledge and understanding of demographics and population dynamics. Population pyramids can be used to graphically represent the age and sex of the population. They are dependent on the birth, death rates and migration, and there are spatio-temporal variations not only for different countries, but also the same country over time. There are three types:

1) Expansive pyramid – broad base with successive decline in population with higher age groups, i.e., more people die at an older age. The pyramid indicates a population in which there are high birth and death rates, lower life expectancy and higher population growth rates. This is typical of developing countries.

2) Stationary pyramid – population remains constant in different age groups over time. There is low birth and death rates, and higher life expectancy. The population is stable or slow growing.
3) Constrictive pyramid – narrow base with low birth and death rates, high life expectancy and an aging population. This is typical of a developed country with high levels of education and a good healthcare system.

The broader the base, the faster the population growth, whereas a narrower base shows population shrinkage. Steeper pyramids equate to a longer life expectancy. Broader bases that decline quickly but are narrower at later age groups indicate high infant mortality and short life expectancy. Yet a more rectangular shape which gets broader at later age groups indicates longer life expectancy. Indentations in the pyramid represent higher death rates than normal or emigration. Bulging in the pyramid represents baby boom from previous years or immigration. Remember population pyramids cannot only be used to display the distribution of a population, but also data such as disease or health characteristics by age and sex.

In this population pyramid, the population is broader for elderly women at the very top which shows women are living longer than men (albeit marginally); hence D is the correct response. There are more males than females aged 25–29. The base is narrower at the base, so the birth rate is lower. The steepness of the sides as age progresses beyond 45 is decreasing which indicates death rate is also declining. There appears to be more younger men immigrating, most likely as a result of work, compared to women. Rapid growth usually indicates a lower standard of living with high birth rates i.e., poor access to birth control and lack of education, and higher death rates i.e., lack of medication/nutrition. This is not seen in this population pyramid.

Index

---

pseudostratified cuboidal epithelium, 91
pseudostratified epithelium, 86
ptosis, 130
pudendal nerve, 159
pulmonary artery, 148
pupillary light reflex, 130
putamen, 121
pyloric sphincter, 69
pyruvate kinase, 8

quadriceps femoris tendon, 162, 163

radial nerve, 138
radioallergosorbent test (RAST), 54
ramipril, 68, 73
randomized controlled trials, 68
reciprocal translocations, 29
red nucleus, 121
reduced FAD, 2
reduced NAD, 2
Reed-Sternberg cells, 55
Reichert's cartilage, 244
relative risk, 270, 271, 273
renal artery stenosis, 68
renal cell carcinoma, 29
renal plexus, 156
reproductive organs, 152–160
respect for persons, 274
retina, 246
retinitis pigmentosa, 33
retroperitoneal structures, 155
retrospective case-control, 267
rhombomeres, 245, 246
ribs, 150, 151
right coronary artery, 144
right gastric artery, 155
risedronate, 71
robertsonian translocation, 29
rocuronium, 69
rostral bifurcation, 126
rotator cuff, component of, 137

sacral plexus, 157
sacrocardinal veins, 244
sample variance, 266
sarcoidosis, 54, 99–100
sarcomere, 4
    ultrastructure of, 5
scapula, 144
sciatic nerve, 161
seborrhoeic keratosis, 98
segregation, 35
self-antigens, 54
semicircular canals, 131
semicircular ducts, 131
semimembranosus, 161
seminal vesicles, 157
semitendinosus, tendon of, 166
sensitivity, 269
septomarginal trabecula, 144

serine, 52
serotonin, 3
serotonin-norepinephrine reuptake inhibitor (SNRI), 72
serratus posterior superior, 145
sertoli cells, 86
severe combined immunodeficiency (SCID), 31
sex chromosome aneuploidies, 29
sickle cell anaemia, 28
sigmoid sinus, 121
sign test, 277
simple cuboidal, 88
single-gene disorder, 34
single-nucleotide polymorphism, 29, 53
sinusoids, 88
sixth rib, 151
Sjögrens syndrome, 2
skeletal muscle, 92
Skene's glands, 158
skin, 246
small intestine, 89
smooth muscle, 92
sodium ions, 2
somatic hypermutation, 53
somitomeres, 242
Southern blot, 3
Spearman's rank correlation coefficient, 278
special senses, 128–135
specificity, 269
spermatic cord, 153
spermatogenesis, 240
sphenoidal sinus, 134
sphenopalatine foramen, 134
spinal cord, 121, 146
spinal segments, 154
spinothalamic tract, 121
spirochete, 8
splanchnic nerves, 156
squamous cell carcinoma *in situ*, 99
standard deviation, 266
stereocilia, 93
sternopericardial ligaments, 145
sternum, 145
stomach, 155
ST-segment elevation, 150
stylohyoid, 120
submandibular gland, 93
submetacentric chromosomes, 29
subscapularis inserts, 138
substrate level phosphorylation, 8
subtalar joint, 165
succinate, 2
superantigens, 53
superficial forearm muscle, 141
superficial inguinal ring, 153
superior fibular, 164
superior gemellus, 161
superior longitudinal muscle, 132
superior mediastinum, 144
superior oblique, 129
superior orbital fissure, 120